THE DIABETES COOKBOOK

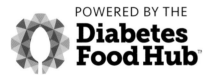

POWERED BY THE
Diabetes Food Hub

300 RECIPES FOR HEALTHY LIVING

Lara Rondinelli-Hamilton, RD, LDN, CDE
& Chef Jennifer Bucko Lamplough

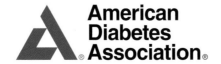

American Diabetes Association.

Associate Publisher, Books, Abe Ogden; *Director, Book Operations*, Victor Van Beuren; *Managing Editor,* John Clark; *Associate Director, Book Marketing,* Annette Reape; *Acquisitions Editor,* Jaclyn Konich; *Senior Manager, Book Editing,* Lauren Wilson; *Project Manager,* Amnet Systems; *Composition,* Amnet Systems; *Cover Design,* Mittera Creative; *Photographer,* Mittera Creative; *Printer,* Imago.

Printed in the Republic of Slovenia
1 3 5 7 9 10 8 6 4 2

The suggestions and information contained in this publication are generally consistent with the *Standards of Medical Care in Diabetes* and other policies of the American Diabetes Association, but they do not represent the policy or position of the Association or any of its boards or committees. Reasonable steps have been taken to ensure the accuracy of the information presented. However, the American Diabetes Association cannot ensure the safety or efficacy of any product or service described in this publication. Individuals are advised to consult a physician or other appropriate health care professional before undertaking any diet or exercise program or taking any medication referred to in this publication. Professionals must use and apply their own professional judgment, experience, and training and should not rely solely on the information contained in this publication before prescribing any diet, exercise, or medication. The American Diabetes Association—its officers, directors, employees, volunteers, and members—assumes no responsibility or liability for personal or other injury, loss, or damage that may result from the suggestions or information in this publication.

Madelyn Wheeler conducted the internal review of this book to ensure that it meets American Diabetes Association guidelines.

⊗ The paper in this publication meets the requirements of the ANSI Standard Z39.48-1992 (permanence of paper).

ADA titles may be purchased for business or promotional use or for special sales. To purchase more than 50 copies of this book at a discount, or for custom editions of this book with your logo, contact the American Diabetes Association at the address below or at booksales@diabetes.org.

American Diabetes Association
2451 Crystal Drive, Suite 900
Arlington, VA 22202

DOI: 10.2337/9781580406802

Library of Congress Cataloging-in-Publication Data
Names: Rondinelli-Hamilton, Lara, 1974- author. | Lamplough, Jennifer, 1974-
    author.
 Title: The diabetes cookbook : 300 recipes for healthy living Powered by the
    Diabetes Food Hub / Lara Rondinelli-Hamilton, RD, LDN, CDE, and Chef Jennifer
    Bucko Lamplough.
 Other titles: Diabetes food hub cookbook
Description: Arlington : American Diabetes Association, 2018. | Includes
    bibliographical references and index.
 Identifiers: LCCN 2018009603 | ISBN 9781580406802 (alk. paper)
 Subjects: LCSH: Diabetes—Diet therapy—Recipes. | LCGFT: Cookbooks.
 Classification: LCC RC662 .R64 2018 | DDC 641.5/6314—dc23
 LC record available at https://lccn.loc.gov/2018009603

dedication

THIS BOOK IS
DEDICATED TO ALL
OF YOU WHO WANT
TO IMPROVE YOUR
HEALTH AND FEEL
GREAT. MAY YOU
LEARN TO USE FOOD
AS MEDICINE WHILE
LOVING, COOKING, AND
ENJOYING REAL FOOD.

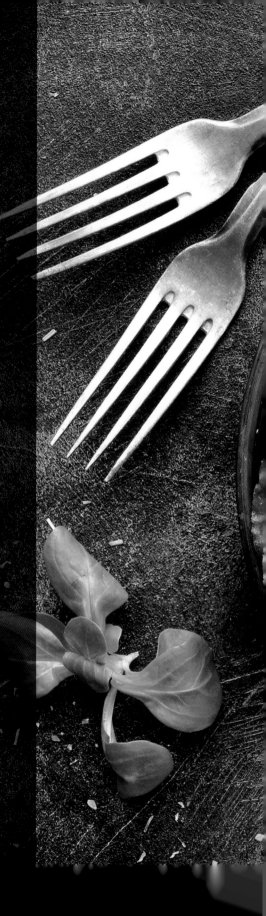

TABLE OF CONTENTS

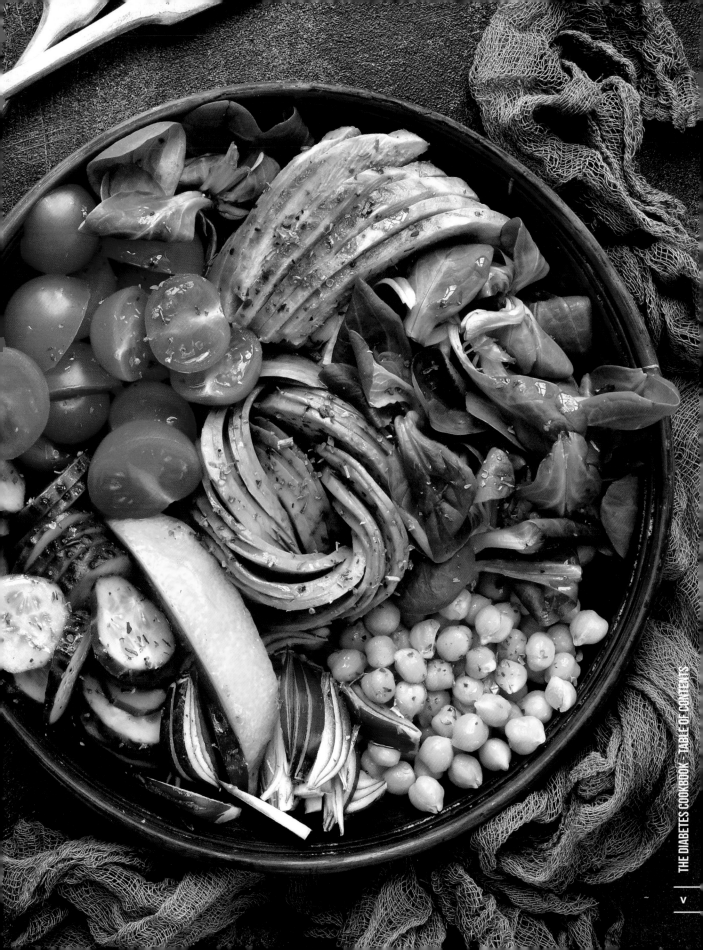

acknowledgments

FIRST AND FOREMOST I MUST THANK GOD, FOR LEADING ME ON THIS CAREER PATH. LITTLE DID I KNOW HOW MUCH I WOULD NEED NUTRITION FOR MY OWN HEALTH ISSUES.

It is very clear to me that I could not have planned this career myself and God is great—I'm so grateful.

Thank you to Abe Ogden, the director of book publishing, for believing in us and always presenting us with such awesome projects. Thank you to Lyn Wheeler, for your nutrition analysis expertise and for answering our million questions. You are amazing, and we are so glad to have you with us on another cookbook. Thank you to Lauren Wilson, senior manager, book editing, for your patience, dedication, and expertise.

Thank you to a wonderful chef, writer, runner, blogger, and best friend, Jennifer Lamplough. It's been so great to grow up together, write cookbooks together, and see our families grow together. We are so blessed to work on this amazing cookbook (I think the best one yet!) and to have even more reasons to talk and get together.

I'm so thankful for my incredible family, who has been by my side, supporting me all the way. Thank you to my husband, Jared, for sharing my love of healthy food, for being adventurous with eating, for making me laugh, and for your constant love and support. There is no one else I would rather have by my side through all the ups and downs of life. Thank you to my two little foodies, Ethan and Penelope, for helping me in the kitchen, for loving food, for eating your veggies, and for making me smile every day. Thank you to my parents, Tom and Jane Rondinelli, for always encouraging me to do anything I dreamed of and always believing in me. It has been a joy to see you transform your lives with healthy eating, too. My sisters, Jennifer Sebring and Kari Mender, have been our biggest cookbook cheerleaders—thank you for all your support. The Italian love of food is a part of our upbringing, and it's always wonderful to share great food, good conversation, and a glass of wine together!

Thank you also to all the people in my life who go out of their way to prepare safe (gluten-free) food for me. As anyone with celiac disease or food allergies knows, eating outside your house can be very stressful. I'm blessed to have my Dinner Club girls, friends, neighbors, and family, including my extended family and in-laws, who are always thinking of feeding me safely.

Thank you to my patients, who continue to inspire me every day with their dedication and healthy lifestyle changes. It is because of all of you that I truly love my job. I hope this cookbook creates many delicious meals in your home and improves your health even more!

Lara Rondinelli-Hamilton

I HAVE SO MUCH GRATITUDE EVERY DAY FOR THE GIFT OF THIS PROJECT AND THE ABILITY I HAVE TO CREATE RECIPES FOR PEOPLE WHO NEED AND WANT TO EAT HEALTHFULLY AND WELL.

Thank you to Abe Ogden, director of book publishing, for always bringing us these awesome projects and for believing in us for all these years. Thank you to Lyn Wheeler for your expertise, knowledge, and unfailing patience in analyzing our recipes and answering our endless questions!

To my lifelong, dearest friend, and co-author, Lara Rondinelli-Hamilton. Your unflappable faith, brilliant mind, talent, patience, and kindness and care for your patients, your family, and your friends are all a constant inspiration to me and have been since we were kids. Not many people I know are allowed to work together, play together, raise families together, and grow as people, authors, mothers, wives, and friends as we have been blessed to be able to do. I am unendingly grateful for that, and for you. I am so proud of the work we have created together now and over the years, and I can't wait to see what's next for us. I hope it includes many glasses of wine.

To my husband, Mike, who supports me no matter what I do and no matter how hard it is. You are my anchor, my heart, my love. Thanks for always being my number one taste tester, my number one source of laughter, my number one person to bounce ideas off of . . . my number one. I love you more than words can say. Thank you for taking care of our beloved little man, Ike, while Mama is constantly testing recipes and stressing over deadlines. And my Ike, my good little eater, my sidekick in the kitchen, and the light of my life. I love you so much my sweet boy. Everything I do is for you and Dada.

Thank you to the rest of my family, especially my mom for her love, encouragement, and always-incredible recipe ideas; my siblings, Jill Kilhefner, Jane DiMartin, Jackie Burke, and Jim Bucko, and their families, who are always excited for me and supportive of our work. You all are some of our best cheerleaders, and I love you dearly for it (and eight million other things!). To my in-laws, Margaret McKenzie, Joel and Laura Lamplough, my brother-in-law, Joel Lamplough, and extended family: I can't believe I got so lucky to have you amazingly funny and smart people in my life.

To my dear friends who are some of my best taste testers and biggest supporters, especially Draga Doolittle, the foundation of our trifecta of BFFs, who makes me laugh more than anyone in the world, and probably believes in me more than that. Since we were little girls, sharing bread at your mom's house, to making cones at the DQ, to the women we are now, your love and support are everything. To the Dinner Club girls and my Batavia neighbors, you are better friends than a girl could ask for! Thanks for the love, laughs, support, and glasses of champagne when I've desperately needed them!

Last, to my coworkers at Northern Illinois Food Bank, with whom I get to work every day in the fight against hunger. Doing this incredible work to feed our neighbors in northern Illinois who are hungry and in need of nutritious, wholesome food has been one of the greatest honors of my life. Thank you for letting me walk alongside you on this journey to end hunger.

Jennifer Bucko Lamplough

introduction

The American Diabetes Association's website Diabetes Food Hub (https://www.diabetesfoodhub.org/) is a tool that was created to make healthy eating and meal planning easier, more realistic, and more delicious. Inspired by the Association's original website Recipes for Healthy Living, the meal plans on Diabetes Food Hub are not only diabetes-friendly but are also tasty enough for the whole family to enjoy.

Now consumers can have many of these recipes conveniently at their fingertips with *The Diabetes Cookbook: 300 Recipes for Healthy Living Powered by the Diabetes Food Hub. The Diabetes Cookbook* offers traditional recipes, such as pizza and lasagna, reimagined into healthy, diabetes-friendly dishes, along with trendy, low-carb recipes using cauliflower rice and zucchini noodles. This cookbook includes all the popular sections that the Diabetes Food Hub website offers, such as Foodie recipes, Quick recipes, Slow-Cooker recipes, and Budget–Friendly recipes, along with exciting new sections, such as Mediterranean and Low Glycemic-Index recipes.

The American Diabetes Association recommends a variety of eating patterns, such as Mediterranean-style and vegetarian diets, for the management of diabetes. Personal preferences along with cultural and religious factors and economic status are considered when recommending eating patterns for people with diabetes. *The Diabetes Cookbook* is the only cookbook to take into account a variety of healthy eating patterns that will appeal to everyone, with or without diabetes. There is something for everyone in this cookbook, and you will soon see that healthy cooking can be done quickly and can taste more delicious than you ever imagined. Turn the pages and get started today!

SYMBOLS KEY

You'll see a few symbols used in the recipes on the following pages. Let this key be your guide to getting the most of these recipes.

- Prep time
- Cooking time
- Number of servings
- Serving size
- GF Gluten-free recipes. But always check to confirm that all ingredients are gluten-free.
- LC Low-carb recipes. These recipes contain 10 g of carbohydrate or less per serving.
- VG Vegetarian recipes. May include eggs and dairy products.

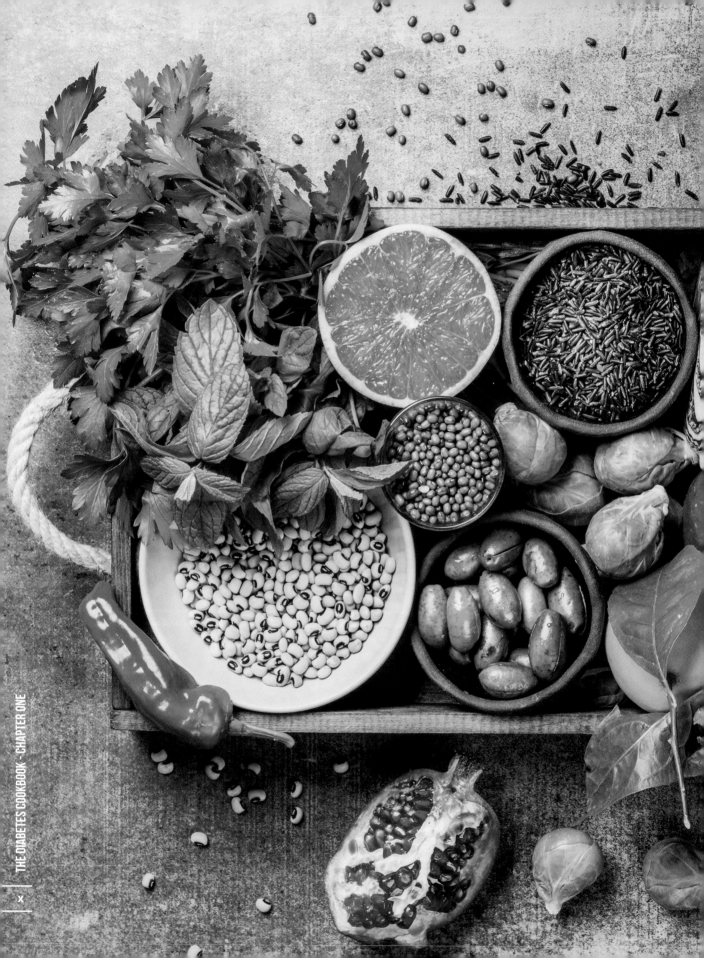

CHAPTER ONE
QUICK RECIPES

THE MAJORITY OF THESE

RECIPES CAN BE PREPARED

IN 30 MINUTES OR LESS

AND DON'T REQUIRE MANY

INGREDIENTS. ALTHOUGH

THEY REQUIRE LESS TIME

AND FEWER INGREDIENTS,

THESE RECIPES ARE STILL

PACKED WITH FLAVOR

AND ARE PERFECT FOR

WEEKNIGHT MEALS.

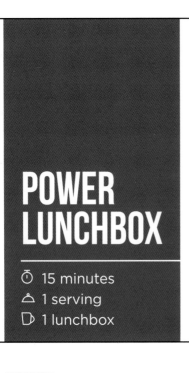

POWER LUNCHBOX

⏱ 15 minutes
🍽 1 serving
🍱 1 lunchbox

PACK YOUR LUNCH THE NIGHT BEFORE TO START YOUR MORNING WITH LESS STRESS!

SANDWICH

1	ounce reduced-sodium deli ham
1/2	ounce reduced-fat colby jack cheese
1/4	avocado, mashed
1	large bibb lettuce leaf

ADDITIONAL LUNCHBOX ITEMS

2	hard-boiled egg whites
12	roasted almonds (unsalted)
1	green apple (such as Granny Smith), sliced into eighths
3	baby carrots

1. Assemble the sandwich by layering the ham, cheese, and avocado on the lettuce leaf; then roll it tightly and wrap in plastic wrap. Serve the sandwich with the egg whites, almonds, and baby carrots.

Nutrition Facts

Serves: 1
Serving Size: 1 lunchbox

Amount per serving
Calories   **360**

Calories from fat 160

Total fat 18.0 g

    Saturated fat 3.5 g

    Trans fat 0.0 g

Cholesterol 20 mg

Sodium 500 mg

Potassium 820 mg

Total carbohydrate 33 g

    Dietary fiber 10 g

    Sugars 19 g

Protein 21 g

Phosphorus 265 mg

Choices/Exchanges: 1 Fruit, 1/2 Carbohydrate, 2 Nonstarchy Vegetable, 3 Lean Protein, 2 Fat

SALAD

- 1 (29-ounce) can gluten-free black beans, rinsed and drained
- 2 cups frozen corn, thawed
- 1 red bell pepper, finely diced
- 1/2 cup red onion, finely diced
- 1/2 cup chopped fresh cilantro

DRESSING

- Juice of 2 small limes
- 3 tablespoons extra-virgin olive oil
- 1/2 teaspoon cumin
- 1/4 teaspoon garlic powder
- 1/4 teaspoon ground black pepper
- 1/4 teaspoon cayenne pepper

1. In a medium bowl, combine beans, corn, red pepper, red onion, and cilantro.

2. In a small bowl, whisk together remaining ingredients and pour over bean salad. Toss to coat.

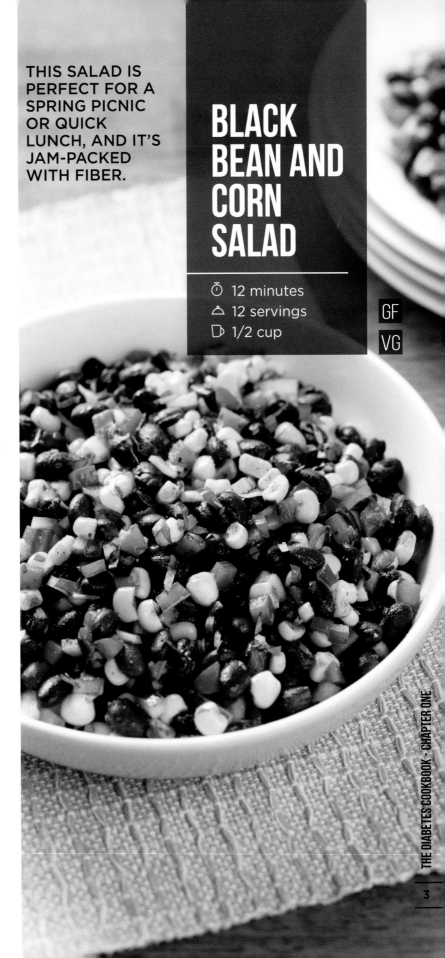

THIS SALAD IS PERFECT FOR A SPRING PICNIC OR QUICK LUNCH, AND IT'S JAM-PACKED WITH FIBER.

BLACK BEAN AND CORN SALAD

- ⏱ 12 minutes
- △ 12 servings
- ▭ 1/2 cup

GF
VG

Nutrition Facts

Serves: 12
Serving Size: 1/2 cup

Amount per serving	
Calories	**110**
Calories from fat 35	
Total fat 4.0 g	
Saturated fat 0.6 g	
Trans fat 0.0 g	
Cholesterol 0 mg	
Sodium 50 mg	
Potassium 230 mg	
Total carbohydrate 16 g	
Dietary fiber 4 g	
Sugars 2 g	
Protein 4 g	
Phosphorus 75 mg	

Choices/Exchanges: 1 Starch, 1/2 Fat

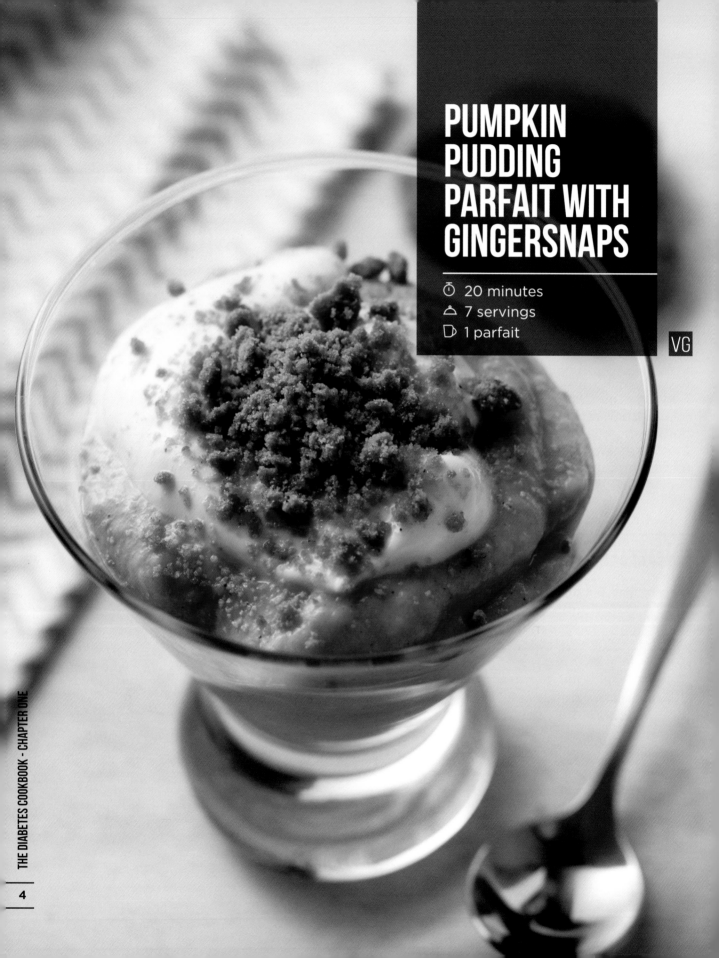

PUMPKIN PUDDING PARFAIT WITH GINGERSNAPS

- ⏱ 20 minutes
- ⌂ 7 servings
- 🥤 1 parfait

VG

THIS NO-COOK DESSERT IS A GREAT SUBSTITUTE FOR PUMPKIN PIE—AND IT'S ONLY 100 CALORIES! FOR A QUICK, HEALTHY, DELICIOUS, PUMPKIN DESSERT, LOOK NO FURTHER—THIS PUDDING PARFAIT IS AMAZING AND READY IN MINUTES. YOU CAN SUBSTITUTE LIGHT WHIPPED CREAM FOR THE GREEK YOGURT HERE IF DESIRED.

1	(1-ounce) package fat-free, sugar-free instant cheesecake pudding mix
1 2/3	cups skim milk
1	cup canned pure pumpkin
1/2	teaspoon cinnamon
1/8	teaspoon nutmeg
1	cup fat-free vanilla Greek yogurt, divided
7	gingersnap cookies, crumbled

1. In a medium mixing bowl, whisk together the pudding mix and milk 2 minutes. Let sit 5 minutes.
2. Fold in the pumpkin, cinnamon, and nutmeg. Fold in 1/2 cup of the yogurt and refrigerate 10 minutes.
3. Scoop 1/2 cup pudding mixture into a parfait glass. Top with 1 heaping tablespoon of the remaining yogurt and 1 crumbled gingersnap cookie.
4. Repeat procedure for remaining 6 parfaits.

Nutrition Facts

Serves: 7
Serving Size: 1 parfait

Amount per serving
Calories   **100**

Calories from fat 15

Total fat 1.5 g

   Saturated fat 0.5 g

   Trans fat 0.0 g

Cholesterol 2 mg

Sodium 250 mg

Potassium 240 mg

Total carbohydrate 16 g

   Dietary fiber 1 g

   Sugars 7 g

Protein 6 g

Phosphorus 215 mg

Choices/Exchanges:
1 Carbohydrate, 1/2 Fat

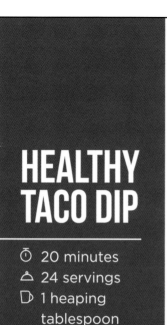

HEALTHY TACO DIP

GF
LC
VG

- ⏱ 20 minutes
- △ 24 servings
- ▭ 1 heaping tablespoon

THE TRADITIONAL VERSION OF THIS TACO DIP IS MUCH HIGHER IN FAT AND USES SOUR CREAM AND CREAM CHEESE. BY USING A HEALTHIER FAT SUCH AS AN AVOCADO AND REDUCED-FAT CHEESE, YOU SAVE A LOT OF CALORIES WITHOUT GIVING UP ANY TASTE.

1	(16-ounce) can fat-free refried beans, put in bowl and let sit at room temperature 10 minutes
2	teaspoons chili powder
1/2	teaspoon cumin
1/4	teaspoon garlic powder
1 1/2	avocados, mashed
1/3	cup salsa
1	cup shredded romaine lettuce
1	large tomato, seeded and diced
1	cup shredded 2%-milk Mexican cheese

1. In a medium bowl, mix together refried beans, chili powder, cumin, and garlic powder.
2. Spread refried beans evenly on a medium serving platter. Spread mashed avocados evenly over beans.
3. Spread salsa evenly over top of avocados. Top with shredded lettuce, tomatoes, and shredded cheese.

CHEF TIP: *Serve the dip with your choice of baked tortilla chips, black bean chips, or jicama slices.*

Nutrition Facts

Serves: 24
Serving Size: 1 heaping tablespoon

Amount per serving

Calories	45

Calories from fat 20	
Total fat 2.5 g	
Saturated fat 0.8 g	
Trans fat 0.0 g	
Cholesterol 3 mg	
Sodium 140 mg	
Potassium 150 mg	
Total carbohydrate 4 g	
Dietary fiber 2 g	
Sugars 1 g	
Protein 3 g	
Phosphorus 55 mg	

Choices/Exchanges:
1/2 Carbohydrate, 1/2 Fat

MEXICAN BLACK BEAN SOUP

⏱ 10 minutes
🍲 25 minutes
🍽 7 servings
🥣 1 cup

THIS FLAVORFUL, LOW-CARB SOUP MAKES A GREAT LUNCH THE NEXT DAY, TOO. IF YOU CAN'T FIND CANNED FIRE-ROASTED TOMATOES, YOU CAN USE CANNED DICED TOMATOES WITH GREEN CHILES INSTEAD.

Nonstick cooking spray
2 teaspoons olive oil
1/2 onion, diced
1 pound boneless skinless chicken breast, cut into 1/2-inch cubes
1/2 teaspoon adobo seasoning (such as Goya), divided
1/4 teaspoon ground black pepper
1 (14.5-ounce) can diced fire-roasted tomatoes
1 tablespoon chili powder
1/2 teaspoon cumin
1/2 cup frozen corn
1 (15-ounce) can black beans, rinsed and drained
40 ounces fat-free low-sodium chicken broth

1. Spray a large soup pot with cooking spray. Add oil and onion and sauté over medium-high heat 3 minutes or until onion is clear.
2. Add chicken and season with 1/4 teaspoon adobo seasoning and the pepper. Cook chicken until slightly brown, about 6–7 minutes.
3. Add remaining ingredients (including the other 1/4 teaspoon adobo seasoning). Reduce heat and simmer 15 minutes.

MAKE IT GLUTEN-FREE: *Use gluten-free chicken broth and verify that the spices and beans are gluten-free.*

Nutrition Facts

Serves: 7
Serving Size: 1 cup

Amount per serving
Calories **170**

Calories from fat 30

Total fat 3.5 g

    Saturated fat 0.7 g

    Trans fat 0.0 g

Cholesterol 40 mg

Sodium 420 mg

Potassium 570 mg

Total carbohydrate 15 g

    Dietary fiber 5 g

    Sugars 4 g

Protein 20 g

Phosphorus 225 mg

Choices/Exchanges: 1/2 Starch, 1 Nonstarchy Vegetable, 2 Lean Protein

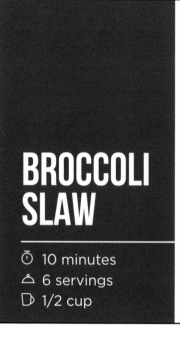

BROCCOLI SLAW

THIS CRUNCHY SIDE DISH IS A TWIST ON TRADITIONAL TANGY-SWEET BROCCOLI SALAD, BUT WITH NO ADDED SUGAR.

⏱ 10 minutes
△ 6 servings
▽ 1/2 cup

GF
LC

BROCCOLI SLAW

1	(12-ounce) bag broccoli slaw
1/4	cup raisins
6	slices cooked turkey bacon, chopped

DRESSING

1/4	cup light mayonnaise
3	tablespoons fat-free plain yogurt
2	tablespoons apple cider vinegar

1. In a salad bowl, mix together the broccoli slaw, raisins, and turkey bacon.
2. In a small bowl, whisk together the dressing ingredients. Pour the dressing over the salad and toss to coat.

DIETITIAN TIP:

This satisfying side dish is quick to make with bagged broccoli slaw, and it is full of fiber and flavor.

Nutrition Facts

Serves: 6
Serving Size: 1/2 cup

Amount per serving
Calories **90**

Calories from fat 40

Total fat 4.5 g

   Saturated fat 0.8 g

   Trans fat 0.0 g

Cholesterol 15 mg

Sodium 260 mg

Potassium 300 mg

Total carbohydrate 10 g

   Dietary fiber 2 g

   Sugars 6 g

Protein 4 g

Phosphorus 90 mg

Choices/Exchanges: 1/2 Fruit, 1 Nonstarchy Vegetable, 1 Fat

ROASTED BABY CARROTS

GF
LC
VG

⏱ 5 minutes
🍲 20 minutes
🍽 8 servings
🥄 1/3 cup

ROASTING BRINGS OUT THE NATURAL FLAVOR AND SWEETNESS IN THE CARROTS. YOU COULD SUBSTITUTE TARRAGON FOR PARSLEY HERE IF DESIRED.

Nonstick cooking spray
1 pound baby carrots
1 1/2 tablespoons olive oil
1 tablespoon honey or 2 packets artificial sweetener
1/2 teaspoon dried parsley

1. Preheat oven to 425°F. Spray a baking sheet with cooking spray.
2. In a small bowl, mix together the carrots and olive oil. Pour the mixture onto the baking sheet.
3. Bake 15–20 minutes, until the carrots are tender.
4. Place the carrots in a bowl and mix with the honey or artificial sweetener. Sprinkle the carrots with parsley.

Nutrition Facts

Serves: 8
Serving Size: 1/3 cup

Amount per serving
Calories 50

Calories from fat 20

Total fat 2.5 g

Saturated fat 0.4 g

Trans fat 0.0 g

Cholesterol 0 mg

Sodium 40 mg

Potassium 180 mg

Total carbohydrate 8 g

Dietary fiber 2 g

Sugars 5 g

Protein 1 g

Phosphorus 20 mg

Choices/Exchanges: 1 Nonstarchy Vegetable, 1/2 Fat

CHICKEN NACHO CASSEROLE

⏱ 5 minutes
🍲 25 minutes
🍽 6 servings
🥄 1 cup

GF

WHO SAID PEOPLE WITH DIABETES CAN'T EAT NACHOS? THIS HEALTHY VERSION HAS ALL THE FLAVOR OF TRADITIONAL NACHOS WITHOUT ALL THE EXTRA FAT AND CARBS.

Nonstick cooking spray
1   pound boneless skinless chicken breasts, cut into small pieces
1/8   teaspoon ground black pepper
1   (14.5-ounce) can fire-roasted diced tomatoes
1   (15-ounce) can no-salt-added black beans, drained and rinsed
2   teaspoons chili powder
1/2   teaspoon cumin
1/2   teaspoon garlic powder
2/3   cup shredded reduced-fat cheddar cheese
1 1/2   ounces (about 24) baked tortilla chips, crushed

1. Preheat oven to 375°F. Spray a 2 1/2-quart baking dish with cooking spray.
2. Season the chicken with pepper. Spray a large sauté pan with cooking spray and heat over medium-high. Add the chicken and cook 8 minutes.
3. Add the diced tomatoes, black beans, chili powder, cumin, and garlic powder to the pan. Reduce the heat to low and simmer 5 minutes.
4. Pour the chicken mixture into the baking dish. Sprinkle cheese on top, and then top with the crushed tortilla chips. Bake 12 minutes or until the cheese is melted.

Nutrition Facts

Serves: 6
Serving Size: 1 cup

Amount per serving
Calories   **230**

Calories from fat 50

Total fat 6.0 g

    Saturated fat 2.3 g

    Trans fat 0.0 g

Cholesterol 50 mg

Sodium 360 mg

Potassium 520 mg

Total carbohydrate 21 g

    Dietary fiber 4 g

    Sugars 3 g

Protein 24 g

Phosphorus 295 mg

Choices/Exchanges: 1 Starch, 1 Nonstarchy Vegetable, 3 Lean Protein

CHICKEN AND BLACK BEAN BURRITOS

⏱ 15 minutes
△ 4 servings
▢ 1 burrito

HERE'S HOW TO MAKE A RESTAURANT-STYLE BURRITO FRESH AT HOME. YOU COULD SUBSTITUTE LEAN BEEF OR PORK FOR THE CHICKEN IN THIS RECIPE.

1   avocado, mashed
4   large low-carb whole-wheat tortillas
1/2   cup pico de gallo or salsa
2   cups shredded cooked chicken breast
1   cup canned no-salt-added black beans, rinsed and drained
6   tablespoons reduced-fat shredded cheddar cheese
1   cup shredded lettuce
1   cup diced tomatoes

1. Spread 3 tablespoons mashed avocado on 1 tortilla. Top with 2 tablespoons pico de gallo, 1/2 cup chicken, 1/4 cup black beans, 1 1/2 tablespoons cheese, 1/4 cup lettuce, and 1/4 cup diced tomatoes.
2. Fold into a burrito. Repeat procedure for remaining 3 burritos.

DIETITIAN TIP: *These mouthwatering burritos are prepared with lean protein from the chicken, healthy carbohydrates from the whole-wheat tortillas and beans, and good-for-you monounsaturated fat from the avocado. Delicious!*

Nutrition Facts

Serves: 4
Serving Size: 1 burrito

Amount per serving
Calories   **370**

Calories from fat 130	
Total fat 14.0 g	
Saturated fat 3.0 g	
Trans fat 0.0 g	
Cholesterol 65 mg	
Sodium 500 mg	
Potassium 770 mg	
Total carbohydrate 36 g	
Dietary fiber 19 g	
Sugars 4 g	
Protein 37 g	
Phosphorus 455 mg	

Choices/Exchanges: 2 Starch, 1 Nonstarchy Vegetable, 4 Lean Protein, 1/2 Fat

BALSAMIC CHICKEN WITH MUSHROOMS

⏱ 20 minutes
🍲 22 minutes
🍽 4 servings
🍽 1 chicken breast with heaping 1/4 cup mushrooms

THIS LOW-COST DISH IS BOTH HEALTHY AND PACKED WITH FLAVOR.

1 pound boneless skinless chicken breasts
1 tablespoon olive oil
1/4 cup flour
1 tablespoon trans fat–free margarine
10 ounces sliced mushrooms
1/4 teaspoon ground black pepper
1/3 cup balsamic vinegar
1/2 cup fat-free reduced-sodium chicken broth

1. Place the chicken breasts in a plastic bag and pound thin with a mallet.
2. Heat olive oil over medium-high heat in a skillet.
3. Dredge the chicken breasts in flour, coating them on both sides. Add the chicken to the pan and sauté 5 minutes per side. Remove the chicken from the pan and set aside.
4. Melt the margarine in the pan. Add the mushrooms and pepper and cook 5 minutes. Add the balsamic vinegar to the pan and bring it to a boil to reduce the liquid.
5. Add the chicken broth to the pan and simmer 2 more minutes. Add the chicken breasts back to the pan and simmer 5 minutes.

Nutrition Facts

Serves: 4

Serving Size: 1 chicken breast with heaping 1/4 cup mushrooms

Amount per serving

Calories **240**

Calories from fat 80	
Total fat 9.0 g	
Saturated fat 1.9 g	
Trans fat 0.0 g	
Cholesterol 65 mg	
Sodium 160 mg	
Potassium 480 mg	
Total carbohydrate 12 g	
Dietary fiber 1 g	
Sugars 5 g	
Protein 27 g	
Phosphorus 255 mg	

Choices/Exchanges:
1 Carbohydrate, 4 Lean Protein

SPINACH SALAD WITH CHICKEN AND AVOCADO

⏱ 15 minutes
🍽 4 servings
🥣 2 cups

GF

A GOOD SALAD NEEDS VEGGIES, PROTEIN, FLAVOR, AND DIFFERENT TEXTURES. THE CHICKEN IN THIS RECIPE PROVIDES THE PROTEIN. WHEN COMBINED WITH AVOCADO AND SUNFLOWER SEEDS, YOU GET THE PERFECT FLAVOR, TEXTURE, AND CRUNCH.

SALAD

12	ounces baby spinach
1	small avocado, cut into thin slices
2	roma tomatoes, diced
1	cup cooked chicken breast
4	tablespoons sunflower seeds

DRESSING

6	tablespoons light ranch dressing

1. In a large salad bowl, combine the salad ingredients.
2. Add the salad dressing and toss to coat.

Nutrition Facts

Serves: 4
Serving Size: 2 cups

Amount per serving
Calories 230

Calories from fat 140

Total fat 15.0 g
  Saturated fat 2.1 g
  Trans fat 0.0 g
Cholesterol 35 mg
Sodium 310 mg
Potassium 860 mg
Total carbohydrate 11 g
  Dietary fiber 5 g
  Sugars 3 g
Protein 16 g
Phosphorus 280 mg

Choices/Exchanges:
1/2 Carbohydrate, 1 Nonstarchy Vegetable, 2 Lean Protein, 2 Fat

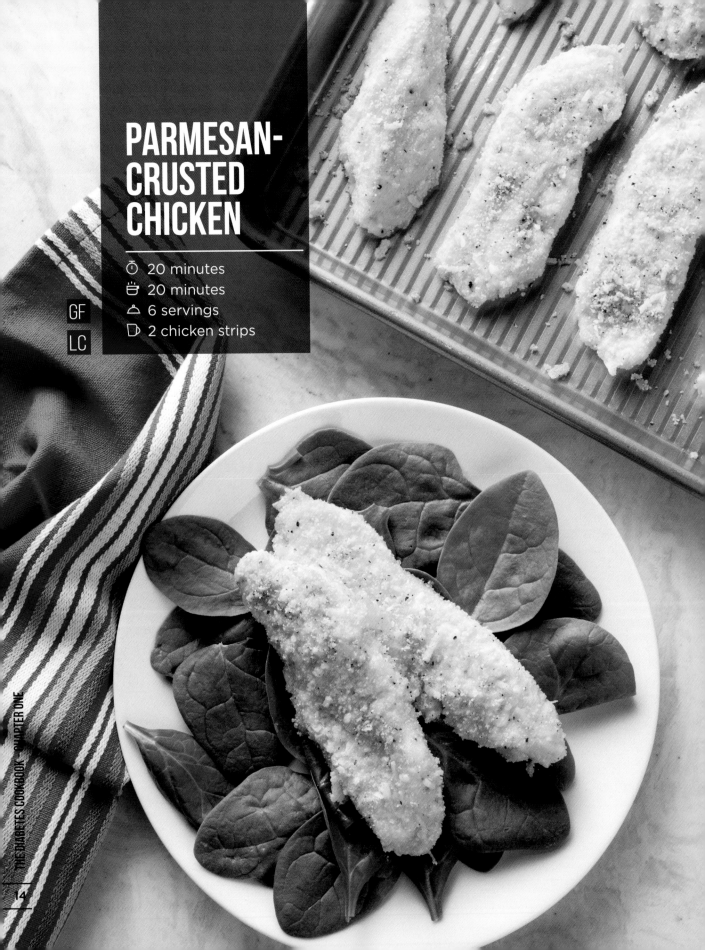

PARMESAN-CRUSTED CHICKEN

- ⏱ 20 minutes
- 🍲 20 minutes
- 🍽 6 servings
- 🥡 2 chicken strips

GF
LC

A FLAVORFUL AND VERSATILE CHICKEN RECIPE, SERVE THIS AS AN ENTRÉE WITH VEGETABLES OR OVER A SALAD. IT'S ALSO KID-FRIENDLY AND MUCH HEALTHIER THAN ANY FROZEN CHICKEN NUGGETS.

Nonstick cooking spray
1/2 cup certified gluten-free cornmeal
1/3 cup freshly grated parmesan cheese
1/2 teaspoon garlic powder
1/4 teaspoon ground black pepper
3 egg whites
1 1/2 pounds boneless skinless chicken breasts, cut into 12 thin strips

1. Preheat oven to 425°F. Spray a baking sheet with cooking spray.
2. In a shallow dish, mix together cornmeal, parmesan cheese, garlic powder, and pepper.
3. In another shallow baking dish, whisk together egg whites.
4. Dip chicken breast strip in egg mixture and then dredge in cornmeal mixture. Coat well and place on baking sheet. Repeat procedure for all chicken strips.
5. Spray chicken strips with cooking spray. Bake 15–20 minutes or until done; turn chicken pieces over halfway through cooking time.

DIETITIAN TIP: *You can keep the chicken breasts whole if you prefer them that way. Just be sure to increase the cooking time if using whole breasts.*

Nutrition Facts

Serves: 6
Serving Size: 2 chicken strips

Amount per serving
Calories **200**

Calories from fat 40	
Total fat 4.5 g	
Saturated fat 1.5 g	
Trans fat 0.0 g	
Cholesterol 70 mg	
Sodium 140 mg	
Potassium 250 mg	
Total carbohydrate 10 g	
Dietary fiber 1 g	
Sugars 0 g	
Protein 28 g	
Phosphorus 220 mg	

Choices/Exchanges: 1/2 Starch, 4 Lean Protein

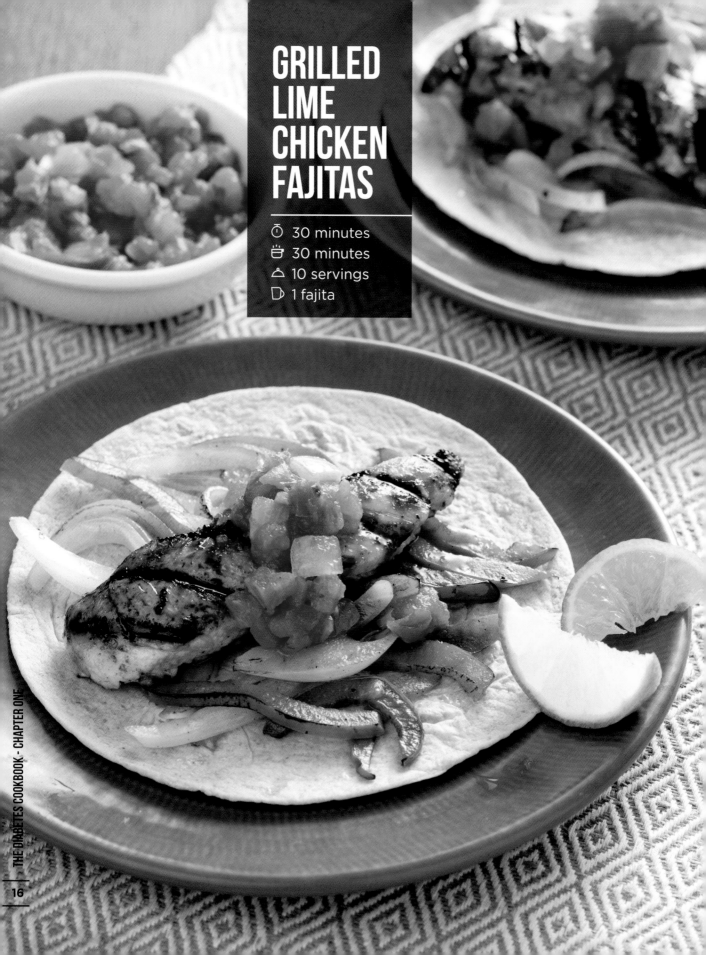

GRILLED LIME CHICKEN FAJITAS

- ⏱ 30 minutes
- ⏲ 30 minutes
- 🍽 10 servings
- 🥡 1 fajita

CHICKEN FAJITAS ARE ONE OF THE BEST CHOICES WHEN IT COMES TO MEXICAN FOOD BECAUSE CHICKEN IS A LEAN MEAT AND GRILLING IS A HEALTHY COOKING METHOD. ALSO, FAJITAS ARE TOPPED WITH LOW-CARB VEGGIES LIKE ONIONS AND GREEN PEPPERS.

MARINADE

Juice of 1 large lime
1   teaspoon lime zest
1   tablespoon honey or 2 packets artificial sweetener
2   tablespoons chopped fresh cilantro
1/2   teaspoon cumin
1   teaspoon chili powder
1/4   teaspoon garlic powder
1/4   teaspoon ground black pepper

FAJITAS

1 1/4   pounds chicken breast tenderloins
1   large onion, sliced into strips
2   green bell peppers, seeded and sliced into strips
10   (soft taco size) low-carb tortillas
10   tablespoons salsa

1. In a medium bowl, mix together the marinade ingredients. Add the chicken breast tenderloins and marinate in the refrigerator 20–60 minutes.
2. Preheat a grill to medium heat. Place the onion and green peppers in a grill basket. Grill the vegetables in the basket, stirring occasionally, about 15–20 minutes until slightly charred.
3. Add the chicken directly to the grill and cook 10–12 minutes until done, turning once.
4. Divide the chicken, green peppers, and onion evenly among 10 tortillas. Top each fajita with 1 tablespoon salsa.

DIETITIAN TIP: *If you don't have a grilling basket, you can purchase an inexpensive one at your local superstore. It's worth the purchase because it makes grilling vegetables a simple task!*

MAKE IT GLUTEN-FREE: *Confirm all ingredients are gluten-free and use corn tortillas.*

Nutrition Facts

Serves: 10
Serving Size: 1 fajita

Amount per serving
Calories   **160**

Calories from fat 35

Total fat 4.0 g
    Saturated fat 1.4 g
    Trans fat 0.0 g
Cholesterol 35 mg
Sodium 370 mg
Potassium 300 mg
Total carbohydrate 22 g
    Dietary fiber 10 g
    Sugars 5 g
Protein 18 g
Phosphorus 195 mg

Choices/Exchanges: 1 Starch, 1 Nonstarchy Vegetable, 1 Lean Protein

BLACK BEAN, MANGO, AND CHICKEN QUESADILLAS WITH SALAD

DON'T UNDERESTIMATE THIS SIMPLE AND LOW-COST DISH. IT'S A GREAT MIX OF FLAVORS WITH BEANS, CHICKEN, AND SWEET MANGO. SERVING THE QUESADILLA OVER SALAD TURNS IT INTO A COMPLETE MEAL.

- ⏱ 15 minutes
- 🍲 20 minutes
- 🍽 4 servings
- 🍴 1 quesadilla plus 2 cups salad

GF

Nonstick cooking spray
- 1 cup canned black beans, rinsed and drained
- 1 cup diced cooked chicken
- 2 tablespoons diced red onion
- 1/4 teaspoon cumin
- 1/2 cup diced mango
- 8 corn tortillas
- 8 tablespoons reduced-fat shredded cheddar cheese
- 8 cups romaine lettuce salad
- 4 tablespoons Hidden Valley Fiesta Salsa Ranch Light salad dressing

1. Spray a pan with cooking spray and heat it over medium-high. Add the black beans, chicken, onion, and cumin; sauté about 5 minutes. Add the mango and sauté 1 minute. Remove the mixture from the pan and set aside in a bowl.
2. Spray the pan with cooking spray. Place 1 tortilla in the pan and spread 2 tablespoons cheese on top of the tortilla. Add 1/2 cup chicken and bean mixture, and place another tortilla on top. Cook 1–2 minutes, flip, and cook 1–2 more minutes, until the cheese is melted.
3. Repeat this procedure for the remaining 3 quesadillas. Cut the quesadillas into triangles.
4. Serve one quesadilla over 2 cups lettuce salad, and top with 1 tablespoon salad dressing. Repeat this procedure for the remaining 3 salads.

Nutrition Facts

Serves: 4
Serving Size: 1 quesadilla plus 2 cups salad

Amount per serving
Calories — **340**

Calories from fat 90	
Total fat 10.0 g	
Saturated fat 3.3 g	
Trans fat 0.0 g	
Cholesterol 40 mg	
Sodium 330 mg	
Potassium 610 mg	
Total carbohydrate 43 g	
Dietary fiber 9 g	
Sugars 6 g	
Protein 22 g	
Phosphorus 410 mg	

Choices/Exchanges: 2 1/2 Starch, 1 Nonstarchy Vegetable, 2 Lean Protein, 1/2 Fat

CHILI LIME CORN ON THE COB

⏱ 10 minutes
🍲 20 minutes
🍽 4 servings
🥫 1 cob

GF

NOTHING SAYS SUMMER LIKE CORN ON THE COB. IT'S AN AMERICAN FAVORITE, AND THIS RECIPE PUTS A NICE TWIST OF FLAVOR INTO IT. REMEMBER, CORN IS A STARCHY VEGETABLE, SO SERVE IT WITH SOME LEAN PROTEIN AND LOW-CARB VEGETABLES LIKE GREEN BEANS, ZUCCHINI, OR A SALAD.

Juice of 1 lime
1   teaspoon lime zest
2   tablespoons light trans fat–free margarine, softened
1   teaspoon chili powder
4   medium ears corn, shucked

1. Preheat a grill to medium-high.
2. In a small bowl, mix together the lime juice, lime zest, margarine, and chili powder.
3. Using a spoon and your hands, spread the margarine mixture evenly over the 4 ears of corn.
4. Wrap each ear of corn individually in aluminum foil. Grill 20 minutes, turning frequently. Serve hot.

Nutrition Facts

Serves: 4
Serving Size: 1 cob

Amount per serving
Calories 130

Calories from fat 35	
Total fat 4.0 g	
Saturated fat 0.8 g	
Trans fat 0.0 g	
Cholesterol 0 mg	
Sodium 50 mg	
Potassium 250 mg	
Total carbohydrate 23 g	
Dietary fiber 3 g	
Sugars 5 g	
Protein 4 g	
Phosphorus 85 mg	

Choices/Exchanges: 1 1/2 Starch, 1/2 Fat

HUEVOS RANCHEROS WITH PINTO BEANS, BROWN RICE, AND CHICKEN SAUSAGE

⏱ 5 minutes
🍲 20 minutes
🍽 4 servings
🥛 1 1/3 cups

Nonstick cooking spray
2 links (3 ounces each) chorizo or other spicy fully cooked chicken sausage, diced
1/2 cup diced onion
1 medium jalapeño pepper, seeded, deveined, and minced
1 cup cooked pinto beans (see Note)
1 tablespoon chili powder
1 teaspoon cumin
1/4 teaspoon cayenne pepper
3/4 cup fat-free low-sodium chicken broth
1 cup cooked brown rice (see Note)

2 eggs
4 egg whites
1/16 teaspoon salt
1/4 teaspoon ground black pepper
2 tablespoons cold water
1/4 cup crumbled queso fresco or feta cheese

1. Spray a medium nonstick sauté pan with cooking spray and heat the pan over medium heat. Add sausage, onion, and jalapeño pepper. Sauté 2–3 minutes.
2. Add beans, chili powder, cumin, cayenne pepper, and broth. Simmer until the broth is absorbed, about 8–9 minutes.
3. Stir in brown rice and set aside.
4. In a small bowl, whisk together eggs, egg whites, salt, pepper, and cold water.
5. Spray another nonstick sauté pan with cooking spray and place the pan over medium heat. Scramble eggs until just set.

SPICE UP YOUR NEXT WEEKEND BREAKFAST OR BRUNCH WITH THIS RECIPE. IT'S A GREAT WAY TO USE LEFTOVER RICE AND BEANS. TO REDUCE CARBS FURTHER, SUBSTITUTE CAULIFLOWER RICE FOR BROWN RICE.

---

6. To serve, scoop 1 cup of sausage mixture into a bowl and top with 1/3 cup scrambled eggs and 1 tablespoon crumbled cheese.

CHEF TIP: *You can make the sausage mixture ahead of time and scramble eggs to order for breakfast.*

NOTE:

BULK COOKING DRY PINTO BEANS

Add 1 pound (16 ounces) dry pinto beans to a large pot of boiling water (at least 6 cups of water). Boil rapidly 2 minutes. Remove from heat and cover. Let sit 1 hour.

Drain and rinse beans. Add 6 fresh cups of water. Bring to a boil; then reduce to a simmer 1 hour or until the beans are soft but not split. Makes 5 cups cooked beans. These beans can be used in any recipe calling for cooked or canned beans. Store in an airtight container in the refrigerator for 7 days, or freeze in 1-cup portions for up to 6 months.

BULK COOKING BROWN RICE

Add 1 pound (16 ounces) of long grain (not instant) brown rice to a large soup pot with 5 cups of water. Bring to a boil then reduce to a simmer. Cover and simmer 45 minutes or until all liquid is absorbed. Makes 10 cups cooked brown rice. This rice can be used in any recipe calling for cooked brown rice. Store in an airtight container in the refrigerator for 7 days, or freeze in 1-cup portions for up to 6 months.

Nutrition Facts

Serves: 4
Serving Size: 1 1/3 cups

Amount per serving
Calories **290**

Calories from fat 80

Total fat 9.0 g

    Saturated fat 3.0 g

    Trans fat 0.1 g

Cholesterol 130 mg

Sodium 440 mg

Potassium 580 mg

Total carbohydrate 31 g

    Dietary fiber 6 g

    Sugars 4 g

Protein 22 g

Phosphorus 310 mg

Choices/Exchanges: 1 1/2 Starch, 1 Nonstarchy Vegetable, 2 Lean Protein, 1 Fat

NO MAYO EGG SALAD

⏱ 5 minutes
🍽 4 servings
🍴 1/2 cup egg salad on top of 1 cup arugula

LC
VG

THIS EGG SALAD HOLDS UP WELL IN THE REFRIGERATOR. IT IS DELICIOUS SERVED OVER FRESH GREENS BUT COULD ALSO BE SERVED ON WHOLE-WHEAT CRACKERS OR IN A WHOLE-WHEAT PITA.

12   hard-boiled egg whites
4   spreadable creamy light Swiss cheese wedges (such as Laughing Cow)
1   tablespoon Dijon mustard
1   teaspoon prepared horseradish
1/4   teaspoon ground black pepper
4   cups arugula

1. In a medium bowl, mash together egg whites, cheese wedges, mustard, horseradish, and pepper using a potato masher or sturdy whisk. You can also use a food processor, but take care not to overprocess the egg salad. Pulse until combined but still slightly chunky.
2. Serve 1/2 cup egg salad mixture on top of 1 cup arugula.

Nutrition Facts

Serves: 4
Serving Size: 1/2 cup egg salad on top of 1 cup arugula

Amount per serving	
Calories	**100**
Calories from fat 20	
Total fat 2.0 g	
Saturated fat 1.0 g	
Trans fat 0.0 g	
Cholesterol 2 mg	
Sodium 440 mg	
Potassium 270 mg	
Total carbohydrate 3 g	
Dietary fiber 1 g	
Sugars 2 g	
Protein 13 g	
Phosphorus 155 mg	

Choices/Exchanges: 2 Lean Protein

MUSHROOM BURGER

⏱ 5 minutes
🍲 15 minutes
🍽 4 servings
🍴 1 burger

IF YOU'D LIKE, YOU CAN ADD A SLICE OF REDUCED-FAT SWISS CHEESE TO THESE BURGERS. CHEESE WILL ADD EXTRA CALORIES AND FAT BUT NOT TOO MANY CARBS. TO LOWER CARBS FURTHER, SERVE THE BURGER IN A LETTUCE WRAP IN PLACE OF THE BUN.

1 pound lean ground turkey
1/2 teaspoon garlic powder
1/4 teaspoon ground black pepper
1 tablespoon trans fat–free margarine
8 ounces sliced mushrooms
4 whole-wheat hamburger buns, about 1 1/2 ounces each
4 slices tomato
4 romaine lettuce leaves

1. Prepare and preheat an indoor or outdoor grill.
2. In a medium bowl, mix together turkey, garlic powder, and pepper. Divide turkey into 4 equal portions, shaping each portion into a patty.
3. Place patties on grill rack, and grill 3–4 minutes per side or until juice runs clear.
4. In a medium sauté pan, heat margarine over medium-high heat. Add mushrooms and sauté 5 minutes until soft. Place each burger on a bun, top with mushrooms, tomato, and lettuce.

MAKE IT GLUTEN-FREE: *Use gluten-free bread and confirm all other ingredients are gluten-free.*

Nutrition Facts

Serves: 4
Serving Size: 1 burger

Amount per serving
Calories 330

Calories from fat 120

Total fat 13.0 g	
Saturated fat 3.3 g	
Trans fat 0.1 g	
Cholesterol 85 mg	
Sodium 330 mg	
Potassium 630 mg	
Total carbohydrate 25 g	
Dietary fiber 4 g	
Sugars 5 g	
Protein 27 g	
Phosphorus 370 mg	

Choices/Exchanges: 1 1/2 Starch, 1 Nonstarchy Vegetable, 3 Lean Protein, 1 Fat

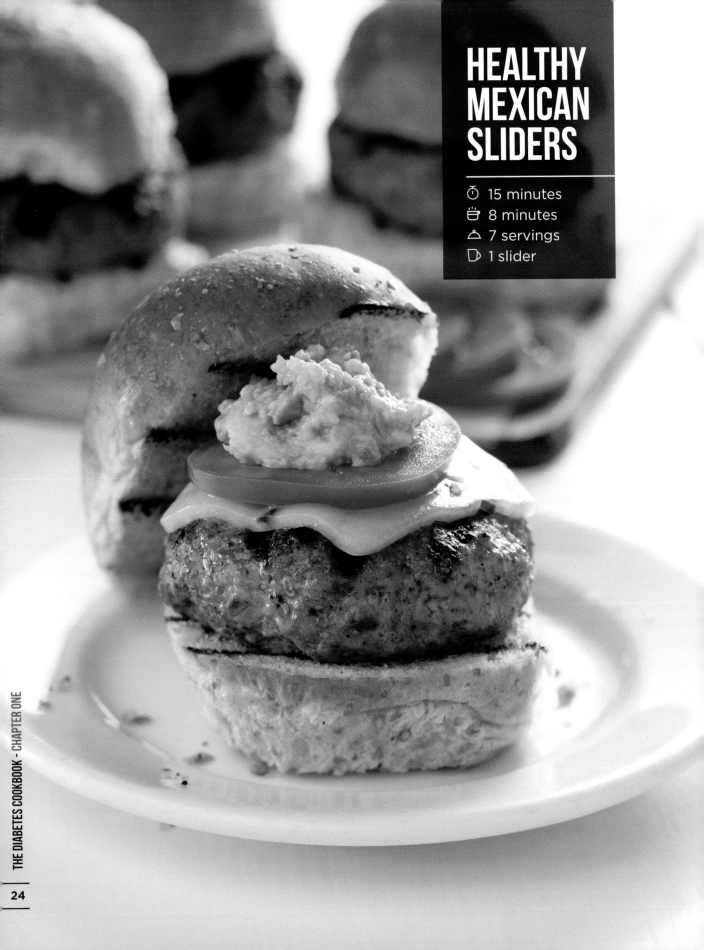

HEALTHY MEXICAN SLIDERS

⏱ 15 minutes
🍲 8 minutes
🍽 7 servings
🥤 1 slider

HEALTHY EATING CAN TASTE DELICIOUS AND DOESN'T HAVE TO BE BORING! SERVE THESE BURGERS AT YOUR NEXT TAILGATE PARTY OR BARBECUE AND YOUR GUESTS WILL HAVE NO IDEA THEY ARE EATING A HEALTHY BURGER.

1	pound lean ground turkey
1	tablespoon chili powder
1/2	teaspoon garlic powder
1/4	teaspoon ground black pepper
7	mini whole-wheat hamburger buns (or gluten-free bread/buns)
1/2	avocado, mashed
7	tomato slices
3 1/2	slices reduced-fat pepper jack cheese, cut 3 slices in half (7 half-slices total)

1. Prepare an indoor or outdoor grill.
2. In a medium bowl, mix together turkey, chili powder, garlic powder, and pepper. Divide turkey into 7 equal portions, shaping each portion into a patty.
3. Place patties on grill rack, and grill 3–4 minutes per side or until juices run clear.
4. Place burger on bun and top with 2 teaspoons avocado, 1 tomato slice, and 1/2 slice cheese. Repeat process for remaining 6 burgers.

MAKE IT GLUTEN-FREE: *Use gluten-free bread and confirm all other ingredients are gluten-free.*

Nutrition Facts

Serves: 7
Serving Size: 1 slider

Amount per serving
Calories 250

Calories from fat 90

Total fat 10.0 g

    Saturated fat 3.2 g

    Trans fat 0.1 g

Cholesterol 55 mg

Sodium 320 mg

Potassium 380 mg

Total carbohydrate 21 g

    Dietary fiber 4 g

    Sugars 4 g

Protein 19 g

Phosphorus 260 mg

Choices/Exchanges: 1 Starch, 1 Nonstarchy Vegetable, 2 Lean Protein, 1 1/2 Fat

CITRUS MAHI-MAHI PACKET WITH BROCCOLI

GF

- ⏱ 5 minutes
- 🍲 25 minutes
- 🍽 2 servings
- 🍴 1 mahi-mahi fillet and 1 cup broccoli

IF YOU'RE NOT SURE HOW TO COOK FISH, TRY A SIMPLE AND DELICIOUS METHOD LIKE THIS PACKET. IT'S FULL OF FRESH FLAVORS FROM LEMON, ORANGE, AND DILL.

Juice of 1/2 lemon
1 tablespoon olive oil
1/4 teaspoon ground black pepper
2 tablespoons chopped fresh dill
1 lemon, sliced
1 orange, sliced
2 mahi-mahi fillets (5 ounces each)
1 head broccoli, cut into florets

1. Preheat oven to 425°F. Place two pieces parchment paper on a baking sheet.
2. In a small bowl, whisk together lemon juice, olive oil, pepper, and dill.
3. Place a few lemon and orange slices in the center of each parchment paper. Place a fish fillet on top of the orange and lemon slices. Drizzle lemon sauce evenly over fish fillets. Top fish with remaining orange and lemon slices. Fold over the top of the parchment paper; then roll the sides in to form a sealed pouch.
4. Place packets on baking sheet and bake 25 minutes or until done.
5. While fish is baking, steam the broccoli 5–6 minutes.
6. Serve the fish packets with steamed broccoli. Be cautious when opening the fish packets, as steam may be hot.

DIETITIAN TIP: *It's best to eat two servings of fish per week for heart health, so mix up your choices! You can substitute another type of fish in the recipe.*

Nutrition Facts

Serves: 2
Serving Size: 1 mahi-mahi fillet and 1 cup broccoli

Amount per serving	
Calories	**270**
Calories from fat 80	
Total fat 9.0 g	
Saturated fat 1.4 g	
Trans fat 0.0 g	
Cholesterol 110 mg	
Sodium 200 mg	
Potassium 1210 mg	
Total carbohydrate 18 g	
Dietary fiber 5 g	
Sugars 7 g	
Protein 32 g	
Phosphorus 330 mg	

Choices/Exchanges: 1/2 Fruit, 2 Nonstarchy Vegetable, 4 Lean Protein

GLUTEN-FREE SPINACH AND MUSHROOM QUESADILLAS AND SALAD

⏱ 10 minutes
🍲 25 minutes
🍽 4 servings
🍴 1 quesadilla and 2 cups salad

GF
VG

DO YOU NEED A 10-MINUTE HEALTHY DINNER? THIS RECIPE IS A GREAT CHOICE—AND IT'S EASY ON THE BUDGET! IF YOU DON'T NEED THESE TO BE GLUTEN-FREE, MAKE THE QUESADILLAS WITH WHOLE-WHEAT TORTILLAS.

QUESADILLA

- 1 tablespoon olive oil
- 2 cups white mushrooms, diced
- 4 cups baby spinach
- 1 clove garlic, minced
- Nonstick cooking spray
- 4 gluten-free whole-grain tortillas (such as La Tortilla Factory gluten-free wraps)
- 1/2 cup shredded reduced-fat mozzarella cheese

SALAD

- 8 cups romaine lettuce salad

DRESSING

- 3 tablespoons extra-virgin olive oil
- 2 tablespoons lime juice
- 1 tablespoon honey or 1/2 packet artificial sweetener

1. Heat the olive oil in a non-stick pan over medium-high heat. Add the mushrooms and spinach, and sauté about 5 minutes, until the spinach wilts. Add the garlic and sauté 30 seconds. Remove the mixture from the pan and set aside in a bowl.
2. Spray the pan with cooking spray. Place 1 tortilla in the pan and spread 1/4 of the spinach-mushroom mixture on one half of the tortilla. Sprinkle 2 tablespoons cheese over each spinach-mushroom mixture. Fold the tortilla in half. Cook 1–2 minutes. Flip the tortilla and cook an additional 1–2 minutes, until golden brown. Cut the quesadilla into triangles.
3. Repeat procedure for remaining 3 quesadillas.
4. Place lettuce in a bowl.
5. In a small bowl or jar, whisk or shake the olive oil, lime juice, and honey. Spoon dressing over salad. Divide salad into four 2-cup servings.

Nutrition Facts

Serves: 4
Serving Size: 1 quesadilla and 2 cups salad

Amount per serving	
Calories	**390**
Calories from fat 200	
Total fat 22.0 g	
Saturated fat 4.7 g	
Trans fat 0.0 g	
Cholesterol 5 mg	
Sodium 480 mg	
Potassium 700 mg	
Total carbohydrate 44 g	
Dietary fiber 6 g	
Sugars 8 g	
Protein 9 g	
Phosphorus 370 mg	

Choices/Exchanges: 2 Starch, 1/2 Carbohydrate, 1 Nonstarchy Vegetable, 1 Lean Protein, 3 Fat

VEGGIE AND CHICKEN PASTA SALAD

- ⏱ 15 minutes
- 🍲 10 minutes
- 🍽 4 servings
- 🥤 1 cup

THE KEY TO INCLUDING PASTA IN YOUR MEAL PLAN WITHOUT GOING OVERBOARD ON CARBOHYDRATES IS TO KEEP THE PORTION SIZE SMALL AND SERVE IT WITH LOTS OF VEGGIES AND SOME PROTEIN. THIS IS A QUICK DINNER THE WHOLE FAMILY CAN ENJOY ANY TIME OF YEAR.

SALAD

1	cup uncooked whole-wheat elbow pasta
1/2	cup diced red bell pepper
1/2	cup peeled and diced cucumber
1/2	cup small broccoli florets
1	large carrot, diced
1	cup diced cooked chicken breast

DRESSING

1/4	cup light mayonnaise
1	tablespoon red wine vinegar
1/8	teaspoon dried oregano
1/8	teaspoon freshly ground black pepper

1. Cook the pasta according to the directions on the package. Drain.
2. In a large bowl, mix together the pasta, red pepper, cucumber, broccoli, carrot, and chicken.
3. In a small bowl, whisk together the dressing ingredients. Pour the dressing over the pasta, vegetables, and chicken, and mix well.

Nutrition Facts

Serves: 4
Serving Size: 1 cup

Amount per serving
Calories 200

Calories from fat 45

Total fat 5.0 g

    Saturated fat 0.7 g

    Trans fat 0.0 g

Cholesterol 30 mg

Sodium 160 mg

Potassium 280 mg

Total carbohydrate 24 g

    Dietary fiber 3 g

    Sugars 3 g

Protein 15 g

Phosphorus 165 mg

Choices/Exchanges: 1 1/2 Starch, 1 Nonstarchy Vegetable, 1 Lean Protein, 1/2 Fat

RUSTIC RED POTATOES AND GREEN BEANS

GF
VG

- ⏱ 10 minutes
- 🍲 35 minutes
- 🍽 6 servings
- 🥄 About 3/4 cup

THIS MIXED VEGGIE DISH IS A GREAT EXAMPLE OF HOW TO INCREASE YOUR VEGETABLE INTAKE WHILE CONTROLLING YOUR CARBOHYDRATE INTAKE. REMEMBER, HALF OF YOUR PLATE SHOULD BE LOW-CARB VEGGIES SUCH AS GREEN BEANS, BROCCOLI, CAULIFLOWER, ASPARAGUS, ZUCCHINI, OR SPINACH.

Nonstick cooking spray
6   small red potatoes, cut into eighths
2   tablespoons olive oil, divided
1/2   teaspoon garlic salt, divided
1/4   teaspoon ground black pepper, divided
1/4   teaspoon dried parsley
1   pound green beans

1. Preheat oven to 400°F. Spray a baking sheet with cooking spray.
2. In a medium bowl mix together potatoes, 1 tablespoon olive oil, 1/4 teaspoon garlic salt, 1/8 teaspoon pepper, and 1/4 teaspoon parsley.
3. Place potatoes on half of the baking sheet and bake 15 minutes.
4. In a medium bowl mix together green beans, 1 tablespoon olive oil, 1/4 teaspoon garlic salt, and 1/8 teaspoon pepper.
5. After potatoes have baked 15 minutes, add green beans to the other half of the baking sheet. Bake potatoes and green beans an additional 20 minutes.
6. Place potatoes and green beans in a serving bowl and mix together.

Nutrition Facts

Serves: 6
Serving Size: About 3/4 cup

Amount per serving
Calories 110

Calories from fat 45	
Total fat 5.0 g	
Saturated fat 0.7 g	
Trans fat 0.0 g	
Cholesterol 0 mg	
Sodium 115 mg	
Potassium 410 mg	
Total carbohydrate 16 g	
Dietary fiber 3 g	
Sugars 2 g	
Protein 3 g	
Phosphorus 60 mg	

Choices/Exchanges: 1/2 Starch, 1 Nonstarchy Vegetable, 1 Fat

INDIVIDUAL S'MORE DESSERTS

VG

⏱ 15 minutes
🍲 4 servings
🥤 1 parfait

IMPRESS YOUR SWEETHEART WITH THIS QUICK AND HEALTHY DESSERT THAT LOOKS GOURMET. INDIVIDUAL DESSERTS CAN HELP WITH PORTION CONTROL AND OVEREATING.

1 (1.4-ounce) box sugar-free instant chocolate pudding
2 cups skim milk
1 1/2 graham cracker sheets
8 tablespoons light whipped cream (such as Cabot Sweetened Light Whipped Cream)
4 teaspoons mini chocolate chips

1. In a medium bowl whisk together pudding and skim milk according to the directions on the package. Cool in refrigerator 5 minutes.
2. Place graham cracker sheets in a small plastic bag. Use a rolling pin to crush the crackers into crumbs.
3. Place 1/4 cup pudding into the bottom of a small juice glass or parfait dish. Top with 1 tablespoon graham cracker crumbs and 1 tablespoon whipped cream. Layer with another 1/4 cup pudding and 1 tablespoon whipped cream. Sprinkle top with 1 teaspoon chocolate chips.
4. Repeat procedure for remaining 3 desserts.

MAKE IT GLUTEN-FREE: *If you need this dessert to be gluten-free, use gluten-free graham crackers and confirm all other ingredients are gluten-free.*

Nutrition Facts

Serves: 4
Serving Size: 1 parfait

Amount per serving
Calories   **140**

Calories from fat 30

Total fat 3.5 g

   Saturated fat 1.8 g

   Trans fat 0.0 g

Cholesterol 5 mg

Sodium 400 mg

Potassium 250 mg

Total carbohydrate 22 g

   Dietary fiber 1 g

   Sugars 11 g

Protein 6 g

Phosphorus 225 mg

Choices/Exchanges: 1/2 Fat-Free Milk, 1 Carbohydrate, 1/2 Fat

SCALLOPS WITH PASTA IN WINE SAUCE

⏱ 5 minutes
🍲 20 minutes
🍽 4 servings
🍴 1 cup spaghetti,
4 ounces scallops, and
1/2 cup sauce

BAY SCALLOPS ARE SMALLER AND SWEETER THAN THEIR SEA SCALLOP COUSINS. PAIRED WITH WHOLE-GRAIN PASTA, THEY MAKE FOR A SIMPLE YET ELEGANT DISH THAT'S HEART HEALTHY AS WELL.

8	ounces whole-wheat spaghetti
1	tablespoon olive oil
1	pound bay scallops
1	clove garlic, minced
1	cup dry white wine
1	cup fat-free reduced-sodium chicken broth
1/2	teaspoon dried basil

1. Cook pasta according to the directions on the package. Drain.
2. Heat olive oil in a skillet over medium-high heat. Add scallops and cook 6–7 minutes, turning once. Remove scallops from pan and cover to keep warm.
3. Add garlic to pan and sauté 30 seconds. Add wine and simmer 3–4 minutes. Add chicken broth and basil to pan and cook 2–3 minutes.
4. Return scallops to skillet. Add spaghetti and cook 30 seconds.

DIETITIAN TIP: *If you want to lower the carbohydrates in this dish you could serve the scallops over zucchini or carrot "noodles" in place of traditional pasta. These "veggie noodles" are now sold in grocery stores in the freezer section with the frozen vegetables.*

Nutrition Facts

Serves: 4
Serving Size: 1 cup spaghetti, 4 ounces scallops, and 1/2 cup sauce

Amount per serving	
Calories	**350**
Calories from fat 45	
Total fat 5.0 g	
Saturated fat 0.7 g	
Trans fat 0.0 g	
Cholesterol 30 mg	
Sodium 340 mg	
Potassium 360 mg	
Total carbohydrate 46 g	
Dietary fiber 6 g	
Sugars 2 g	
Protein 25 g	
Phosphorus 435 mg	

Choices/Exchanges: 3 Starch, 3 Lean Protein

SHRIMP FAJITAS

- ⏱ 15 minutes
- 🍲 15 minutes
- 🍽 5 servings
- 🍴 2 fajitas

GF

SERVE THIS DISH WITH JICAMA STICKS AND FRESH GUACAMOLE. IF YOU'D LIKE, YOU CAN MAKE THIS COLORFUL DISH EVEN MORE VIBRANT BY USING DIFFERENT COLOR PEPPERS OR PURPLE ONION.

Nonstick cooking spray
1	pound medium shrimp, peeled and deveined
1	teaspoon olive oil
1	red bell pepper, sliced into thin strips
1	green bell pepper, sliced into thin strips
1	medium onion, sliced into thin strips
1/4	cup water
1/2	tablespoon chili powder
1/4	teaspoon cayenne pepper
1/4	teaspoon cumin
1/2	teaspoon salt
1/2	teaspoon ground black pepper
10	corn tortillas

1. Coat a large nonstick skillet with cooking spray. Cook the shrimp over medium heat about 2 minutes. Remove the shrimp from the pan and set aside.
2. Add the oil to the pan and heat. Add the bell peppers and onions and cook about 7 minutes or until they begin to brown. Add the shrimp and any juices back to the pan.
3. Add the water and spices, including salt and pepper. Bring the mixture to a boil; reduce heat and simmer until the water evaporates. Serve the shrimp and peppers in the corn tortillas.

NOTE: *If possible, use fresh (never frozen) shrimp, or shrimp that are free of preservatives (for example, shrimp that have not been treated with salt or STPP [sodium tripolyphosphate]).*

Nutrition Facts

Serves: 5
Serving Size: 2 fajitas

Amount per serving
Calories 230

Calories from fat 25

Total fat 3.0 g

    Saturated fat 0.4 g

    Trans fat 0.0 g

Cholesterol 150 mg

Sodium 340 mg

Potassium 470 mg

Total carbohydrate 31 g

    Dietary fiber 5 g

    Sugars 4 g

Protein 23 g

Phosphorus 380 mg

Choices/Exchanges: 1 1/2 Starch, 1 Nonstarchy Vegetable, 2 Lean Protein

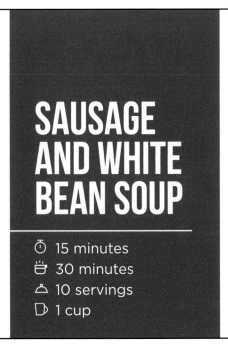

SAUSAGE AND WHITE BEAN SOUP

- ⏱ 15 minutes
- 🍲 30 minutes
- 🍽 10 servings
- 🥣 1 cup

LC

THIS ONE-POT SOUP RECIPE PROVIDES HEALTHY CARBS FROM THE BEANS, PROTEIN FROM THE TURKEY SAUSAGE, AND VEGGIES FROM THE SPINACH AND TOMATOES. YOU CAN ALSO ADD A LITTLE GRATED PARMESAN CHEESE WHEN YOU ADD THE SPINACH FOR SOME ADDED CREAMINESS; IT WILL INCREASE THE FAT A BIT, BUT NOT THE CARBS. HEALTHY EATING AND COOKING CAN BE EASY AND DELICIOUS!

Nonstick cooking spray
1   medium onion, finely diced
3   Italian turkey sausage links (about 12 ounces total)
32   ounces fat-free low-sodium chicken broth
1 1/2 cups water
1 1/2 cups canned crushed tomatoes
1   (15-ounce) can no-salt-added great northern beans, drained and rinsed
1/2 tablespoon dried basil
1/4 teaspoon dried oregano
1/4 teaspoon ground black pepper
6   ounces baby spinach

1. Spray a large soup pot with cooking spray. Add onion and sauté over medium-high heat 3 minutes or until clear.
2. Squeeze sausage meat from casings and discard casings. Add sausage to pot and break up into pieces with a spoon. Cook until brown, about 7–8 minutes.
3. Add remaining ingredients, except baby spinach. Reduce heat and simmer 15 minutes.
4. Add baby spinach and cook an additional 1–2 minutes.

MAKE IT GLUTEN-FREE: *Use gluten-free chicken broth and verify the spices and beans are gluten-free.*

Nutrition Facts

Serves: 10
Serving Size: 1 cup

Amount per serving
Calories   **110**

Calories from fat 30	
Total fat 3.5 g	
Saturated fat 0.8 g	
Trans fat 0.1 g	
Cholesterol 20 mg	
Sodium 390 mg	
Potassium 480 mg	
Total carbohydrate 10 g	
Dietary fiber 3 g	
Sugars 3 g	
Protein 11 g	
Phosphorus 140 mg	

Choices/Exchanges: 1/2 Starch, 1 Nonstarchy Vegetable, 1 Lean Protein

POWER LUNCH SALAD

- ⏱ 10 minutes
- 🍴 4 servings
- 🥣 About 3 cups

THIS SALAD MAKES A NUTRITIOUS AND FLAVOR-PACKED LUNCH THAT YOU ARE BOUND TO LOVE. IT'S A GREAT EXAMPLE OF HOW A SALAD CAN BE A MEAL WHEN YOU INCLUDE VEGETABLES, PROTEIN, AND HEALTHY CARBS.

SALAD

12	cups organic baby spinach and spring mix blend
1/4	cup sliced raw unsalted almonds
1/3	cup dry-roasted unsalted pepitas
1/2	cup dried cranberries
2	small organic apples, cored and diced
1/3	cup crumbled reduced-fat feta cheese
7	ounces reduced-sodium deli turkey breast, sliced into 1/2-inch strips

DRESSING

1/3	cup balsamic vinegar
1 1/2	tablespoons extra-virgin olive oil

1. In a salad bowl, mix together all salad ingredients.
2. In a small bowl, whisk together dressing ingredients. Pour over salad and toss to coat.

DIETITIAN TIP:

This recipe uses organic spinach, lettuce, and apples because they are among the "dirty dozen" list of foods that tend to contain the most pesticides. So if you are trying to figure out what foods to buy organic, these are a few to start with. If you can't find pepitas, substitute sunflower seeds. Dried fruits, such as cranberries, are high in carbs, but it's good to eat them with other low-carb foods such as spinach, salad, and almonds.

MAKE IT GLUTEN-FREE:

Confirm the ingredients you use are gluten-free.

Nutrition Facts

Serves: 4
Serving Size: About 3 cups

Amount per serving

Calories   310

Calories from fat 140

Total fat 15.0 g

    Saturated fat 2.8 g

    Trans fat 0.0 g

Cholesterol 25 mg

Sodium 440 mg

Potassium 530 mg

Total carbohydrate 28 g

    Dietary fiber 4 g

    Sugars 19 g

Protein 18 g

Phosphorus 320 mg

Choices/Exchanges: 1 Fruit, 1 Carbohydrate, 2 Lean Protein, 2 Fat

SPINACH ARTICHOKE DIP

GF
LC
VG

⏱ 15 minutes
🍲 15 minutes
🍽 12 servings
🥄 2 tablespoons

THIS LOW-CARB APPETIZER IS A MUCH LIGHTER VERSION OF TRADITIONAL SPINACH ARTICHOKE DIP, BUT IT STILL PACKS IN GREAT FLAVOR. WHIP UP THIS DIP IN NO TIME FOR YOUR NEXT PARTY.

1	cup chopped frozen spinach, thawed
1 1/2	cups frozen artichoke hearts, chopped and thawed
5	spreadable creamy light Swiss cheese wedges (such as Laughing Cow Garlic & Herb)
	Juice of 1/2 lemon
2	tablespoons light mayonnaise
3	tablespoons grated parmesan cheese
1/4	teaspoon red pepper flakes

1. In a small pot, boil spinach and artichoke hearts in 1 cup water until tender. Discard liquid, drain well, and set the vegetables aside in a bowl.
2. In the same pot, melt the cheese wedges over low heat. Add remaining ingredients, mix well, and continue to cook an additional 1–2 minutes.
3. Add the spinach and artichoke mixture to the pot and stir. Cook an additional 2 minutes.
4. Serve warm with your choice of vegetables or whole-wheat crackers.

Nutrition Facts

Serves: 12
Serving Size: 2 tablespoons

Amount per serving
Calories   **40**

Calories from fat 15	
Total fat 1.5 g	
Saturated fat 0.7 g	
Trans fat 0.0 g	
Cholesterol 2 mg	
Sodium 150 mg	
Potassium 115 mg	
Total carbohydrate 3 g	
Dietary fiber 2 g	
Sugars 1 g	
Protein 2 g	
Phosphorus 80 mg	

Choices/Exchanges: 1/2 Fat

SPINACH AND HAM ENGLISH MUFFIN PIZZAS

○ 10 minutes
🍽 8 minutes
🍲 4 servings
☕ 1 pizza

NEED A DINNER IN LESS THAN 20 MINUTES? HERE'S YOUR ANSWER! IT'S NOT FANCY, BUT IT PROVIDES SOME VEGETABLES AND IS HEALTHIER AND LESS EXPENSIVE THAN ORDERING OUT.

2 high-fiber english muffins, split in half
4 tablespoons frozen chopped spinach, thawed and drained
6 tablespoons pizza sauce
2 ounces lower-sodium deli-style ham
1/2 cup shredded reduced-fat mozzarella cheese

1. Preheat oven to 425°F.
2. Top each english muffin half with 1 tablespoon spinach, 1 1/2 tablespoons pizza sauce, 1/2 ounce ham, and 2 tablespoons mozzarella cheese.
3. Bake pizzas 8 minutes or until cheese is golden brown on top.

DIETITIAN TIP: *Wondering what to do with the leftover spinach? Use it to make an omelet or scrambled eggs the next morning, or add it to soup or pasta for dinner.*

Nutrition Facts
Serves: 4
Serving Size: 1 pizza

Amount per serving
Calories **110**

Calories from fat 30	
Total fat 3.5 g	
Saturated fat 1.5 g	
Trans fat 0.0 g	
Cholesterol 15 mg	
Sodium 430 mg	
Potassium 220 mg	
Total carbohydrate 17 g	
Dietary fiber 5 g	
Sugars 2 g	
Protein 9 g	
Phosphorus 190 mg	

Choices/Exchanges: 1 Starch, 1 Lean Protein

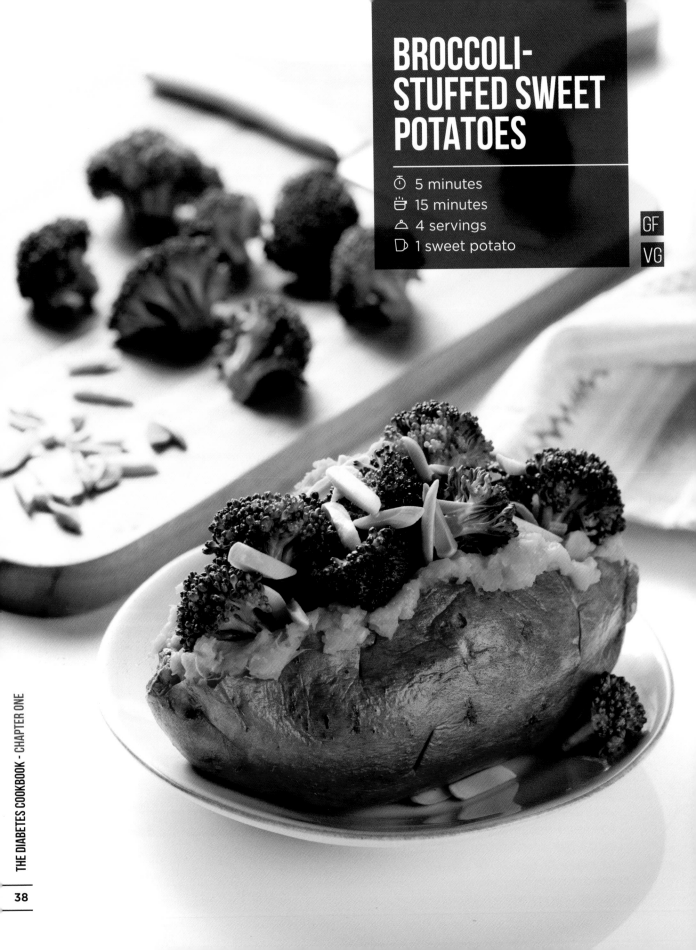

BROCCOLI-STUFFED SWEET POTATOES

- ⏱ 5 minutes
- 🍲 15 minutes
- 🍽 4 servings
- 🥣 1 sweet potato

GF
VG

SWEET POTATOES ARE A HEALTHY CARBOHYDRATE FULL OF FIBER AND VITAMIN A. THEY MAKE A GREAT, QUICK SIDE DISH! YOU COULD ALSO STUFF THIS SWEET POTATO WITH SPINACH AND PINE NUTS.

4 medium sweet potatoes
3 cups broccoli florets
4 teaspoons trans fat–free margarine
4 tablespoons slivered almonds, toasted

1. Pierce each sweet potato with a fork in a few spots. Arrange the potatoes on a microwave-safe plate and microwave until soft, about 12 minutes.

2. Place 3/4 to 1 inch of water in a saucepan with a steamer and bring to a boil. (If you don't have a steamer, you can simply put the broccoli directly into 1 inch of boiling water.) Add the broccoli to the steamer and cover; reduce the heat to medium and let cook 6 minutes.

3. Using a knife, slit each sweet potato in half and pinch the sides to open it up. Fill each sweet potato with 1 teaspoon margarine, 2/3 cup broccoli, and 1 tablespoon toasted almonds.

Nutrition Facts

Serves: 4
Serving Size: 1 sweet potato

Amount per serving
Calories **190**

Calories from fat 60	
Total fat 7.0 g	
Saturated fat 1.2 g	
Trans fat 0.0 g	
Cholesterol 0 mg	
Sodium 85 mg	
Potassium 770 mg	
Total carbohydrate 28 g	
Dietary fiber 6 g	
Sugars 9 g	
Protein 6 g	
Phosphorus 135 mg	

Choices/Exchanges: 1 1/2 Starch, 1 Nonstarchy Vegetable, 1 Fat

PAD THAI FLATBREAD PIZZA WITH SALAD

⏱ 10 minutes
🍲 20 minutes
🍽 2 servings
🍴 1 flatbread pizza and about 2 cups salad

VG

TAKEOUT PIZZA IS USUALLY HIGH IN CALORIES AND CARBOHYDRATES. HERE'S A HEALTHIER PIZZA THAT YOU CAN MAKE AT HOME USING THIN-CRUST FLATBREADS. BY SKIPPING HIGH-FAT MEATS SUCH AS PEPPERONI AND SAUSAGE, YOU'LL CUT BACK ON UNHEALTHY FATS AS WELL.

2   thin-crust wheat flatbreads
1   teaspoon olive oil
5   ounces firm tofu, drained and diced
2 1/3   tablespoons pad thai sauce
1/4   teaspoon crushed red pepper flakes
3   cups coleslaw mix (shredded cabbage and carrots)
1   green onion, chopped
4   tablespoons shredded reduced-fat mozzarella cheese

SALAD

4   cups spring mix
1/2   cucumber, sliced
1   carrot, diced

DRESSING

1/4   cup red wine vinegar
1 1/2   tablespoons extra-virgin olive oil
1/8   teaspoon ground black pepper

1. Preheat oven to 350°F. Place the flatbreads on a pizza pan and bake 4 minutes. Remove the flatbreads from the oven and set aside.
2. In a large nonstick skillet or wok, heat the oil over medium-high heat. Add the tofu and cook 5 minutes or until lightly golden. Add the pad thai sauce and red pepper flakes, and cook 2 more minutes.
3. Add the coleslaw mix and green onion, and cook 2–4 more minutes.
4. Divide the cabbage-tofu mixture in half and spread evenly onto 2 flatbreads. Sprinkle 2 tablespoons cheese on each flatbread. Bake 4 minutes, and serve hot.
5. Place salad ingredients in a small bowl. Whisk together dressing ingredients. Pour dressing over salad.

Nutrition Facts

Serves: 2
Serving Size: 1 flatbread pizza and about 2 cups salad

Amount per serving	
Calories	**450**
Calories from fat 190	
Total fat 21.0 g	
Saturated fat 3.9 g	
Trans fat 0.0 g	
Cholesterol 10 mg	
Sodium 660 mg	
Potassium 740 mg	
Total carbohydrate 49 g	
Dietary fiber 8 g	
Sugars 12 g	
Protein 19 g	
Phosphorus 265 mg	

Choices/Exchanges: 2 Starch, 1/2 Carbohydrate, 2 Nonstarchy Vegetable, 1 Medium-Fat Protein, 3 Fat

TURKEY TACOS

- ⏱ 10 minutes
- 🍽 10 minutes
- 🍴 8 servings
- 🍴 1 taco

THIS MEAT MIXTURE ALSO MAKES A GREAT TOPPING FOR NACHOS (USING BAKED TORTILLA CHIPS AND REDUCED-FAT CHEESE). TOP NACHOS WITH LETTUCE, TOMATOES, CILANTRO, AND GREEK YOGURT FOR A TASTY PARTY SNACK.

Nonstick cooking spray
1   teaspoon olive oil
1   pound lean ground turkey (93% fat-free)
1   packet (1 ounce) lower-sodium (50% less sodium) taco seasoning mix
1   (15-ounce) can no-salt-added petite diced tomatoes
1   (15-ounce) can fat-free or vegetarian refried beans
8   (6-inch) corn tortillas
2   cups shredded iceberg lettuce
2   medium tomatoes, diced
1/4 cup minced fresh cilantro
1/2 cup fat-free plain Greek yogurt
2   limes, quartered

1. Spray a large sauté pan with cooking spray, add olive oil, and place pan over high heat.
2. Sauté the turkey until just cooked through, about 6–7 minutes.
3. Add the taco seasoning packet and the canned tomatoes with the juice. The seasoning packet says to add water, but use the juice from the tomatoes instead. Bring to a simmer.
4. Simmer 3 minutes; then stir in the refried beans until incorporated.
5. Build the tacos with 1/3 cup meat and bean mixture, top with lettuce, tomato, a sprinkling of cilantro, 1 tablespoon Greek yogurt, and lime wedge on the side.

MAKE IT GLUTEN-FREE: *Verify that the seasoning packet, refried beans, and tortillas you are using are gluten-free.*

Nutrition Facts

Serves: 8
Serving Size: 1 taco

Amount per serving
Calories **230**

Calories from fat 50	
Total fat 6.0 g	
Saturated fat 1.5 g	
Trans fat 0.1 g	
Cholesterol 45 mg	
Sodium 460 mg	
Potassium 600 mg	
Total carbohydrate 27 g	
Dietary fiber 5 g	
Sugars 5 g	
Protein 17 g	
Phosphorus 305 mg	

Choices/Exchanges: 1 1/2 Starch, 1 Nonstarchy Vegetable, 2 Lean Protein

TURKEY AND AVOCADO WRAP

⏱ 5 minutes
🍽 4 servings
🍴 1 wrap

TIRED OF THE SAME BORING LUNCH? TRY THIS QUICK AND DELICIOUS WRAP. WHEN MAKING A WRAP, ADD LOTS OF DIFFERENT TEXTURES, AS IS DONE HERE, FOR MAXIMUM FLAVOR AND SATISFACTION.

1/2	avocado, mashed
2	tablespoons fat-free plain Greek yogurt
4	large low-carb tortillas
12	ounces no-salt-added deli-style turkey breast
4	teaspoons sunflower seeds
1	tomato, sliced
1	cup shredded lettuce

1. In a small bowl, mix avocado and yogurt.
2. Spread mixture evenly onto 4 tortillas.
3. Top each tortilla with 3 ounces turkey, 1 teaspoon sunflower seeds, 2 slices tomato, and 1/4 cup lettuce.

MAKE IT GLUTEN-FREE: *Use gluten-free tortillas and confirm all other ingredients are gluten-free.*

Nutrition Facts

Serves: 4
Serving Size: 1 wrap

Amount per serving
Calories **250**

Calories from fat 80

Total fat 9.0 g

    Saturated fat 1.1 g

    Trans fat 0.0 g

Cholesterol 60 mg

Sodium 440 mg

Potassium 550 mg

Total carbohydrate 23 g

    Dietary fiber 15 g

    Sugars 3 g

Protein 33 g

Phosphorus 405 mg

Choices/Exchanges: 1 Starch, 1 Nonstarchy Vegetable, 4 Lean Protein

TURKEY AND BARLEY SOUP

⏱ 15 minutes
🍲 25 minutes
🍽 5 servings
🥣 2 cups

BUYING PRECOOKED TURKEY AND PRESLICED MUSHROOMS IS A HUGE TIME-SAVER IN THIS RECIPE.

1   tablespoon olive oil
1   medium onion, peeled and diced
2   medium carrots, diced (about 1 1/2 cups diced)
2   stalks celery, diced
8   ounces sliced mushrooms
1/2 cup quick-cooking barley
4   cups fat-free low-sodium chicken broth
2   cups water
2   cups (about 10 ounces) shredded or diced cooked turkey breast
1/2 teaspoon salt
1/2 teaspoon ground black pepper

1. Add olive oil to a soup pot over medium-high heat.
2. Add onion, carrots, celery, and mushrooms to the pot. Sauté 8–10 minutes or until onions start to turn clear.
3. Add barley, broth, and water. Bring to a boil; then reduce to a simmer and simmer 15 minutes.
4. Add cooked turkey. Season with salt and pepper.

Nutrition Facts

Serves: 5
Serving Size: 2 cups

Amount per serving
Calories **220**

Calories from fat 40

Total fat 4.5 g

   Saturated fat 0.8 g

   Trans fat 0.0 g

Cholesterol 45 mg

Sodium 440 mg

Potassium 720 mg

Total carbohydrate 21 g

   Dietary fiber 4 g

   Sugars 5 g

Protein 25 g

Phosphorus 280 mg

Choices/Exchanges: 1 Starch, 1 Nonstarchy Vegetable, 3 Lean Protein

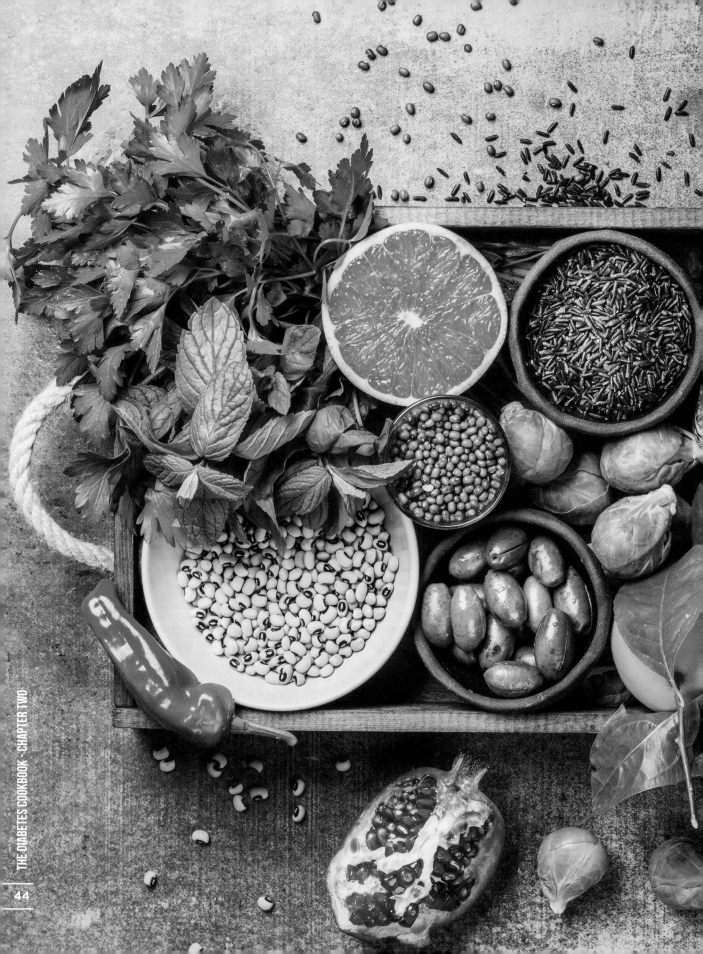

CHAPTER TWO
FOODIE RECIPES

THESE DISHES ARE NOT MEANT TO INTIMIDATE BUT TO PROVE THAT ANYONE CAN CREATE A GOURMET RESTAURANT-STYLE DISH AT HOME THAT IS HEALTHY, TOO!

BARLEY, MUSHROOM, AND HERB RISOTTO

ADD COOKED CHICKEN OR SHRIMP TO THIS DISH TO MAKE IT A MEAL!

- 10 minutes
- 45 minutes
- 6 servings
- 1/2 cup

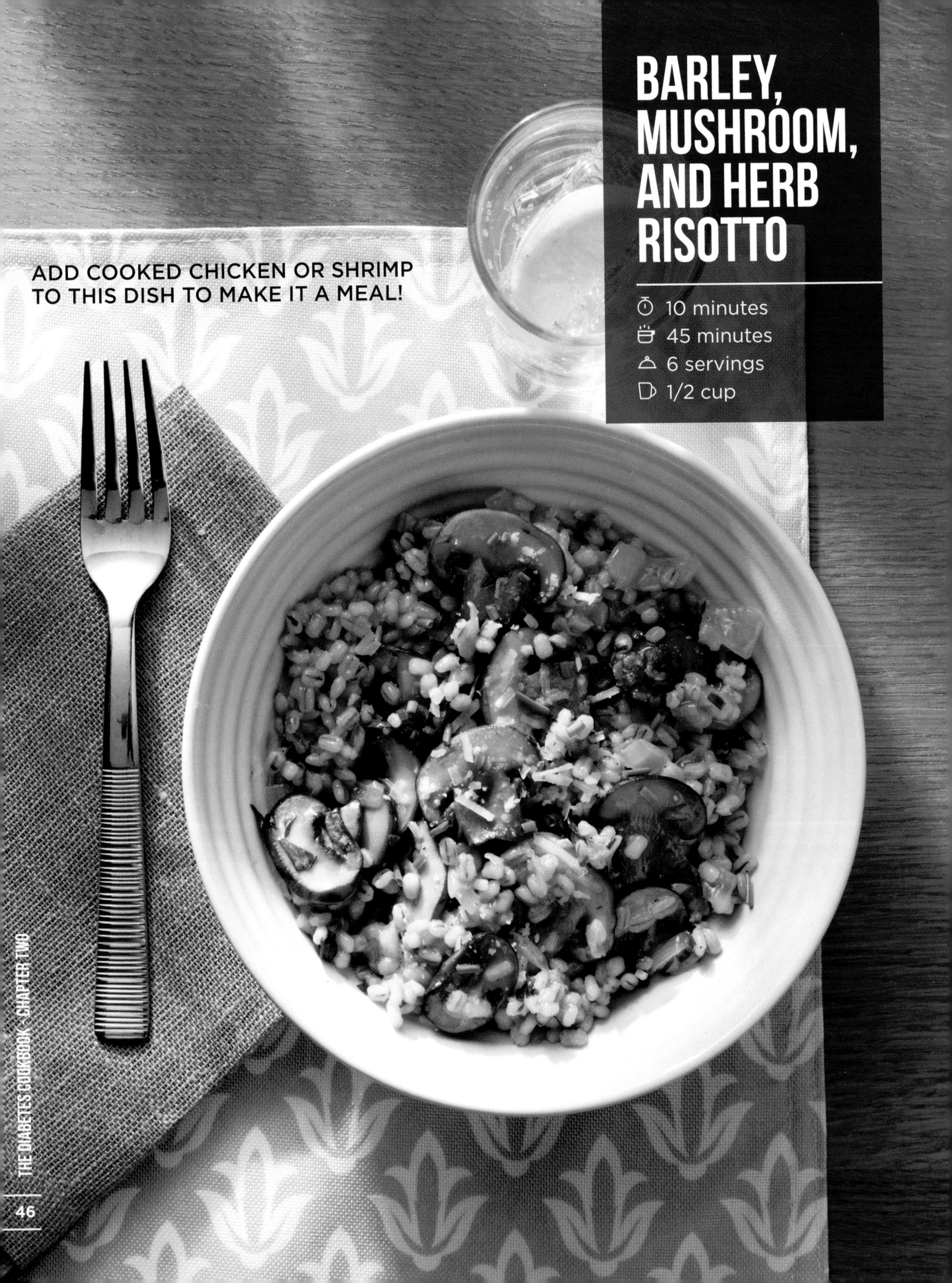

4	cups fat-free reduced-sodium chicken broth
2	cups water
3	teaspoons olive oil, divided
1	small onion, diced (1 cup)
1	cup pearl barley
1	pound fresh mushrooms, sliced
1	clove garlic, minced
2	teaspoons chopped fresh parsley
2	teaspoons chopped fresh chives
1/4	teaspoon ground black pepper
1/4	cup grated parmesan cheese

1. In a saucepan, bring chicken broth and water to a simmer over medium heat. Set aside but keep warm on low heat.

2. In a medium saucepan, add 1 teaspoon olive oil over medium heat. Sauté onion until clear. Add barley and sauté 2 minutes.

3. Ladle 1/2 cup hot broth into barley mixture and stir constantly until liquid is absorbed. Continue to add broth, one 1/2 cup at a time, until the barley is cooked and has a creamy texture.

4. Add 2 teaspoons olive oil to a medium sauté pan over medium-high heat. Add mushrooms and sauté until all the liquid from the mushrooms is expelled and mushrooms begin to brown. Add garlic and sauté 1 minute.

5. Add sautéed mushrooms and garlic to barley mixture; then stir in parsley, chives, pepper, and parmesan cheese. Serve immediately.

6. If the barley risotto gets too thick, add more hot broth, stirring until creamy.

Nutrition Facts

Serves: 6
Serving Size: 1/2 cup

Amount per serving
Calories   190

Calories from fat 30

Total fat 3.5 g

   Saturated fat 0.9 g

   Trans fat 0.0 g

Cholesterol 4 mg

Sodium 430 mg

Potassium 510 mg

Total carbohydrate 32 g

   Dietary fiber 6 g

   Sugars 4 g

Protein 9 g

Phosphorus 195 mg

Choices/Exchanges: 1 1/2 Starch, 1 Nonstarchy Vegetable, 1 Fat

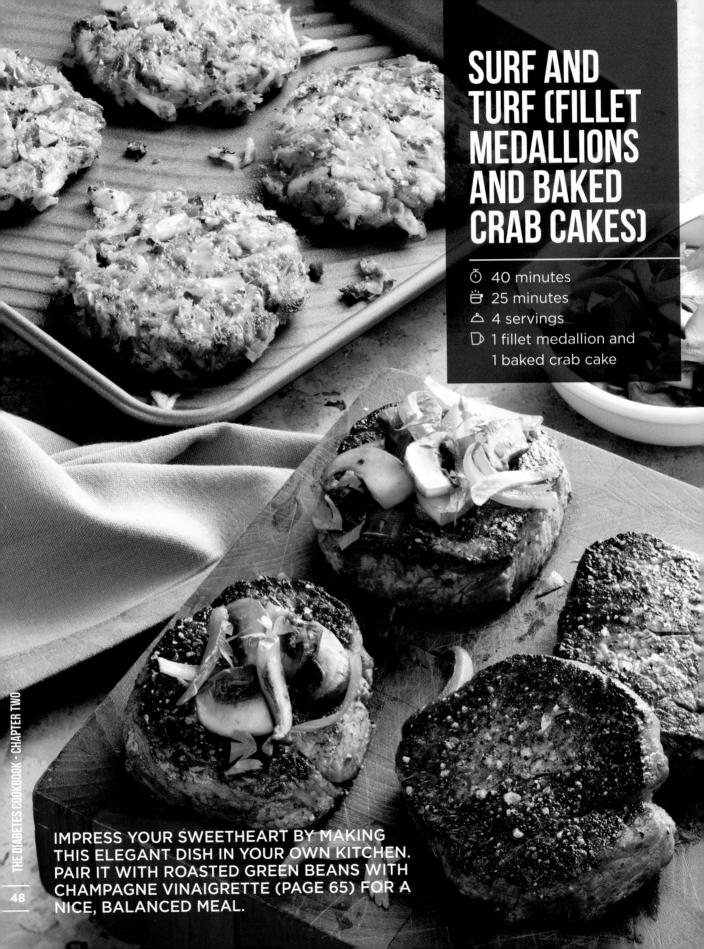

SURF AND TURF (FILLET MEDALLIONS AND BAKED CRAB CAKES)

- ⏱ 40 minutes
- 🍲 25 minutes
- 🍽 4 servings
- 🍴 1 fillet medallion and 1 baked crab cake

IMPRESS YOUR SWEETHEART BY MAKING THIS ELEGANT DISH IN YOUR OWN KITCHEN. PAIR IT WITH ROASTED GREEN BEANS WITH CHAMPAGNE VINAIGRETTE (PAGE 65) FOR A NICE, BALANCED MEAL.

CRAB CAKES

Nonstick cooking spray
1/2 small onion, minced
1/2 red bell pepper, seeded and minced
1 (6-ounce) can lump crabmeat, drained
1/4 cup whole-wheat bread crumbs
2 egg whites
1/2 teaspoon hot sauce
1/4 teaspoon ground black pepper

FILLET MEDALLIONS

1 tablespoon olive oil
4 (3-ounce) beef tenderloin steaks
3/8 teaspoon salt
1 tablespoon cracked black pepper
2 cups sliced mushrooms
1 small onion, thinly sliced
1/2 cup fat-free reduced-sodium beef broth

1. Preheat oven to 375°F. Coat a small baking sheet with cooking spray. Set aside.
2. Coat a small nonstick skillet with cooking spray and place over medium-high heat. Add onion and red pepper and sauté 2–3 minutes or until onions are clear. Set aside to cool.
3. In a medium bowl combine crabmeat, bread crumbs, egg whites, hot sauce, and pepper. Mix well until all ingredients are incorporated. Stir in onion and red pepper mixture. Refrigerate mixture 30 minutes.
4. Form crab mixture into four 1/2-inch-thick patties. Place patties on the prepared baking sheet. Coat the top of each crab cake with cooking spray, and bake 25 minutes on the top rack, turning once halfway through.
5. While crab cakes are baking, heat olive oil in large skillet over high heat.
6. Season both sides of the fillets with salt and cracked black pepper.

7. When pan is very hot (oil should start to smoke slightly), sear steaks on one side 4 minutes. Turn steaks and sear 3 minutes on other side. Remove from pan, set aside, and cover loosely with foil.
8. Turn down heat in the pan and add the mushrooms and onions. Sauté until both are slightly caramelized. Deglaze the pan with the broth and continue to cook until almost all the liquid is reduced.
9. Remove the crab cakes from the oven and serve the steaks with 1/4 of the mushroom and onion mixture on top and a crab cake on the side.

CHEF TIP: *Splurge on high-quality meat for this recipe. It's worth it. If you like your meat more well done, cook a few minutes longer on each side until it's to your preferred doneness.*

Nutrition Facts

Serves: 4
Serving Size: 1 fillet medallion and 1 baked crab cake

Amount per serving
Calories 220

Calories from fat 80

Total fat 9.0 g

Saturated fat 2.3 g

Trans fat 0.0 g

Cholesterol 70 mg

Sodium 480 mg

Potassium 600 mg

Total carbohydrate 12 g

Dietary fiber 3 g

Sugars 4 g

Protein 24 g

Phosphorus 265 mg

Choices/Exchanges: 1/2 Starch, 1 Nonstarchy Vegetable, 3 Lean Protein, 1/2 Fat

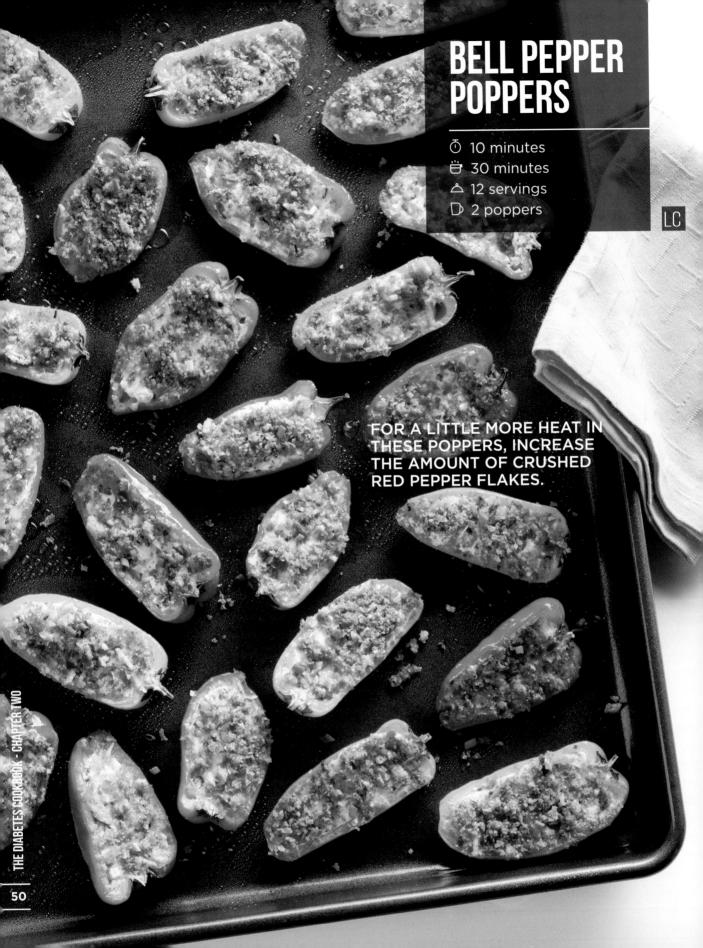

BELL PEPPER POPPERS

- ⏱ 10 minutes
- ⏲ 30 minutes
- ⌒ 12 servings
- ▽ 2 poppers

LC

FOR A LITTLE MORE HEAT IN THESE POPPERS, INCREASE THE AMOUNT OF CRUSHED RED PEPPER FLAKES.

Nonstick cooking spray
12   mini sweet peppers
2   slices turkey bacon, diced
1/2   cup diced onion
4   ounces fat-free cream cheese, room temperature
2   ounces goat cheese, room temperature
1/4   teaspoon crushed red pepper flakes
1   slice whole-wheat bread, toasted
1   clove garlic, minced
1   tablespoon grated parmesan cheese

1. Preheat oven to 375°F. Coat a baking sheet with cooking spray. Set aside.
2. Slice each pepper in half lengthwise; then scoop out the seeds and membrane.
3. Spray a nonstick sauté pan with cooking spray, and cook bacon over medium heat until crisp. Place on a paper towel and set aside.
4. Add onion to the pan used to cook the bacon and add more cooking spray if needed. Cook the onion until clear, stirring occasionally. Set aside to cool.
5. In a small bowl, mix the cream cheese and goat cheese. Add the bacon, onion, and red pepper flakes. Stir until combined.
6. Grind toasted bread in a food processor with the garlic and parmesan cheese. Set aside in a small bowl.
7. Spoon the cheese mixture into each pepper half (1 teaspoon of mixture per popper), and then press the cheese side of the popper into the bread crumb, garlic, and parmesan mixture. Place peppers bread crumb side up on the prepared baking sheet and spray each lightly with cooking spray.
8. Bake about 20 minutes or until the peppers have softened and the bread crumbs are golden brown.

Nutrition Facts

Serves: 12
Serving Size: 2 poppers

Amount per serving
Calories   **45**

Calories from fat 15

Total fat 1.5 g

   Saturated fat 0.9 g

   Trans fat 0.0 g

Cholesterol 5 mg

Sodium 135 mg

Potassium 85 mg

Total carbohydrate 4 g

   Dietary fiber 1 g

   Sugars 1 g

Protein 3 g

Phosphorus 80 mg

Choices/Exchanges: 1 Nonstarchy Vegetable, 1/2 Fat

BUTTERNUT SQUASH GRATIN

○ 15 minutes
⏲ 70 minutes
△ 8 servings
▷ 1/8 of casserole [1 (3 1/4" x 4 1/2") rectangle]

VG

THIS RICH SIDE DISH IS OH-SO-CREAMY AND SATISFYINGLY CHEESY, BUT ONE SERVING IS STILL ONLY 120 CALORIES.

1   (2-pound) butternut squash
1   cup water
Nonstick cooking spray
1   tablespoon olive oil
2   tablespoons flour
2   cups fat-free half-and-half
1/2   cup shredded parmesan cheese, divided
1/2   teaspoon ground black pepper
1   tablespoon chopped fresh thyme
1/4   cup chopped walnuts

1. Preheat oven to 375°F. Cut the squash in half lengthwise and place it facedown in a 9-by-13-inch baking dish. Pour water over the squash and bake 45 minutes.
2. Remove squash from the pan and drain the water. Coat the baking dish with cooking spray.
3. Remove the seeds and scoop the flesh of the squash out of the skin. Place the squash flesh in the prepared baking dish, breaking it up into even-size pieces.
4. Add oil to a sauté pan over medium heat. Add the flour and stir to combine. Cook the oil and flour mixture 2 minutes; then whisk in the half-and-half. Bring to a boil, whisking frequently.
5. Reduce heat to low, stir in 1/4 cup of the parmesan cheese, the pepper, and the thyme. Stir until cheese is melted.

6. Pour the sauce over the butternut squash and sprinkle the remaining 1/4 cup of cheese and walnuts over the top. Bake 25 minutes, or until golden brown and bubbling.

Nutrition Facts

Serves: 8
Serving Size: 1/8 of casserole [1 (3 1/4" x 4 1/2") rectangle]

Amount per serving
Calories **120**

Calories from fat 50

Total fat 6.0 g

Saturated fat 1.3 g

Trans fat 0.0 g

Cholesterol 6 mg

Sodium 95 mg

Potassium 330 mg

Total carbohydrate 14 g

Dietary fiber 3 g

Sugars 4 g

Protein 4 g

Phosphorus 140 mg

Choices/Exchanges: 1/2 Starch, 1/2 Fat-Free Milk, 1 Fat

LOW-CARB ARTICHOKE CHICKEN WRAPS

GF
LC

- ⏱ 10 minutes
- ☕ 20 minutes
- △ 6 servings
- ☕ 1 wrap

THESE WRAPS ARE A GREAT MAKE-AHEAD ITEM FOR YOUR LUNCHBOX.

WRAP

1	egg
4	egg whites
1/2	cup skim milk
1/4	cup coconut flour, sifted
	Nonstick cooking spray

FILLING

2	cups shredded cooked boneless skinless chicken breast
1/2	cup artichoke hearts (drained and rinsed), chopped
1/4	cup minced red onion
2	cups chopped baby spinach
1/4	cup fat-free Italian salad dressing

1. Whisk the egg, egg whites, and milk until well combined and slightly frothy. Sift the coconut flour into the mixture and whisk again until well combined. Let the batter rest at room temperature 15 minutes. **2.** While the wrap batter is resting, toss together the chicken, artichoke hearts, onion, spinach, and Italian dressing. Keep the filling refrigerated until needed. **3.** Spray a 10-inch nonstick sauté pan with cooking spray and place over medium heat. Let the pan heat until a drop of water sizzles in the pan. **4.** Rewhisk the wrap batter, and then pour 1/4 cup of the batter to thinly coat the bottom of the pan (add a little more if needed to coat the bottom of the pan). Let the wrap cook until the edges begin to brown. Using a spatula, flip the wrap and continue to cook another minute. Slide the wrap onto a plate, and repeat this process to make 5 more wraps. Let the wraps cool.

5. Divide the chicken mixture evenly among the wraps (about 1/2 cup filling per wrap), and roll up the wraps.

Nutrition Facts

Serves: 6
Serving Size: 1 wrap

Amount per serving

Calories 140

Calories from fat 25	
Total fat 3.0 g	
Saturated fat 1.2 g	
Trans fat 0.0 g	
Cholesterol 70 mg	
Sodium 260 mg	
Potassium 320 mg	
Total carbohydrate 8 g	
Dietary fiber 3 g	
Sugars 3 g	
Protein 21 g	
Phosphorus 180 mg	

Choices/Exchanges:
1/2 Carbohydrate, 3 Lean Protein

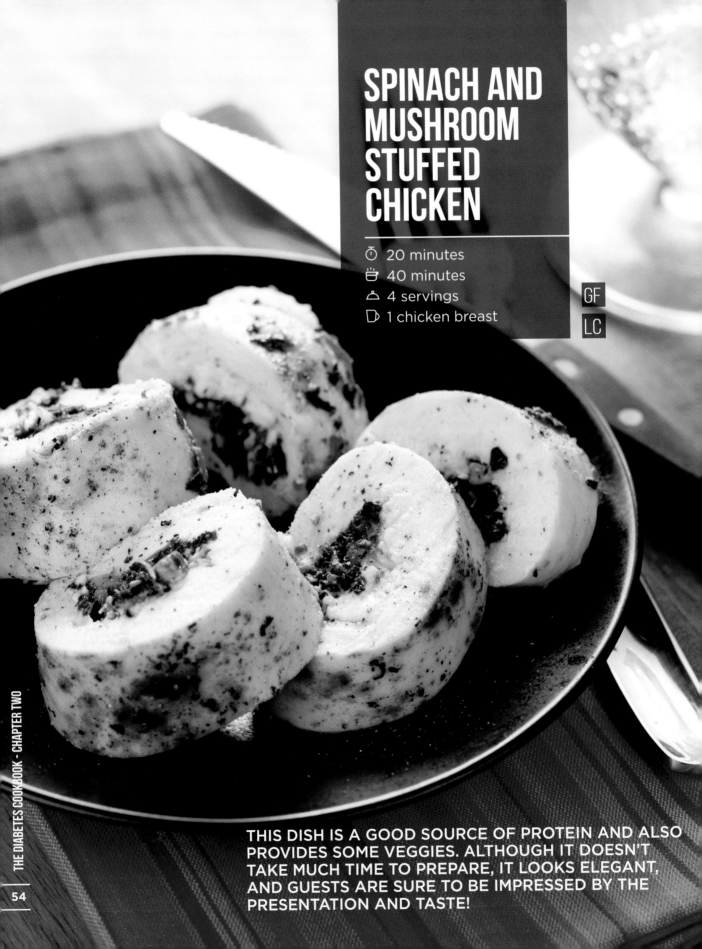

SPINACH AND MUSHROOM STUFFED CHICKEN

- ⏱ 20 minutes
- 🍲 40 minutes
- 🍽 4 servings
- 🥘 1 chicken breast

GF
LC

THIS DISH IS A GOOD SOURCE OF PROTEIN AND ALSO PROVIDES SOME VEGGIES. ALTHOUGH IT DOESN'T TAKE MUCH TIME TO PREPARE, IT LOOKS ELEGANT, AND GUESTS ARE SURE TO BE IMPRESSED BY THE PRESENTATION AND TASTE!

Nonstick cooking spray
1   tablespoon olive oil
1/2 cup frozen chopped spinach, thawed and drained
1   cup finely chopped button mushrooms
1   clove garlic, minced
4   (4-ounce) boneless skinless chicken breasts
4   spreadable creamy light Swiss cheese wedges (such as Laughing Cow Garlic & Herb)
1/4 teaspoon ground black pepper
1/2 teaspoon paprika

1. Preheat oven to 350°F. Spray a baking dish with cooking spray.
2. Add the oil to a medium sauté pan over medium-high heat. Add the spinach and sauté 3 minutes. Add the mushrooms and cook an additional 4–5 minutes. Add the garlic and sauté 30 seconds.
3. Place 1 chicken breast on a cutting board and cover it with plastic wrap. Pound the chicken with a meat tenderizer or rolling pin until it is about 1/4 inch thick. Repeat this process for the other 3 chicken breasts.
4. Spread 1 cheese wedge on one side of a chicken breast. Spread 1/4 cup of the spinach-mushroom mixture on top of the cheese. Roll the chicken breast and secure the seam with a toothpick. Repeat this procedure for the 3 remaining chicken breasts.
5. Sprinkle the chicken breasts with pepper and paprika. Place the rolled chicken breasts on a baking dish and bake 30–40 minutes or until done.
6. To serve, remove the toothpicks and slice each breast into 5 medallions.

Nutrition Facts

Serves: 4
Serving Size: 1 chicken breast

Amount per serving
Calories   **200**

Calories from fat 70	
Total fat 8.0 g	
Saturated fat 2.3 g	
Trans fat 0.0 g	
Cholesterol 70 mg	
Sodium 260 mg	
Potassium 370 mg	
Total carbohydrate 3 g	
Dietary fiber 1 g	
Sugars 2 g	
Protein 27 g	
Phosphorus 375 mg	

Choices/Exchanges: 4 Lean Protein

THIS IS A GREAT PARTY APPETIZER. SERVE THE DIP IN A BOWL ON A LARGE PLATTER AND SURROUND IT WITH THE SKEWERS.

CHICKEN SATAY

- ⏱ 1 hour
- 🍲 10 minutes
- 🍽 4 servings
- 🍴 2 skewers and 2 tablespoons sauce

LC

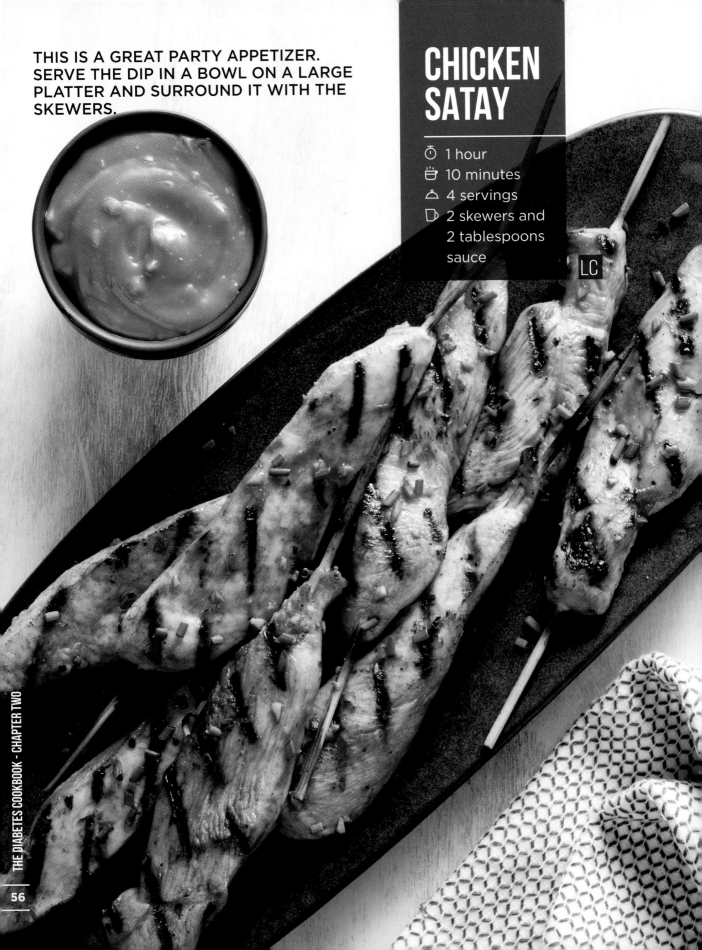

CHICKEN SATAY

8	bamboo skewers
1	pound boneless skinless chicken breasts
1	tablespoon low-calorie brown sugar blend (such as Splenda)
1	tablespoon reduced-sodium soy sauce
1	clove garlic, minced
1	teaspoon minced fresh ginger
2	tablespoons lime juice
1/2	teaspoon Asian-style hot sauce (sriracha)

SATAY SAUCE

1	tablespoon low-calorie brown sugar blend (such as Splenda)
1	tablespoon reduced-sodium soy sauce
1	clove garlic, minced
2	tablespoons creamy peanut butter
1/4	cup unsweetened coconut milk beverage

1. Prepare an indoor or outdoor grill.

2. Soak bamboo skewers in warm water for at least 30 minutes. While skewers are soaking, slice chicken breasts lengthwise into eight strips.

3. In a medium bowl, whisk together Chicken Satay ingredients: brown sugar blend, soy sauce, garlic, ginger, lime juice, and hot sauce. Add chicken strips to the marinade and place in the refrigerator 1 hour.

4. While the chicken is marinating, whisk together the Sauce ingredients (brown sugar blend, soy sauce, garlic, peanut butter, and coconut milk) in a microwave-safe bowl. Set aside.

5. Thread chicken strips lengthwise onto the soaked bamboo skewers and discard the marinade. Grill chicken 4–5 minutes on each side.

6. Right before serving, microwave sauce 30 seconds. Remove from microwave and whisk again to combine. Serve 2 skewers with 2 tablespoons sauce.

Nutrition Facts

Serves: 4
Serving Size: 2 skewers and 2 tablespoons sauce

Amount per serving	
Calories	**220**
Calories from fat 60	
Total fat 7.0 g	
Saturated fat 1.9 g	
Trans fat 0.0 g	
Cholesterol 65 mg	
Sodium 380 mg	
Potassium 290 mg	
Total carbohydrate 10 g	
Dietary fiber 1 g	
Sugars 4 g	
Protein 27 g	
Phosphorus 220 mg	

Choices/Exchanges:
1/2 Carbohydrate, 4 Lean Protein

BAKED HOT WINGS WITH CILANTRO LIME DIP

⏱ 15 minutes
🍲 25 minutes
🍽 4 servings
🥡 3 whole wings (or 6 wings and drumettes) and 1/4 cup dip

THIS IS A HEALTHIER VERSION OF HOT WINGS THAT YOU AND OTHER FOOTBALL FANS WILL LOVE! INSTEAD OF BLUE CHEESE DRESSING, WE SUGGEST THIS TASTY CILANTRO LIME DIP.

2 pounds whole chicken wings
1/2 cup reduced-sugar apricot preserves
1 tablespoon minced garlic, reserve 1/2 teaspoon
1 tablespoon reduced-sodium soy sauce
1 teaspoon Thai-style chili garlic sauce
2 tablespoons lime juice, divided
1/2 teaspoon ground black pepper, divided
1 cup fat-free plain Greek yogurt
1/4 cup chopped fresh cilantro

1. Preheat oven to 375°F. Coat a baking sheet with cooking spray.
2. Remove skin from chicken wings. Place chicken wings in a single layer on the baking sheet and spray again with cooking spray.
3. Bake 10 minutes. While the chicken is baking, whisk together apricot preserves, 2 1/2 teaspoons of garlic, soy sauce, chili garlic sauce, 1 tablespoon lime juice, and 1/4 teaspoon pepper, and set aside.
4. After the wings have been in the oven 10 minutes, coat them generously with the apricot preserve mixture. Return to the oven for another 15 minutes, or until wings are cooked through and glaze is caramelized.
5. In a small bowl, whisk together yogurt, 1 tablespoon lime juice, cilantro, and 1/4 teaspoon pepper. Serve dipping sauce with hot wings.

MAKE IT GLUTEN-FREE: *Verify that the soy sauce and all other ingredients you are using are gluten-free.*

CHEF TIP: *Although it's hard to remove the skin from chicken wings, it's worth the effort because it reduces fat and saturated fat.*

CHEF TIP 2: *If you don't like cilantro, you can substitute 1/4 cup chopped fresh basil or parsley in the dip.*

Nutrition Facts

Serves: 4
Serving Size: 3 whole wings (or 6 wings and drumettes) and 1/4 cup dip

Amount per serving	
Calories	**220**
Calories from fat 45	
Total fat 5.0 g	
Saturated fat 1.5 g	
Trans fat 0.0 g	
Cholesterol 55 mg	
Sodium 240 mg	
Potassium 330 mg	
Total carbohydrate 16 g	
Dietary fiber 0 g	
Sugars 12 g	
Protein 26 g	
Phosphorus 200 mg	

Choices/Exchanges:
1 Carbohydrate, 3 Lean Protein

GREEK YOGURT CHOCOLATE MOUSSE

Ō 10 minutes
Ö 5 minutes
△ 6 servings
▷ Heaping 1/3 cup and 1/3 cup raspberries

VG

MAKING DESSERT FOR A SPECIAL OCCASION? THIS SATISFYING TREAT CAN BE PREPARED AHEAD OF TIME AND REFRIGERATED. JUST BEFORE SERVING, PORTION IT OUT AND TOP WITH THE WHIPPED TOPPING.

6   mini Hershey Sugar-Free Special Dark chocolate bars, chopped
2   cups fat-free plain Greek yogurt
2   tablespoons honey or 4 packets artificial sweetener
1   teaspoon vanilla extract
1/4 cup skim milk
2   cups fresh raspberries
6   tablespoons light whipped cream (such as Cabot Sweetened Light Whipped Cream)

1. Place the chopped chocolate in a microwave-safe bowl. Microwave the chocolate on high 1 minute, then stir. If not completely melted, microwave an additional 30 seconds, and stir. If chocolate is still not melted, microwave another 30 seconds and stir again, just until the chunks in the chocolate are melted. Do not overcook.

2. In a medium mixing bowl, whip the Greek yogurt with an electric mixer until fluffy. Add the honey, vanilla, and milk, and whip; then add the chocolate, a small amount at a time, beating between additions.

3. Once all the chocolate is mixed into the yogurt, divide the mousse into 6 portions and top each portion with 1/3 cup raspberries and 1 tablespoon light whipped cream.

Nutrition Facts

Serves: 6
Serving Size: Heaping 1/3 cup and 1/3 cup raspberries

Amount per serving	
Calories	**130**

Calories from fat 35	
Total fat 4.0 g	
Saturated fat 2.1 g	
Trans fat 0.0 g	
Cholesterol 5 mg	
Sodium 35 mg	
Potassium 220 mg	
Total carbohydrate 17 g	
Dietary fiber 3 g	
Sugars 11 g	
Protein 9 g	
Phosphorus 145 mg	

Choices/Exchanges: 1/2 Fruit, 1/2 Fat-Free Milk, 1/2 Carbohydrate, 1/2 Fat

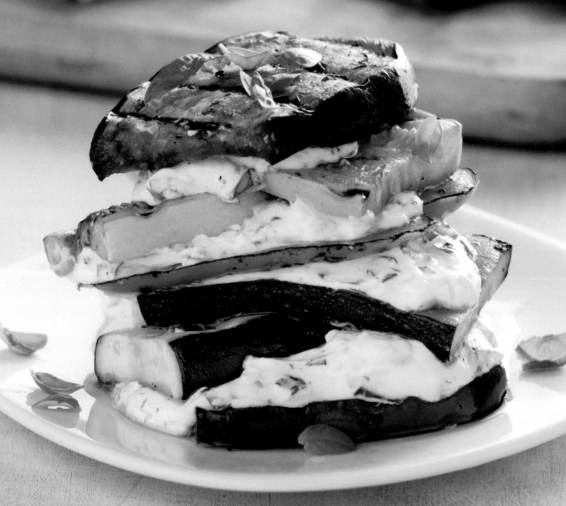

GRILLED VEGETABLE NAPOLEON

- ⏱ 20 minutes
- 🍲 15 minutes
- △ 4 servings
- 🍽 1 napoleon

GF
VG

THIS RECIPE USES FAT-FREE PLAIN GREEK YOGURT TO STRETCH THE GOAT CHEESE. THIS ALSO WORKS FOR CREAM CHEESE! YOU GET THE GREAT FLAVOR AND TEXTURE OF THE CHEESE WITHOUT ALL THE EXTRA FAT AND CALORIES.

1	tablespoon olive oil
2	tablespoons balsamic vinegar
1/2	teaspoon ground black pepper, divided
1	medium zucchini, sliced lengthwise into 4 slices
1	medium yellow squash, sliced lengthwise into 4 slices
1	orange bell pepper, sliced lengthwise into 4 slices
1	small eggplant, sliced lengthwise into 4 slices
1/4	cup goat cheese, softened
1	cup fat-free plain Greek yogurt
1	clove garlic, minced or grated
1	tablespoon minced fresh oregano
1/4	cup chopped fresh basil

1. Preheat an indoor or outdoor grill.
2. In a large bowl, whisk together olive oil, vinegar, and 1/4 teaspoon pepper.
3. Add sliced zucchini, squash, bell pepper, and eggplant, and let sit 5 minutes.
4. Grill the vegetables about 2–3 minutes on both sides.
5. Once grilled, cut the zucchini, squash, and eggplant in half widthwise so you have 8 pieces of each, and set aside to cool.
6. In a medium bowl, whisk together goat cheese, yogurt, garlic, oregano, and 1/4 teaspoon pepper.

7. Place 1 piece of eggplant on a plate, top with 1 heaping tablespoon of cheese mixture, top that with 2 slices of zucchini, followed by another heaping tablespoon of cheese mixture. Top that with 1 slice of bell pepper, then another heaping tablespoon of cheese mixture. Top that with two slices of yellow squash, then another heaping tablespoon of cheese mixture, and then the other slice of eggplant. Sprinkle with 1 tablespoon chopped fresh basil. Repeat process for 3 more napoleons.

Nutrition Facts

Serves: 4
Serving Size: 1 napoleon

Amount per serving
Calories 170

Calories from fat 60

Total fat 7.0 g

Saturated fat 2.8 g

Trans fat 0.0 g

Cholesterol 10 mg

Sodium 80 mg

Potassium 580 mg

Total carbohydrate 19 g

Dietary fiber 4 g

Sugars 10 g

Protein 11 g

Phosphorus 180 mg

Choices/Exchanges: 3 Nonstarchy Vegetable, 1 Lean Protein, 1 Fat

BAKED FALAFEL

⏱ 30 minutes
🍳 30 minutes
🍽 8 servings
🍴 1/2 pita, 2 pieces of falafel, and 2 tablespoons sauce

FALAFEL PATTIES

1   tablespoon minced garlic
1   small onion, chopped
1   tablespoon curry powder
1/4   teaspoon cayenne pepper
2   tablespoons minced fresh cilantro
1   tablespoon minced fresh parsley
1   tablespoon olive oil
2   (15-ounce) cans chickpeas (garbanzo beans), drained and rinsed
1 1/2 tablespoons flour (whole wheat or all-purpose)
2   teaspoons baking powder
1/4   teaspoon salt
1/2   teaspoon ground black pepper
    Nonstick cooking spray
1   tablespoon sesame seeds

SAUCE

1   cup fat-free plain Greek yogurt
1/4   cup tahini
1   tablespoon garlic, minced
1   tablespoon minced fresh parsley

SANDWICH

4   whole-wheat pita pockets, cut in half
2   tomatoes, cut into 8 slices each
1/2   red onion, thinly sliced

1. Preheat oven to 450°F. Line a large baking sheet with a silicone mat or parchment paper. If using parchment paper, coat generously with cooking spray. Set aside.

2. In a food processor or blender, combine garlic, onion, curry powder, cayenne pepper, cilantro, parsley, and olive oil. Blend into a paste.

3. Add chickpeas (garbanzo beans) and pulse to roughly chop beans and combine with paste. Do not overblend; the falafel should be slightly chunky.

4. Add flour, baking powder, salt, and pepper. Pulse just until incorporated.

5. Refrigerate falafel mixture 15–20 minutes. While the falafel is chilling, whisk together yogurt, tahini, garlic, and parsley in a small bowl. Keep yogurt sauce in the refrigerator until ready to use.

6. Scoop falafel into balls that are about 2 tablespoons of mixture (or 1/8 cup). Place on baking sheet, and repeat to make 16 falafel balls.

TO REDUCE THE CARBOHYDRATES IN THIS RECIPE, SERVE THE FALAFEL SANDWICHES IN LETTUCE CUPS INSTEAD OF WHOLE-WHEAT PITAS.

---

7. Spray the falafel balls with cooking spray and sprinkle with sesame seeds.

8. Bake on bottom rack of oven 15 minutes. Turn the oven down to 350°F and move the baking sheet to the top rack. Bake an additional 15 minutes.

9. Once the falafel is done baking, stuff 2 falafel balls into half of a pita, add 2 tablespoons yogurt tahini sauce, 2 slices of tomato, and 3–4 slices of red onion.

Nutrition Facts

Serves: 8

Serving Size: 1/2 pita, 2 pieces of falafel, and 2 tablespoons sauce

Amount per serving

Calories 290

Calories from fat 80	
Total fat 9.0 g	
Saturated fat 1.3 g	
Trans fat 0.0 g	
Cholesterol 0 mg	
Sodium 440 mg	
Potassium 460 mg	
Total carbohydrate 42 g	
Dietary fiber 9 g	
Sugars 6 g	
Protein 14 g	
Phosphorus 395 mg	

Choices/Exchanges: 2 1/2 Starch, 1 Nonstarchy Vegetable, 1 Lean Protein, 1 Fat

SAVORY CREPES

⏱ 20 minutes
🍲 25 minutes
🍽 4 servings
🍽 2 crepes

THESE WHOLE-WHEAT CREPES MAKE A DELICIOUS SAVORY BREAKFAST OR LUNCH, AND THEY PROVIDE A GOOD BALANCE OF WHOLE GRAINS, PROTEIN, AND NONSTARCHY VEGETABLES.

CREPES

2   eggs
2/3   cup fat-free milk
1/2   cup water
1   tablespoon olive oil
1/4   teaspoon salt
1   cup whole-wheat flour
Nonstick cooking spray

FILLING

4   cups broccoli florets
Nonstick cooking spray
1/2   small onion, diced small
8   slices lower-sodium deli ham (1/2 ounce each), diced
4   egg whites
1/4   cup fat-free half-and-half
1/4   teaspoon ground black pepper
1/4   cup shredded parmesan cheese

1. In a large bowl, whisk together all the crepe ingredients except the cooking spray. Blend the mixture in a blender or with an immersion blender. Let the crepe batter rest at room temperature for 20 minutes.
2. Coat a 10-inch nonstick sauté pan with cooking spray and place over medium heat. Let the pan heat until a drop of water sizzles in the pan.
3. Pour 1/4 cup of the crepe batter to thinly coat the bottom of the pan. Let the crepe cook until the edges begin to brown. Using a spatula, flip the crepe and continue to cook another minute. Slide the crepe onto a plate and continue this process to make 8 crepes.
4. Steam the broccoli florets in the microwave or in a saucepan in an inch of water. Steam until the florets are fork-tender.
5. Coat a nonstick sauté pan with cooking spray and place over medium-high heat. Sauté the onion and ham until the onion is soft and beginning to caramelize.
6. Add the steamed broccoli, and use a spatula to break up the broccoli into small pieces, stirring it with the ham and onions.
7. In a small bowl, whisk together the egg whites, fat-free half-and-half, and pepper. Add the mixture and the parmesan cheese to the vegetables and stir to scramble.
8. Fill each crepe with 1/2 cup egg-and-vegetable scramble and fold.

CHEF TIP: *The scramble may have a little liquid from the steamed broccoli. Try to leave the liquid behind when scooping out the scramble to fill the crepes.*

Nutrition Facts

Serves: 4
Serving Size: 2 crepes

Amount per serving

Calories	**260**
Calories from fat 70	
Total fat 8.0 g	
Saturated fat 1.9 g	
Trans fat 0.0 g	
Cholesterol 110 mg	
Sodium 530 mg	
Potassium 610 mg	
Total carbohydrate 29 g	
Dietary fiber 6 g	
Sugars 5 g	
Protein 21 g	
Phosphorus 325 mg	

Choices/Exchanges: 1 1/2 Starch, 1 Nonstarchy Vegetable, 2 Lean Protein, 1/2 Fat

ROASTED GREEN BEANS WITH CHAMPAGNE VINAIGRETTE

IMPRESS GUESTS BY WHIPPING UP THIS SIMPLE YET ELEGANT SIDE DISH TO GO WITH ANY CHICKEN, FISH, OR BEEF ENTRÉE.

GF
LC
VG

⏱ 15 minutes
🍲 25 minutes
🍽 6 servings
🥄 3/4 cup

ROASTED GREEN BEANS

Nonstick cooking spray
1 1/2   pounds fresh green beans, trimmed
1   teaspoon olive oil
1/4   teaspoon salt
1/4   teaspoon ground black pepper
1   tablespoon garlic, minced

CHAMPAGNE VINAIGRETTE

1   tablespoon extra-virgin olive oil
2   tablespoons champagne vinegar
1   teaspoon Dijon mustard
1   teaspoon zero-calorie granulated sweetener (such as Splenda)
1/4   teaspoon crushed red pepper flakes

1. Preheat oven to 450°F. Coat a baking sheet with cooking spray. Set aside.
2. In a large bowl, toss green beans with 1 teaspoon olive oil, salt, black pepper, and garlic. Pour onto prepared baking sheet and roast 25 minutes or until cooked through and starting to brown.
3. While green beans are roasting, whisk together 1 tablespoon olive oil, champagne vinegar, Dijon mustard, zero-calorie granulated sweetener, and crushed red pepper flakes. Set aside.
4. When green beans are done roasting, drizzle with champagne vinaigrette and toss to coat.

CHEF TIP: *If you can't find champagne vinegar, use a good-quality white wine vinegar instead.*

Nutrition Facts

Serves: 6
Serving Size: 3/4 cup

Amount per serving
Calories 70

Calories from fat 30

Total fat 3.5 g

  Saturated fat 0.5 g

  Trans fat 0.0 g

Cholesterol 0 mg

Sodium 120 mg

Potassium 150 mg

Total carbohydrate 9 g

  Dietary fiber 3 g

  Sugars 2 g

Protein 2 g

Phosphorus 30 mg

Choices/Exchanges: 2 Nonstarchy Vegetable, 1/2 Fat

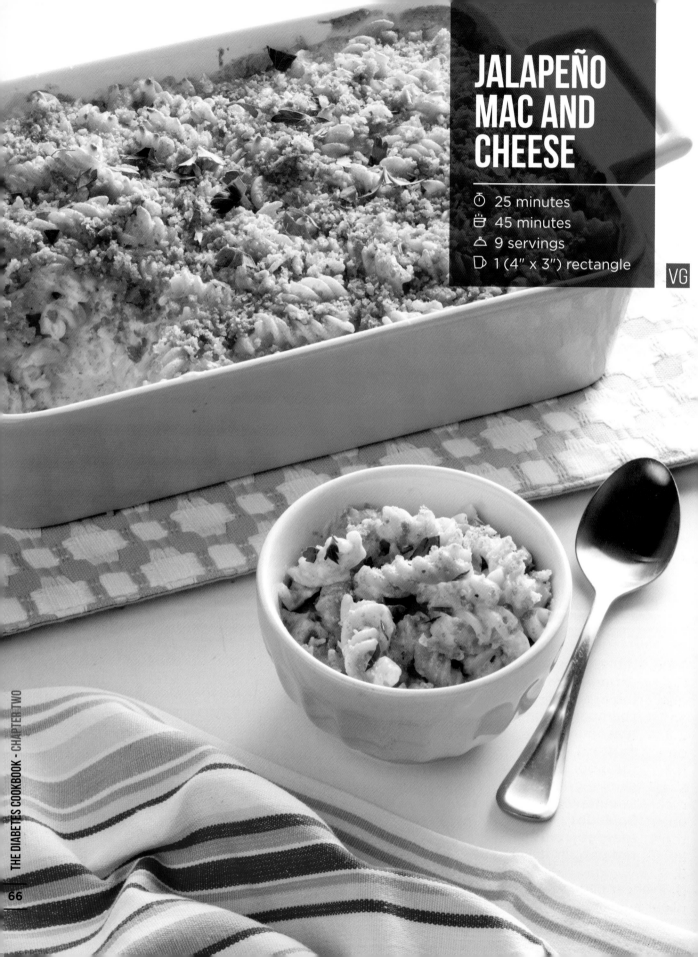

JALAPEÑO MAC AND CHEESE

- ⏱ 25 minutes
- 🍲 45 minutes
- 🍽 9 servings
- 🍴 1 (4" x 3") rectangle

VG

TO MAKE THIS RECIPE A LITTLE MORE QUICKLY, USE A JALAPEÑO SALSA OR HOT SAUCE INSTEAD OF ROASTING THE PEPPERS. USE ABOUT 1/4 CUP OR ADJUST TO THE SPICINESS THAT YOU PREFER.

Nonstick cooking spray
2 small jalapeño peppers
1 tablespoon olive oil
2 tablespoons whole-wheat flour
3 cups skim milk
6 spreadable creamy light Swiss cheese wedges (such as Laughing Cow)
1/4 cup plus 2 tablespoons freshly grated parmesan cheese, divided
1/8 teaspoon ground nutmeg
1/2 teaspoon salt
1/2 teaspoon ground black pepper
1 slice whole-wheat bread
1 clove garlic
16 ounces whole-grain rotini

1. Preheat oven to 450°F. Coat a 9-by-13-inch baking dish with cooking spray and set aside.
2. Lay jalapeño peppers on a piece of aluminum foil or a small baking sheet. Place on the top rack of the oven and roast until the skin is blackened, turning occasionally, about 20–30 minutes.
3. Remove the blackened peppers from the oven, place in a bowl, and imme-diately cover with plastic wrap. Let sit 10–15 minutes to cool. Once the peppers have cooled, peel and seed the peppers. Set aside. Note: Protect your hands with gloves or even plastic sandwich bags to avoid getting pepper juices on your hands.
4. Turn the oven down to 350°F.
5. While jalapeños are roasting and cooling, add olive oil to a medium saucepan over medium heat. Stir in flour and cook 1–2 minutes, taking care not to brown it. Stir constantly.
6. Slowly whisk in the skim milk and bring to a boil, whisking constantly.
7. Add cheese wedges, 1/4 cup parmesan cheese, nutmeg, salt, and pepper, still whisking constantly.
8. Add the jalapeño peppers to the cheese mixture, and use an im-mersion blender or up-right blender to blend until smooth. There will be some texture from the peppers. Set aside.
9. Using a food processor, blend the whole-wheat bread, garlic, and 2 table-spoons grated parmesan cheese to make the crum-ble topping. Set aside.
10. Cook pasta according to directions on the pack-age, omitting salt. Drain pasta and immediately add it to the cheese mix-ture, stirring well to incor-porate.
11. Pour the macaroni and cheese into the prepared baking dish, sprinkle the top with the bread crumb mixture, and bake 15–20 minutes or until bubbly and topping is golden brown.

Nutrition Facts

Serves: 9
Serving Size: 1 (4" x 3") rectangle

Amount per serving
Calories 250

Calories from fat 45

Total fat 5.0 g

Saturated fat 1.7 g

Trans fat 0.0 g

Cholesterol 5 mg

Sodium 360 mg

Potassium 420 mg

Total carbohydrate 43 g

Dietary fiber 7 g

Sugars 6 g

Protein 13 g

Phosphorus 380 mg

Choices/Exchanges: 2 1/2 Starch, 1/2 Fat-Free Milk, 1/2 Fat

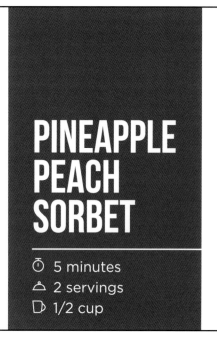

PINEAPPLE PEACH SORBET

⏱ 5 minutes
△ 2 servings
▭ 1/2 cup

WHEN FRESH PRODUCE IS IN SEASON, YOU CAN CUT UP AND FREEZE THE FRUIT YOURSELF. OTHERWISE, YOU CAN FIND AN ABUNDANCE OF FROZEN FRUIT IN THE GROCER'S FREEZER. PLAY AROUND WITH OTHER FRUIT COMBINATIONS LIKE MANGO-STRAWBERRY, PEACH-RASPBERRY, OR PINEAPPLE-BANANA.

1/2 cup frozen peaches
1/2 cup frozen pineapple chunks
1/4 cup sugar-free lemonade

1. Place all the ingredients in a blender and blend until smooth.
2. Place the sorbet in a container and freeze immediately.

Nutrition Facts

Serves: 2
Serving Size: 1/2 cup

Amount per serving

Calories	**40**
Calories from fat 0	
Total fat 0.0 g	
Saturated fat 0.0 g	
Trans fat 0.0 g	
Cholesterol 0 mg	
Sodium 0 mg	
Potassium 130 mg	
Total carbohydrate 10 g	
Dietary fiber 1 g	
Sugars 8 g	
Protein 1 g	
Phosphorus 10 mg	

Choices/Exchanges: 1/2 Fruit

PORK TACOS

⏱ 45 minutes
🍲 30 minutes
🍽 12 servings
🥡 1 taco

THIS RECIPE CALLS FOR PORK TENDERLOIN—ONE OF THE LEANER CUTS OF PORK. YOU CAN ALSO TOP THESE TACOS WITH AVOCADO AND FRESH SALSA.

Juice of 2 limes
2 cloves garlic, minced
1 1/2 tablespoons chili powder
1 teaspoon cumin
1 teaspoon oregano
1/2 teaspoon salt
1/2 teaspoon ground black pepper
2 pork tenderloins (1 1/4 pounds total)
12 low-carb whole-wheat tortillas (10 grams carb per tortilla), heated
2 tomatoes, diced
1 1/2 cups shredded lettuce
1 cup shredded reduced-fat cheddar cheese

1. In a large bowl combine lime juice, garlic, chili powder, cumin, oregano, salt, and pepper. Add pork and coat well. Marinate in refrigerator 30 minutes or up to 4 hours.
2. Preheat oven to 375°F. Place tenderloins in a shallow baking dish and bake 30 minutes or until pork is done.
3. Remove pork from oven and let rest 10 minutes. Cut pork into 1-inch chunks.
4. Serve pork in warm tortillas topped with 1 tablespoon tomatoes, 2 tablespoons lettuce, and 1 1/3 tablespoons cheese.

Nutrition Facts

Serves: 12
Serving Size: 1 taco

Amount per serving
Calories 140

Calories from fat 50

Total fat 6.0 g

Saturated fat 1.6 g

Trans fat 0.0 g

Cholesterol 30 mg

Sodium 410 mg

Potassium 270 mg

Total carbohydrate 13 g

Dietary fiber 8 g

Sugars 1 g

Protein 17 g

Phosphorus 190 mg

Choices/Exchanges: 1 Starch, 2 Lean Protein

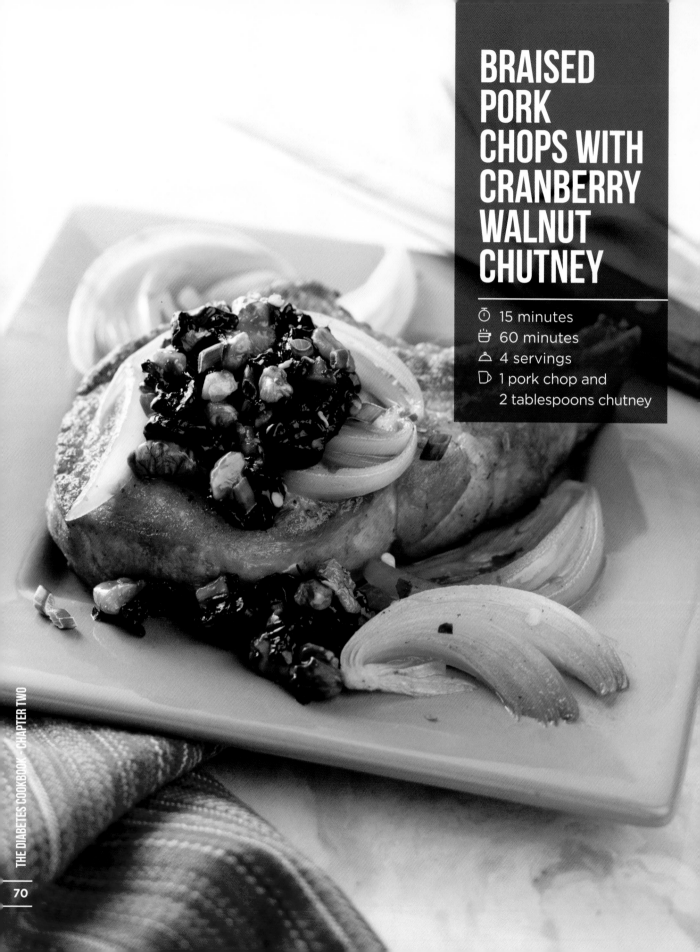

BRAISED PORK CHOPS WITH CRANBERRY WALNUT CHUTNEY

- ⏱ 15 minutes
- 🍲 60 minutes
- 🍽 4 servings
- 🥄 1 pork chop and 2 tablespoons chutney

PORK CHOPS

4	loin-cut bone-in pork chops
1	tablespoon salt-free all-purpose seasoning (such as Spike or Mrs. Dash)
1/2	teaspoon ground black pepper
1	tablespoon olive oil, divided
	Nonstick cooking spray
1	large onion, sliced
1 1/2	cups fat-free low-sodium chicken broth

CHUTNEY

1	small onion, diced
1/3	cup dried cranberries
1	tablespoon maple syrup
2	tablespoons balsamic vinegar
	Dash crushed red pepper flakes
1/3	cup water
1/2	cup unsalted chopped walnuts

1. Preheat oven to 375°F.
2. Trim any visible fat from the pork chops and pat dry with a paper towel. Season both sides of each chop with the salt-free seasoning and black pepper.
3. Add 1 1/2 teaspoons of olive oil and a generous amount of cooking spray to an oven-safe dutch oven or large skillet heated over high heat.
4. Once the oil is hot, sear the 4 pork chops until golden brown on each side.
5. Spread the onion slices over the pork chops and pour the broth on top.
6. Cover and bake 45 minutes or until the pork chops are fork-tender.
7. While the pork chops are braising, add the remaining 1 1/2 teaspoons of olive oil to a small nonstick skillet over medium heat. Add the onion and sauté until it begins to caramelize.
8. Add the remaining chutney ingredients except the nuts and simmer until almost all the liquid evaporates and the chutney is thick and syrupy.
9. Stir in the nuts and remove from the heat. Set aside to cool slightly. The chutney should be served at room temperature.
10. Once the pork chops are done braising, remove the chops from the dutch oven and set aside, leaving the onion and liquid in the pan. Put the dutch oven back on the stove over medium high heat. Simmer until almost all the liquid is evaporated. Pour over the pork chops.
11. Serve one pork chop with 1/4 of the onion and 2 tablespoons of the chutney.

CHEF TIP: *The chutney is also excellent served cold. Use it as you would any other condiment.*

Nutrition Facts

Serves: 4
Serving Size: 1 pork chop and 2 tablespoons chutney

Amount per serving	
Calories	**320**

Calories from fat 130	
Total fat 14.0 g	
Saturated fat 2.3 g	
Trans fat 0.0 g	
Cholesterol 65 mg	
Sodium 120 mg	
Potassium 680 mg	
Total carbohydrate 21 g	
Dietary fiber 3 g	
Sugars 14 g	
Protein 29 g	
Phosphorus 340 mg	

Choices/Exchanges: 1 Fruit, 1 Nonstarchy Vegetable, 4 Lean Protein, 1 1/2 Fat

BANGERS AND MASH

- ⏱ 10 minutes
- 🍳 45 minutes
- 🍽 6 servings
- 🍴 1 piece of sausage and 2/3 cup mashed sweet potatoes

BANGERS AND MASH IS A TRADITIONAL IRISH PUB FOOD THAT IS USUALLY VERY HIGH IN FAT AND CARBS. THIS HEALTHIER VERSION WILL HAVE YOU SAYING *SLAINTE!* TO THE TASTE AND TO THE SCALE THE NEXT MORNING!

MASH (MASHED SWEET POTATOES)

Nonstick cooking spray
2   pounds sweet potatoes, washed and dried
1   tablespoon olive oil
1/4   teaspoon salt
1/4   teaspoon ground black pepper

BANGERS (TURKEY SAUSAGE)

1   slice whole-wheat bread, crusts removed
1/4   cup egg substitute
20   ounces lean ground turkey
1/2   teaspoon ground thyme
1/2   teaspoon ground sage
1   teaspoon garlic powder
1/4   teaspoon cayenne pepper
1/2   teaspoon salt
1/4   teaspoon ground black pepper

1. Preheat oven to 375°F. Coat a baking sheet with cooking spray.
2. Arrange the washed and dried whole sweet potatoes (with the skins on) on the baking sheet and bake 45 minutes or until tender when pierced with a fork. Set aside to cool slightly.
3. While the sweet potatoes are cooling, combine the bread and egg in a bowl until bread is softened and a paste forms. Stir in the remaining Bangers (turkey sausage) ingredients and mix well to incorporate.
4. Divide the sausage mixture into 6 equal-size patties and sauté in a medium nonstick sauté pan coated with cooking spray about 4–5 minutes on each side or until the center of the patty reaches an internal temperature of 165°F.
5. Once the sweet potatoes have cooled slightly, peel the skins off (they should be easy to peel off by hand) and add the peeled sweet potatoes to a bowl with the olive oil, salt, and pepper.

Mash with a potato masher or sturdy whisk until fluffy.
6. Serve one sausage patty on top of a scoop of the mashed sweet potatoes.

Nutrition Facts

Serves: 6

Serving Size: 1 piece of sausage and 2/3 cup mashed sweet potatoes

Amount per serving

Calories	**280**

Calories from fat 90

Total fat 10.0 g

    Saturated fat 2.5 g

    Trans fat 0.1 g

Cholesterol 75 mg

Sodium 430 mg

Potassium 760 mg

Total carbohydrate 25 g

    Dietary fiber 4 g

    Sugars 7 g

Protein 22 g

Phosphorus 250 mg

Choices/Exchanges: 1 1/2 Starch, 3 Lean Protein, 1/2 Fat

SPINACH AND SWEET POTATO CURRY (SAAG ALOO)

⏱ 15 minutes
🍲 15 minutes
🍽 6 servings
🥣 3/4 cup

VG

THIS RECIPE FOR A SPICED INDIAN SPINACH DISH REPLACES REGULAR POTATOES WITH SWEET POTATOES FOR A DELICIOUS AND HEALTHFUL TAKE ON CURRY.

2 (6-ounce) medium sweet potatoes, peeled and cut into 1-inch chunks
1 tablespoon olive oil
1 medium onion, peeled and thinly sliced
2 cloves garlic, grated or minced
1/2 teaspoon salt
1/2 teaspoon ground black pepper
1 teaspoon cumin
1 teaspoon ground turmeric
1 teaspoon ground ginger
1 tablespoon chili powder
1 cup water or fat-free low-sodium vegetable broth
5 ounces baby spinach

CHEF TIP: *If you don't have all the spices for this recipe in your spice rack, substitute a heaping tablespoon of curry powder for the cumin, turmeric, ginger, and chili powder. Make it spicy with cayenne pepper to taste!*

1. Add sweet potatoes and 1/2 cup water to a microwave-safe container or steamer with a lid. Microwave 7–8 minutes or until sweet potatoes are fork tender. Don't overcook them.
2. While the sweet potatoes are steaming, add olive oil to a large sauté pan over medium heat. Add the onion and sauté 3–4 minutes or until onion turns clear. Add the garlic and sauté 2 more minutes.
3. Add the salt, pepper, cumin, turmeric, ginger, chili powder, and water or broth. Bring to a simmer.
4. Add the spinach and cook until wilted, about 5 minutes.
5. Stir in the sweet potatoes to heat through.

Nutrition Facts

Serves: 6
Serving Size: 3/4 cup

Amount per serving

Calories	**80**
Calories from fat 25	
Total fat 3.0 g	
Saturated fat 0.4 g	
Trans fat 0.0 g	
Cholesterol 0 mg	
Sodium 240 mg	
Potassium 390 mg	
Total carbohydrate 12 g	
Dietary fiber 3 g	
Sugars 4 g	
Protein 2 g	
Phosphorus 45 mg	

Choices/Exchanges: 1/2 Starch, 1 Nonstarchy Vegetable, 1/2 Fat

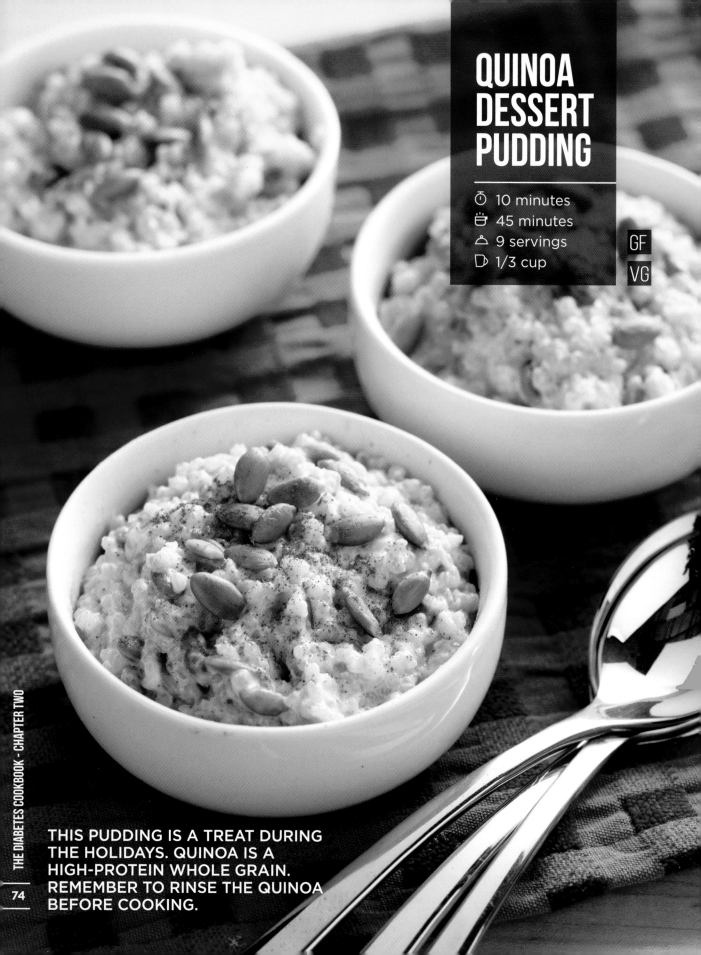

QUINOA DESSERT PUDDING

- ⏱ 10 minutes
- 🍲 45 minutes
- 🍽 9 servings
- 🥣 1/3 cup

GF
VG

THIS PUDDING IS A TREAT DURING
THE HOLIDAYS. QUINOA IS A
HIGH-PROTEIN WHOLE GRAIN.
REMEMBER TO RINSE THE QUINOA
BEFORE COOKING.

1 cup quinoa
1 1/2 cups skim milk
1 1/2 cups fat-free half-and-half
1/4 cup low-calorie brown sugar blend (such as Truvia or Splenda)
1 teaspoon vanilla extract
1/2 teaspoon ground cinnamon
1/4 teaspoon ground nutmeg
1/2 cup pumpkin seeds, toasted

1. Rinse quinoa under cold water for 2 minutes.
2. Whisk together milk, fat-free half-and-half, brown sugar blend, vanilla, cinnamon, and nutmeg in a medium saucepan over medium heat. Bring to a simmer.
3. Once the milk mixture is simmering, stir in quinoa and reduce heat to a low simmer. Partially cover the pan and cook 40 minutes, stirring every 10 minutes.
4. When quinoa is done cooking, stir in toasted pumpkin seeds and serve.

CHEF TIP: *Rinsing the quinoa is an important step. It helps avoid any bitter taste.*

Nutrition Facts

Serves: 9
Serving Size: 1/3 cup

Amount per serving
Calories 150

Calories from fat 45

Total fat 5.0 g

Saturated fat 1.0 g

Trans fat 0.0 g

Cholesterol 5 mg

Sodium 60 mg

Potassium 300 mg

Total carbohydrate 21 g

Dietary fiber 2 g

Sugars 7 g

Protein 7 g

Phosphorus 265 mg

Choices/Exchanges: 1 Starch, 1/2 Fat-Free Milk, 1/2 Fat

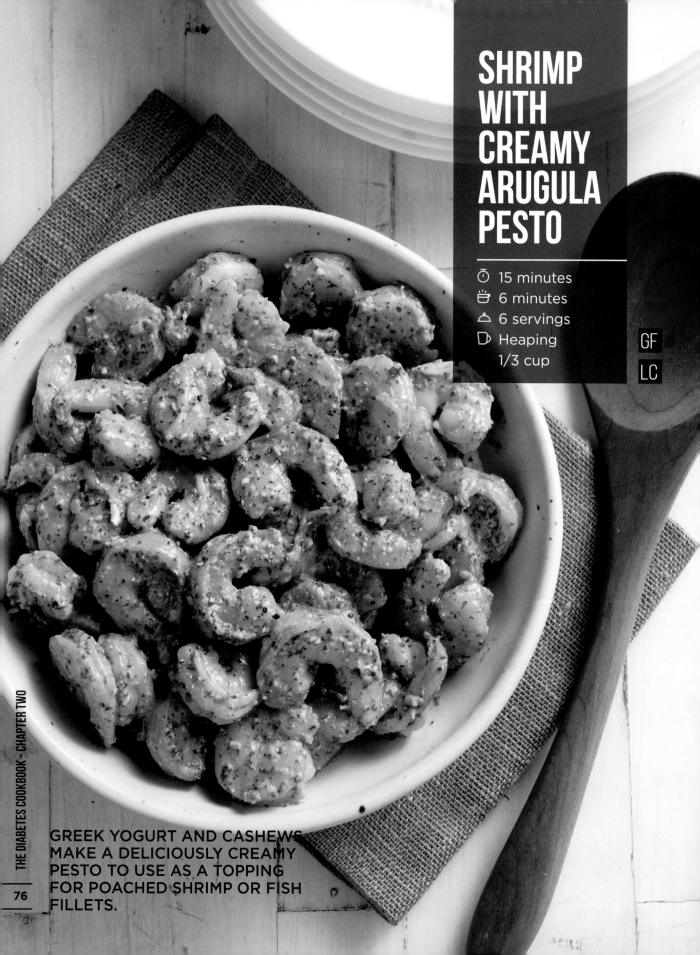

SHRIMP WITH CREAMY ARUGULA PESTO

- ⏱ 15 minutes
- 🍲 6 minutes
- 🍽 6 servings
- ☕ Heaping 1/3 cup

GF
LC

GREEK YOGURT AND CASHEWS MAKE A DELICIOUSLY CREAMY PESTO TO USE AS A TOPPING FOR POACHED SHRIMP OR FISH FILLETS.

3 cups water
1 tablespoon salt-free all-purpose seasoning (such as Spike or Mrs. Dash)
1 1/4 pounds medium peeled and deveined shrimp
4 cups packed arugula
1/4 cup fat-free plain Greek yogurt
2 cloves garlic
1 tablespoon olive oil
1/4 cup unsalted cashews
1/4 cup shredded parmesan cheese
1/4 teaspoon ground black pepper

1. Bring water and salt-free seasoning to a boil in a medium saucepan. Reduce heat to barely a simmer and add shrimp. Cook 6 minutes or until shrimp are pink and just cooked through.
2. While shrimp are cooking, add the arugula, yogurt, garlic, olive oil, cashews, parmesan cheese, and black pepper to a blender or food processor. Blend until smooth.
3. Drain shrimp and toss with the pesto while the shrimp are still hot.

CHEF TIP: *Shrimp can be served hot over cooked whole-wheat pasta, or chilled over salad greens.*

NOTE: *If possible use fresh (never frozen) shrimp, or shrimp that are free of preservatives (for example, shrimp that have not been treated with salt or STPP [sodium tripolyphosphate]).*

Nutrition Facts

Serves: 6
Serving Size: Heaping 1/3 cup

Amount per serving
Calories **130**

Calories from fat 50

Total fat 6.0 g

  Saturated fat 1.2 g

  Trans fat 0.0 g

Cholesterol 115 mg

Sodium 100 mg

Potassium 280 mg

Total carbohydrate 3 g

  Dietary fiber 1 g

  Sugars 1 g

Protein 17 g

Phosphorus 205 mg

Choices/Exchanges: 3 Lean Protein

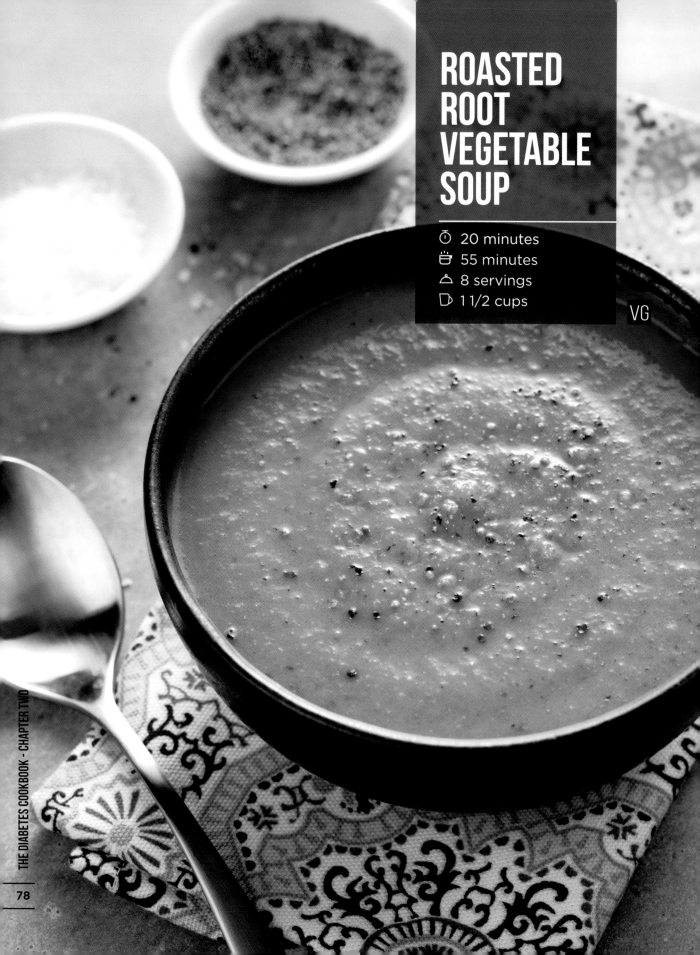

ROASTED ROOT VEGETABLE SOUP

- ⏱ 20 minutes
- 🍲 55 minutes
- 🍽 8 servings
- 🥣 1 1/2 cups

VG

ROASTING THE VEGETABLES IN THIS RECIPE MAXIMIZES THE FLAVOR OF THE SOUP. ALL THESE VEGGIES ARE ABUNDANT AND AVAILABLE DURING THE WINTER MONTHS. HERBS DE PROVENCE IS A DRIED HERB MIXTURE USUALLY MADE UP OF THYME, MARJORAM, ROSEMARY, OREGANO, SAVORY, AND SOMETIMES LAVENDER. IF YOU CAN'T FIND IT, YOU CAN SUBSTITUTE DRIED THYME IN THIS RECIPE.

Nonstick cooking spray
1 small butternut squash (about 1 pound), peeled, seeded, and cut into 1-inch chunks
2 small turnips, peeled and cut into 1-inch chunks
2 parsnips, peeled and cut into 1-inch chunks
2 carrots, peeled and cut into 1-inch chunks
1 large onion, peeled and diced
3 stalks celery, diced
1/2 small head green cabbage, chopped
4 cloves garlic, chopped
1 tablespoon olive oil
1 tablespoon herbes de Provence
2 quarts fat-free low-sodium vegetable broth
1 tablespoon sherry vinegar
1/4 teaspoon salt
1/2 teaspoon ground black pepper

1. Preheat oven to 400°F. Coat a large baking sheet (or 2 medium-size baking sheets) with cooking spray. Set aside.
2. In a large bowl, toss all the vegetables, including the garlic, with the olive oil and herbes de Provence. Pour onto prepared baking sheet(s) and roast 45 minutes or until cooked through and starting to brown.
3. After vegetables are done roasting, put them in a large soup pot. Mix with the vegetable broth and bring to a boil. Reduce heat and simmer 10 minutes.

4. Purée the soup in the pot with an immersion blender or in batches in an upright blender.
5. Season the soup with sherry vinegar, salt, and pepper.

CHEF TIP: *If you can't find sherry vinegar, use a good-quality red wine vinegar instead.*

MAKE IT GLUTEN-FREE: *Ensure the ingredients you are using, such as the broth, are gluten-free.*

Nutrition Facts

Serves: 8
Serving Size: 1 1/2 cups

Amount per serving
Calories   **90**

Calories from fat 20	
Total fat 2.0 g	
Saturated fat 0.3 g	
Trans fat 0.0 g	
Cholesterol 0 mg	
Sodium 250 mg	
Potassium 550 mg	
Total carbohydrate 18 g	
Dietary fiber 6 g	
Sugars 8 g	
Protein 2 g	
Phosphorus 135 mg	

Choices/Exchanges: 1 Starch, 1 Nonstarchy Vegetable

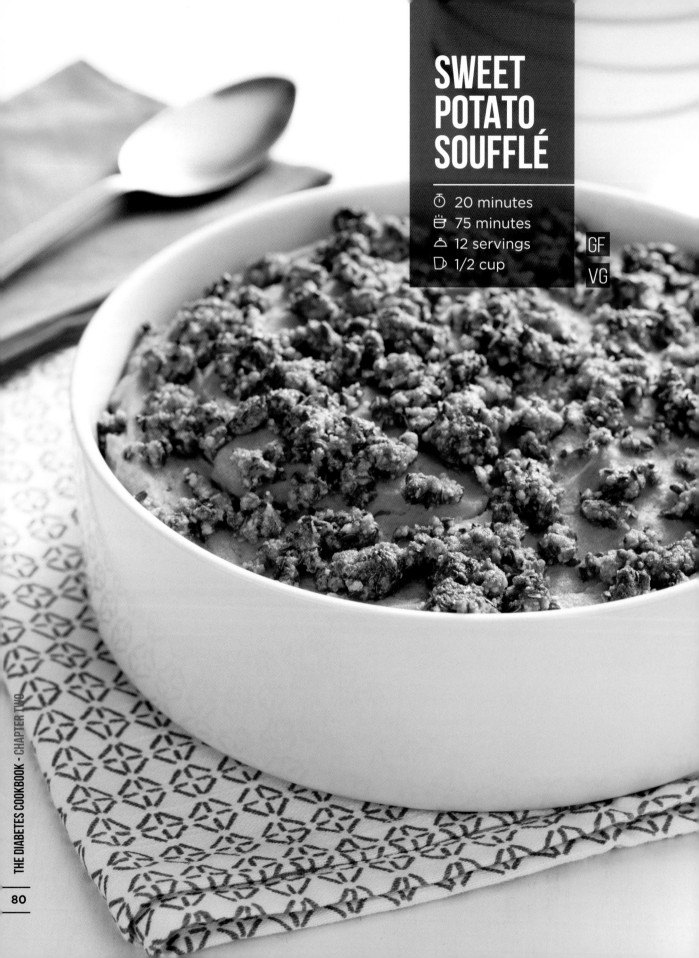

SWEET POTATO SOUFFLÉ

- ⏱ 20 minutes
- 🍳 75 minutes
- 🍽 12 servings
- 🥄 1/2 cup

GF
VG

LOOKING FOR A NEW SWEET POTATO DISH TO SERVE YOUR GUESTS DURING THE HOLIDAY SEASON? THIS SWEET POTATO SOUFFLÉ IS JUST THE TICKET!

Nonstick cooking spray
3 pounds whole sweet potatoes, washed and dried
1/4 cup plus 2 tablespoons low-calorie brown sugar blend (such as Splenda), divided
1/4 cup low-sugar (or freshly squeezed) orange juice
1/2 teaspoon salt
1/2 cup shelled walnut pieces
1/4 cup ground flaxseed
2 tablespoons trans fat–free margarine
6 egg whites
1/4 teaspoon cream of tartar

1. Preheat oven to 400°F. Coat a deep 8-inch round or square casserole dish with cooking spray. Set aside.

2. Coat a baking sheet with cooking spray. Arrange the washed and dried whole sweet potatoes (with the skins on) on the sheet and coat generously with cooking spray. Bake 50–60 minutes or until tender (check their tenderness by spearing the largest one with a paring knife or fork).

3. Remove sweet potatoes from the oven and peel off the skin. In a large bowl, combine (or blend with a mixer) the roasted sweet potatoes with 1/4 cup brown sugar blend, orange juice, and salt. Set aside to cool.

4. Using a food processor or chopper, grind the walnuts, flaxseed, and 2 tablespoons brown sugar blend together until it is the consistency of wet sand. Add the margarine to the mixture and pulse to incorporate (do not overmix or it will turn into a paste). Set aside.

5. Combine egg whites and cream of tartar in a large glass or metal bowl and beat with an electric mixer on medium speed or with a stand mixer using the whisk attachment until egg whites form soft peaks with tips that curl over when the beaters are lifted.

6. Working in batches, incorporate 1/3 of the egg whites into the sweet potato mixture using a large flat rubber spatula, gently folding them in until combined. Repeat this process two more times until all the egg whites are incorporated into the sweet potatoes.

7. Pour sweet potato soufflé mixture into the prepared casserole dish and top with the walnut mixture.

8. Place the soufflé in the oven and bake at 400°F for 20 minutes. Reduce the temperature to 350°F and continue to bake 15 more minutes. Serve hot.

NOTE: *The soufflé may deflate a little bit after baking, so it's best served immediately but is still okay to hold in a warming oven for service.*

CHEF TIP: *Do not open the oven during baking or the soufflé may not rise as high as it should.*

Nutrition Facts

Serves: 12
Serving Size: 1/2 cup

Amount per serving	
Calories	**160**
Calories from fat 50	
Total fat 6.0 g	
Saturated fat 0.8 g	
Trans fat 0.0 g	
Cholesterol 0 mg	
Sodium 170 mg	
Potassium 480 mg	
Total carbohydrate 25 g	
Dietary fiber 4 g	
Sugars 9 g	
Protein 5 g	
Phosphorus 75 mg	

Choices/Exchanges: 1 Starch, 1/2 Carbohydrate, 1 Fat

ROOT VEGETABLE CAKES

- ⏱ 20 minutes
- 🍲 35 minutes
- 🍽 10 servings
- 🍰 1 cake

VG

THESE CAKES MAKE A GREAT SIDE DISH OR SNACK AND ARE EXCELLENT WHEN PAIRED WITH BEEF AND SWEET POTATO STEW (PAGE 237).

1 large sweet potato (about 10 ounces), peeled and shredded
1 medium rutabaga (about 10 ounces), peeled and shredded
2 medium parsnips (about 3 ounces each), peeled and shredded
1 egg
3 egg whites
1/4 cup chopped fresh parsley
2 cloves garlic, minced
1/2 cup whole-wheat flour
1/2 teaspoon salt
1/2 teaspoon ground black pepper
Nonstick cooking spray

1. Preheat oven to 375°F. Line a large baking sheet with parchment paper or a silicone mat.
2. Combine all ingredients except the cooking spray in a large mixing bowl and mix well.
3. Pack the root vegetable mixture into a 1/2 cup measure and turn out onto the baking sheet. Press lightly to form a cake. Repeat this process for remaining 9 cakes (depending on the size of your baking sheet, you may need to make these in batches or use two baking sheets).
4. Spray the tops of the cakes with cooking spray and bake 35 minutes.
5. Let the cakes cool slightly before removing them from the baking sheet.

Nutrition Facts

Serves: 10
Serving Size: 1 cake

Amount per serving
Calories 70

Calories from fat 5	
Total fat 0.5 g	
Saturated fat 0.2 g	
Trans fat 0.0 g	
Cholesterol 20 mg	
Sodium 150 mg	
Potassium 270 mg	
Total carbohydrate 13 g	
Dietary fiber 2 g	
Sugars 3 g	
Protein 3 g	
Phosphorus 65 mg	

Choices/Exchanges: 1 Starch

MODERN TUNA NOODLE CASSEROLE

THIS RECIPE USES VEGETABLES TO BULK UP A DISH THAT IS TYPICALLY HIGH IN CARBS AND FAT.

⏱ 5 minutes
🍲 40 minutes
🍽 8 servings
🥣 1 cup

Nonstick cooking spray
12   ounces whole-grain penne or farfalle pasta
1   tablespoon olive oil
8   ounces button mushrooms, sliced
1   small yellow onion, diced (about 3/4 cup)
5   ounces baby spinach
1/2   teaspoon salt-free all-purpose seasoning (such as Spike or Mrs. Dash)
3   tablespoons flour
2   cups skim milk
1/2   teaspoon salt
1/4   teaspoon ground black pepper
1   (5-ounce) can tuna packed in water, drained
1/2   cup shredded parmesan cheese

1. Preheat oven to 375°F. Coat a 9-by-13-inch baking dish with cooking spray. Set aside.
2. Cook the pasta according to directions on the package, minus two minutes (the pasta should be slightly undercooked).
3. While the pasta is cooking, add the olive oil to a large sauté pan and place over medium-high heat. Add the mushrooms and onion and sauté until the onion turns clear, about 5 minutes.
4. Add the spinach and salt-free seasoning and sauté until the spinach is wilted and soft, about 3 minutes.

5. In a small bowl, whisk together the flour, milk, salt, and pepper until there are no flour lumps. Pour over the vegetables and bring to a boil. Stir in the tuna and pasta and pour into the prepared baking pan.
6. Sprinkle the parmesan cheese on top of the casserole and bake 15 minutes.

Nutrition Facts
Serves: 8
Serving Size: 1 cup

Amount per serving
Calories   **250**

Calories from fat 35

Total fat 4.0 g

    Saturated fat 1.2 g

    Trans fat 0.0 g

Cholesterol 10 mg

Sodium 300 mg

Potassium 380 mg

Total carbohydrate 42 g

    Dietary fiber 6 g

    Sugars 6 g

Protein 13 g

Phosphorus 235 mg

Choices/Exchanges: 2 1/2 Starch, 1 Nonstarchy Vegetable, 1 Lean Protein

TURKEY TOSTADAS

⏱ 30 minutes
🍲 30 minutes
🍽 6 servings
🍴 1 tostada

SERVE THIS DISH WITH A SALAD AND YOUR FAVORITE SALSA.

Nonstick cooking spray
1   pound lean ground turkey (93% fat-free)
1   (15-ounce) can no-salt-added black beans, drained and rinsed
1   tablespoon chili powder
1   teaspoon cumin
1/4 teaspoon crushed red pepper flakes
2   cloves garlic, minced
1/2 teaspoon salt
1/2 teaspoon ground black pepper
1   (6-ounce) bag baby spinach
2   spreadable creamy light Swiss cheese wedges (such as Laughing Cow)
1/4 cup shredded reduced-fat Mexican-style cheese
1/4 cup fat-free reduced-sodium chicken broth
6   corn tortillas
6   cups shredded lettuce
3   tomatoes, seeded and diced
6   tablespoons fat-free plain Greek yogurt

1. Preheat oven to 375°F. Coat a baking sheet with cooking spray. Set aside.
2. Coat a large sauté pan with cooking spray and place over high heat. Add turkey and sauté until turkey begins to brown, about 7–9 minutes. Add the black beans and heat through.
3. Add chili powder, cumin, red pepper flakes, garlic, salt, and pepper. Sauté an additional 2–3 minutes. Add spinach and cook until wilted, about 3 minutes.

4. Add both cheeses and chicken broth and stir until cheese is melted.
5. Lay 6 corn tortillas on the prepared baking sheet. Spoon the turkey mixture evenly onto each tortilla. Bake 15 minutes or until tortilla is crispy.
6. Top each tostada with 1 cup lettuce, 1/2 tomato, and 1 tablespoon Greek yogurt.

MAKE IT GLUTEN-FREE: *Verify that the ingredients you are using, such as the chicken broth, are gluten-free.*

Nutrition Facts

Serves: 6
Serving Size: 1 tostada

Amount per serving	
Calories	**300**
Calories from fat 70	
Total fat 8.0 g	
Saturated fat 2.8 g	
Trans fat 0.1 g	
Cholesterol 60 mg	
Sodium 430 mg	
Potassium 890 mg	
Total carbohydrate 31 g	
Dietary fiber 6 g	
Sugars 5 g	
Protein 25 g	
Phosphorus 430 mg	

Choices/Exchanges: 1 1/2 Starch, 1 Nonstarchy Vegetable, 3 Lean Protein, 1/2 Fat

STUFFED ITALIAN MEAT LOAF BALLS

🕐 20 minutes
🍲 55 minutes
🍽 8 servings
🍴 1 meatball

GF

FILLING

Nonstick cooking spray
1 tablespoon olive oil
8 ounces cremini (baby bella) mushrooms, chopped
1/2 medium onion, chopped
2 cloves garlic, chopped
1 teaspoon dried oregano
1/4 teaspoon ground black pepper
1/4 cup grated parmesan cheese

MEAT LOAF

1 pound lean ground turkey
1/2 cup certified gluten-free oats
2 egg whites
2 cloves garlic, minced
1/2 medium onion, minced
1 medium zucchini, shredded
1/2 teaspoon salt
1/4 teaspoon ground black pepper

GLAZE

1/2 cup ketchup
1/4 cup balsamic vinegar

1. Preheat oven to 375°F. Coat a large baking sheet with cooking spray.
2. Heat olive oil in a medium sauté pan over medium-high heat. Add to the pan all the filling ingredients except the parmesan cheese and sauté until mushrooms and onion are tender and have expelled all their liquid. Remove from heat, stir in the parmesan cheese, and set aside to cool.
3. In a mixing bowl, combine the meat loaf ingredients until incorporated.
4. Once the filling is cool, pulse the filling in a food processor until minced but still slightly chunky. Do not overprocess into a paste.
5. Divide meat loaf mixture into 8 equal portions. Flatten one portion onto

THESE STUFFED MEAT LOAF BALLS AREN'T YOUR GRANDMOTHER'S MEAT LOAF. THEY ARE A FUN PARTY FOOD, AND KIDS LOVE THEM, TOO. SERVE WITH A GREEN SALAD AND POLENTA FOR A FANCY ITALIAN MEAL.

your hand to form a patty. Place 1 heaping tablespoon of mushroom mixture in the center of the patty and close your hand to form a ball around the mushroom mixture. Repeat for remaining meat loaf balls. Place meat loaf balls on the sprayed baking sheet and bake 35 minutes.

6. In a small bowl, whisk together ketchup and balsamic vinegar. After the meat loaf balls have baked 35 minutes, brush the meat loaf balls generously with half the glaze. Return to the oven for 5 minutes, then brush the remaining glaze on the meat loaf balls and bake 5 more minutes.

Nutrition Facts

Serves: 8
Serving Size: 1 meatball

Amount per serving
Calories 180

Calories from fat 60	
Total fat 7.0 g	
Saturated fat 1.9 g	
Trans fat 0.1 g	
Cholesterol 45 mg	
Sodium 400 mg	
Potassium 450 mg	
Total carbohydrate 13 g	
Dietary fiber 1 g	
Sugars 7 g	
Protein 15 g	
Phosphorus 200 mg	

Choices/Exchanges:
1/2 Carbohydrate, 1 Nonstarchy Vegetable, 2 Lean Protein, 1/2 Fat

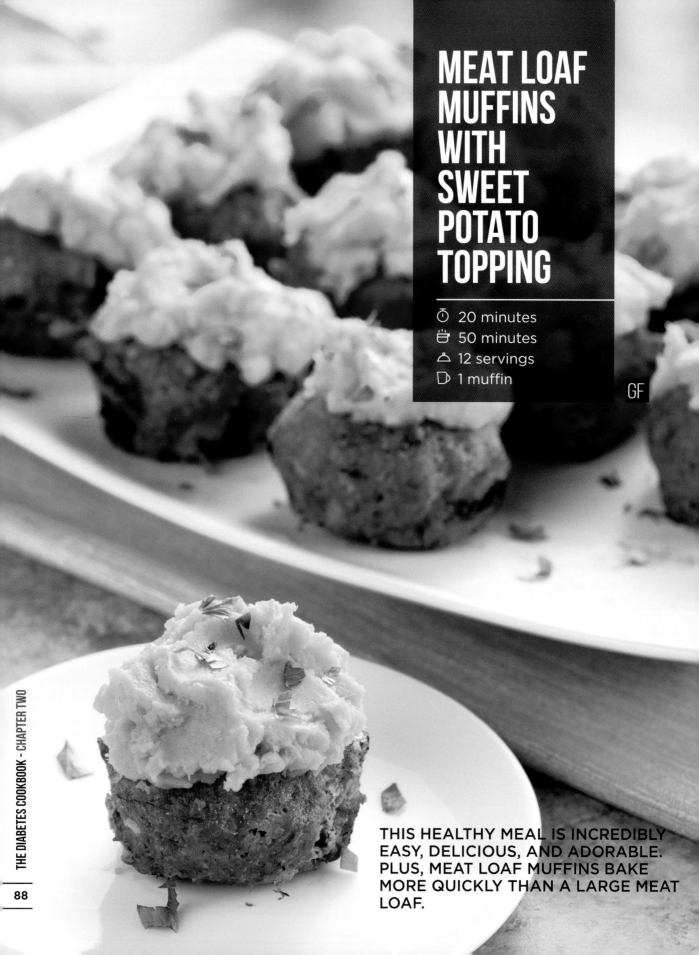

MEAT LOAF MUFFINS WITH SWEET POTATO TOPPING

- ⏱ 20 minutes
- 🍲 50 minutes
- 🍽 12 servings
- 🍴 1 muffin

GF

THIS HEALTHY MEAL IS INCREDIBLY EASY, DELICIOUS, AND ADORABLE. PLUS, MEAT LOAF MUFFINS BAKE MORE QUICKLY THAN A LARGE MEAT LOAF.

SWEET POTATO TOPPING

2	(12-ounce) sweet potatoes
1	tablespoon trans fat–free margarine

MEAT LOAF

20	ounces lean ground turkey
1	egg, slightly beaten
1	tablespoon chili powder
1/4	teaspoon ground black pepper
1	teaspoon garlic powder
1/3	cup finely diced onion
1/2	cup certified gluten-free cornmeal or oats
2	tablespoons ketchup

1. Preheat oven to 425°F. Line a muffin pan with muffin papers.

2. Clean the potatoes and prick them several times with a fork. Bake the potatoes 20 minutes. Remove the potatoes from the oven and microwave them an additional 5 minutes or until soft. Remove the skins from the potatoes and place the potatoes in a medium bowl. Mash with a potato masher and stir in the margarine. Mix well.

3. In a medium bowl, mix together the meat loaf ingredients.

4. Fill each lined muffin cup with about 1/4 cup meat loaf mixture. Bake 25 minutes.

5. Top each cooked meat loaf muffin with a scoop of sweet potatoes.

Nutrition Facts

Serves: 12
Serving Size: 1 muffin

Amount per serving
Calories 150

Calories from fat 45	
Total fat 5.0 g	
Saturated fat 1.4 g	
Trans fat 0.1 g	
Cholesterol 50 mg	
Sodium 100 mg	
Potassium 350 mg	
Total carbohydrate 15 g	
Dietary fiber 2 g	
Sugars 4 g	
Protein 11 g	
Phosphorus 130 mg	

Choices/Exchanges: 1 Starch, 1 Lean Protein, 1/2 Fat

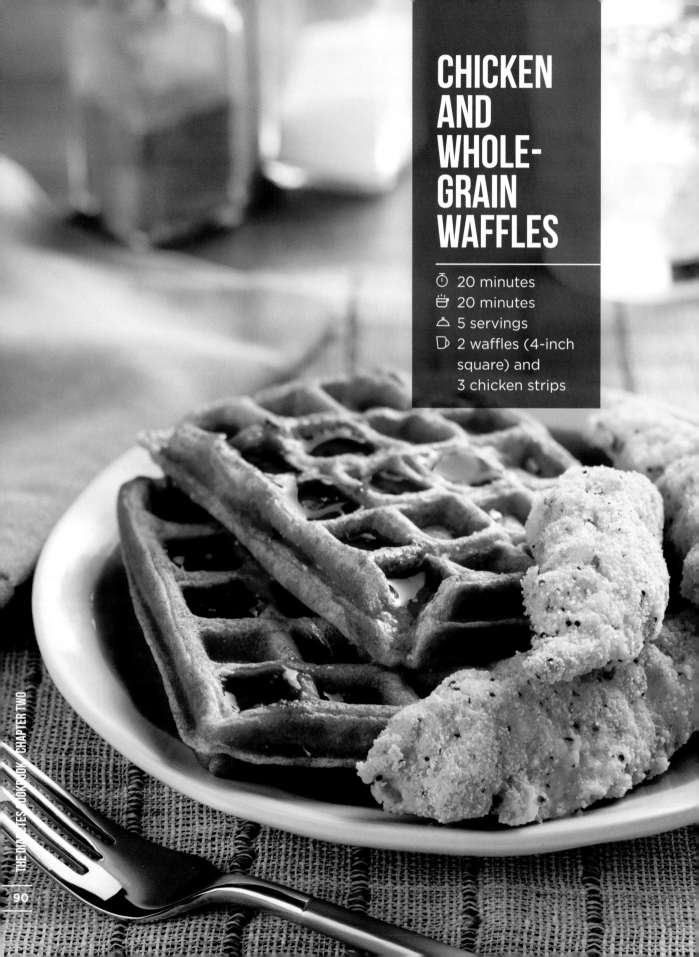

CHICKEN AND WHOLE-GRAIN WAFFLES

- ⏱ 20 minutes
- ⏲ 20 minutes
- 🍽 5 servings
- 🍴 2 waffles (4-inch square) and 3 chicken strips

HERE'S A LIGHTER VERSION OF WHAT IS USUALLY A DEEP-FRIED, HIGH-CARBOHYDRATE, HIGH-CALORIE MEAL. YOU'LL NEED A WAFFLE IRON TO MAKE THIS DISH.

CHICKEN

Nonstick cooking spray
1/4	cup whole-wheat flour
3	egg whites
1	tablespoon hot sauce
1/2	cup cornmeal
1	teaspoon salt-free all-purpose seasoning (such as Spike or Mrs. Dash)
1/2	teaspoon ground black pepper
1	pound boneless skinless chicken breasts

WAFFLES

1	large egg
1	cup skim milk
1/2	cup fat-free plain Greek yogurt
2	tablespoons olive oil
1/2	teaspoon baking soda
1 1/2	cups whole-wheat flour
1 1/2	teaspoons baking powder
3	egg whites

1. Preheat oven to 375°F. Coat a baking sheet with cooking spray. Set aside.
2. Place the flour in a small bowl. In a second small bowl, whisk together the egg whites and hot sauce. In a third small bowl, mix together the cornmeal, salt-free seasoning, and pepper.
3. Slice chicken breasts lengthwise into 1-inch strips (this should make 15 strips). Dredge each strip in the flour, shake off the excess, dip in the egg whites, then coat with the cornmeal, and place on the prepared baking sheet.
4. Once all the chicken strips are coated, spray each strip with cooking spray on both sides. Bake 20 minutes.
5. While the chicken is cooking, preheat a waffle iron according to the manufacturer's directions, and set to high. In a small bowl, whisk together the egg, milk, yogurt, and oil.
6. In a large bowl, sift together the baking soda, flour, and baking powder.
7. In another bowl, whip the egg whites to stiff peaks.
8. Mix the wet ingredients into the dry ingredients until combined. Gently fold in the whipped egg whites until combined. Cook the waffles according to your waffle iron instructions. For 4-inch waffles, use 1/2 cup batter. Cook the waffles until they are dark golden brown.
9. Serve 2 waffles with 3 strips of chicken.

CHEF TIP: *For an additional topping, mix 5 tablespoons 100% pure maple syrup and 1 teaspoon Thai chili garlic sauce (or any hot sauce) in a microwave-safe bowl. Microwave, covered, 45 seconds. Drizzle each serving of chicken and waffles with 1 tablespoon of topping.*

Nutrition Facts

Serves: 5
Serving Size: 2 waffles (4-inch square) and 3 chicken strips

Amount per serving	
Calories	**410**

Calories from fat 90	
Total fat 10.0 g	
Saturated fat 2.0 g	
Trans fat 0.0 g	
Cholesterol 90 mg	
Sodium 450 mg	
Potassium 540 mg	
Total carbohydrate 44 g	
Dietary fiber 5 g	
Sugars 5 g	
Protein 35 g	
Phosphorus 530 mg	

Choices/Exchanges: 3 Starch, 4 Lean Protein

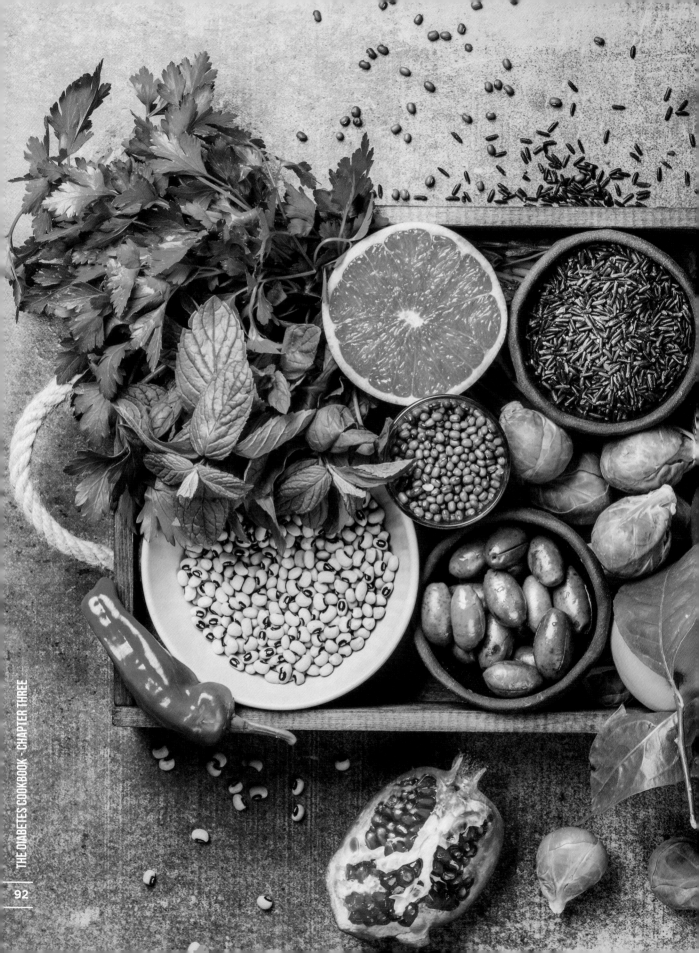

CHAPTER THREE

BUDGET-FRIENDLY RECIPES

THESE MEALS WILL FEED A FAMILY OF FOUR AND WON'T BREAK THE BANK AT AROUND TEN DOLLARS PER MEAL. OF COURSE, THEY ARE MADE WITH HEALTHY CARBS, LEAN PROTEINS, AND HEALTHY FATS FOR GOOD BLOOD SUGAR CONTROL, TOO.

BARLEY HOPPIN' JOHN WITH TURKEY KIELBASA

⏱ 15 minutes
🍲 20 minutes
🍽 6 servings
🥄 1 cup
Recipe Cost: $7.50

IT'S A TRADITION TO EAT BLACK-EYED PEAS ON NEW YEAR'S DAY FOR GOOD LUCK. WHY STOP THERE? ENJOY THIS HEARTY TAKE ON HOPPIN' JOHN ANY DAY OF THE YEAR!

2   teaspoons olive oil
1   medium onion, diced
1   red bell pepper, seeded and diced
2   cloves garlic, minced
8   ounces turkey kielbasa, diced
1   cup fat-free low-sodium chicken broth
1/4 teaspoon crushed red pepper flakes (or to taste)
1/2 teaspoon ground black pepper
1   (15.5-ounce) can black-eyed peas, drained and rinsed
1   cup cooked barley (see Note)
2   scallions, thinly sliced (green and white parts)

1. Add oil to a large sauté pan and place over medium heat. Add onion, bell pepper, and garlic. Sauté 5 minutes. Add kielbasa and sauté another 2 minutes.

2. Add broth, red pepper flakes, black pepper, and black-eyed peas. Bring to a boil; then reduce to a low simmer. Simmer 7 minutes. Stir in cooked barley and simmer 2 minutes.

3. Top with sliced scallions.

NOTE:

BULK COOKING BARLEY: *Add 11 ounces dry pearled (quick-cooking) barley to a pot of 4 cups boiling water. Cover, reduce heat, and simmer 10–12 minutes. Remove from heat, and keep pot covered 5 minutes. This makes 6 cups cooked barley. This barley can be used in any recipe calling for cooked barley. Store in an airtight container in the refrigerator for 7 days, or freeze in 1-cup portions for up to 6 months.*

CHEF TIP: *This dish typically is made with white rice, but using barley adds more fiber and an interesting texture.*

Nutrition Facts

Serves: 6
Serving Size: 1 cup

Amount per serving
Calories 190

Calories from fat 45

Total fat 5.0 g

Saturated fat 1.0 g

Trans fat 0.0 g

Cholesterol 20 mg

Sodium 450 mg

Potassium 380 mg

Total carbohydrate 25 g

Dietary fiber 6 g

Sugars 5 g

Protein 12 g

Phosphorus 190 mg

Choices/Exchanges: 1 1/2 Starch, 1 Nonstarchy Vegetable, 1 Lean Protein

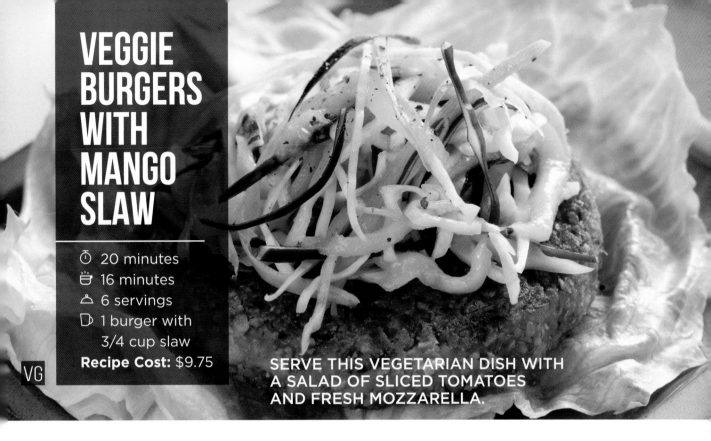

VEGGIE BURGERS WITH MANGO SLAW

- ⏱ 20 minutes
- 🍳 16 minutes
- 🍽 6 servings
- 🍴 1 burger with 3/4 cup slaw

Recipe Cost: $9.75

VG

SERVE THIS VEGETARIAN DISH WITH A SALAD OF SLICED TOMATOES AND FRESH MOZZARELLA.

Nonstick cooking spray
1   (15-ounce) can cannellini (white kidney) beans, rinsed and drained
1/2 cup diced onion
1   clove garlic, minced
1   cup diced mushrooms
1   cup shredded carrots
1   tablespoon Worcestershire sauce
1   tablespoon reduced-sodium soy sauce
1   cup oatmeal
2   teaspoons Montreal steak seasoning
1   mango (unripened or not soft), peeled, seeded, and shredded
1   (9-ounce) bag coleslaw mix
2   tablespoons rice wine vinegar
1   tablespoon olive oil
6   large lettuce leaves (such as bibb or butter)

1. Coat a large nonstick sauté pan with cooking spray. Set aside.
2. Combine cannellini beans, onion, garlic, mushrooms, carrots, Worcestershire sauce, soy sauce, oatmeal, steak seasoning, and salt in a food processor. Pulse several times until mixture is combined but stop before it forms a paste.
3. Divide burger mixture into 6 equal portions and form into patties.
4. Heat prepared sauté pan over medium-high heat. Sauté burgers on each side 6–8 minutes. Set aside.
5. In a large bowl, combine shredded mango, coleslaw mix, vinegar, and olive oil. Toss to coat.
6. Add a burger to a lettuce leaf, and top each with 3/4 cup coleslaw mixture.

Nutrition Facts

Serves: 6
Serving Size: 1 burger with 3/4 cup slaw

Amount per serving	
Calories	**180**

Calories from fat 30	
Total fat 3.5 g	
Saturated fat 0.5 g	
Trans fat 0.0 g	
Cholesterol 0 mg	
Sodium 430 mg	
Potassium 540 mg	
Total carbohydrate 32 g	
Dietary fiber 7 g	
Sugars 8 g	
Protein 7 g	
Phosphorus 155 mg	

Choices/Exchanges: 1 Starch, 1/2 Fruit, 1 Nonstarchy Vegetable, 1/2 Fat

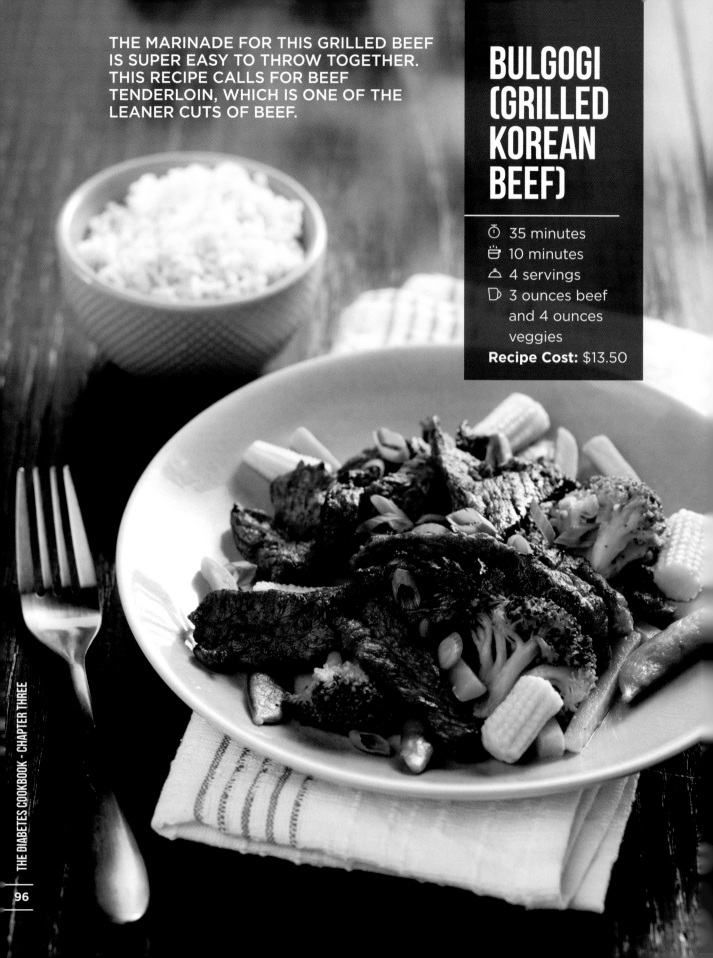

THE MARINADE FOR THIS GRILLED BEEF IS SUPER EASY TO THROW TOGETHER. THIS RECIPE CALLS FOR BEEF TENDERLOIN, WHICH IS ONE OF THE LEANER CUTS OF BEEF.

BULGOGI (GRILLED KOREAN BEEF)

- 35 minutes
- 10 minutes
- 4 servings
- 3 ounces beef and 4 ounces veggies

Recipe Cost: $13.50

12	ounces lean boneless beef tenderloin
3	scallions (white and green parts), chopped
2	cloves garlic, minced
2	teaspoons rice wine vinegar
2	tablespoons water
3	tablespoons reduced-sodium soy sauce
1	tablespoon honey or 2 packets artificial sweetener
1/2	teaspoon ground black pepper
1	(16-ounce) steamer bag frozen stir-fry vegetables

1. Wrap the beef in plastic wrap and freeze until firm (but not rock hard). Once firm, slice beef thinly into long strips. Place in a baking dish.

2. In a small bowl, whisk together the scallions, garlic, vinegar, water, soy sauce, honey, and pepper. Pour the mixture over the beef and let it marinate in the refrigerator for at least 30 minutes, up to 2 hours. While the beef is marinating, preheat an indoor or outdoor grill.

3. Remove the beef from the marinade and shake off any excess marinade. Grill beef 2–3 minutes on each side or until it is cooked to a medium-well doneness.

4. Steam the vegetables and serve the beef over the steamed vegetables.

Nutrition Facts

Serves: 4
Serving Size: 3 ounces beef and 4 ounces veggies

Amount per serving	
Calories	**180**

Calories from fat 40	
Total fat 4.5 g	
Saturated fat 1.6 g	
Trans fat 0.0 g	
Cholesterol 45 mg	
Sodium 200 mg	
Potassium 460 mg	
Total carbohydrate 13 g	
Dietary fiber 3 g	
Sugars 6 g	
Protein 17 g	
Phosphorus 195 mg	

Choices/Exchanges: 2 Nonstarchy Vegetable, 2 Lean Protein

ROASTED BEETS HAVE A TOTALLY DIFFERENT FLAVOR THAN THE CANNED BEETS YOU MAY BE USED TO. THEY ARE RICHER IN FLAVOR AND HAVE A GREAT TEXTURE. PAIRED WITH THE GOAT CHEESE, THIS IS A WONDERFULLY EASY, BUT GOURMET TASTING, SALAD!

ROASTED BEET AND CHICKEN SALAD WITH GOAT CHEESE

- ⏱ 20 minutes
- ⏲ 50 minutes
- 🍽 4 servings
- 🍴 1 salad

Recipe Cost: $9.75

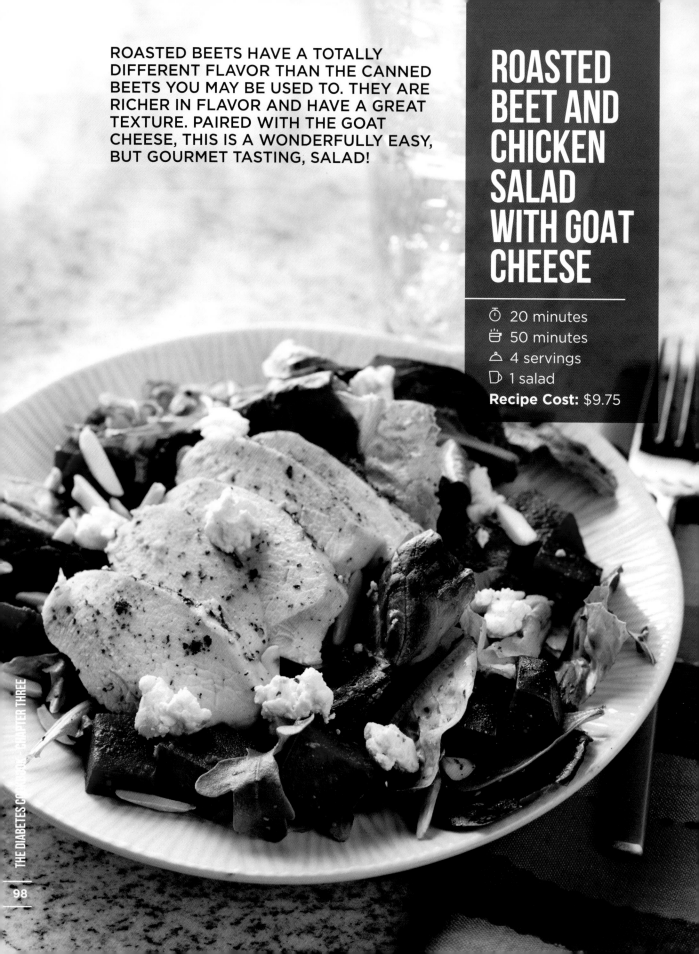

Nonstick cooking spray
4   small beets, greens removed
2   (6-ounce) boneless skinless chicken breasts
1/4 teaspoon ground black pepper
1/4 cup balsamic vinegar
1   tablespoon extra-virgin olive oil
2   tablespoons fat-free reduced-sodium vegetable broth
1   tablespoon honey or 2 packets artificial sweetener
2   teaspoons Dijon mustard
1   clove garlic, minced or grated
8   cups mesclun salad mix
2   tablespoons crumbled goat cheese
1/3 cup slivered almonds, toasted

1. Preheat oven to 375°F. Coat a baking sheet with cooking spray. Set aside.
2. Wrap the beets in aluminum foil and place them on the baking sheet. Lay the chicken breasts on the baking sheet next to the beets. Coat the chicken with cooking spray and season with black pepper. Roast the chicken and beets 25–30 minutes or until internal temperature of the chicken is 165°F. Remove the chicken breasts from the oven and set aside. Once slightly cool, cut chicken into thin slices.
3. Continue to roast the beets until tender, another 15–20 minutes. Remove the beets from the oven and set aside.
4. Once the beets are cool, peel off the skin and cut each beet into 1/2-inch chunks.
5. In a medium bowl, whisk together the vinegar, olive oil, broth, honey, mustard, and garlic.

6. Add the salad mix and beet chunks to a large bowl. Pour the dressing over the salad and toss to coat.
7. Divide the salad among 4 plates. Top each salad with 1/4 of the chicken breast slices, 1 tablespoon goat cheese, and 1 heaping tablespoon slivered almonds.

CHEF TIP: *To save time, use the chicken breast meat from a deli rotisserie chicken to make this recipe.*

Nutrition Facts

Serves: 4
Serving Size: 1 salad

Amount per serving	
Calories	**270**

Calories from fat 110	
Total fat 12.0 g	
Saturated fat 2.0 g	
Trans fat 0.0 g	
Cholesterol 55 mg	
Sodium 200 mg	
Potassium 660 mg	
Total carbohydrate 19 g	
Dietary fiber 4 g	
Sugars 14 g	
Protein 23 g	
Phosphorus 245 mg	

Choices/Exchanges:
1/2 Carbohydrate, 2 Nonstarchy Vegetable, 3 Lean Protein, 1 1/2 Fat

POWER VEGGIE TACOS

⏱ 15 minutes
🍲 12 minutes
🍽 5 servings
🌮 1 taco

Recipe Cost: $10.35

VG

TRYING TO EAT MORE VEGETABLES? THESE TACOS ARE A GREAT PLACE TO START! THIS MEAL IS FULL OF FLAVOR AND FIBER.

2	teaspoons olive oil
3	large carrots, diced small
1	cup small-diced broccoli
1	cup small-diced cauliflower
1	(15-ounce) can black beans, rinsed and drained
1	tablespoon chili powder
1	teaspoon cumin
1/4	teaspoon ground black pepper
1/2	teaspoon garlic powder
5	(6-inch) whole-wheat low-carb tortillas
10	tablespoons shredded reduced-fat cheddar cheese
1 1/4	cup shredded lettuce
1	large tomato, diced
1/2	avocado, thinly sliced

1. Heat oil in sauté pan over medium high heat. Add the carrots, broccoli, and cauliflower and sauté 5–7 minutes. Add the beans, chili powder, cumin, pepper, and garlic powder and stir to incorporate. Cook 5 more minutes.

2. Scoop 1/5 of the veggie mixture into a tortilla. Top with 2 tablespoons cheese, 1/4 cup lettuce, 1 tablespoon diced tomatoes, and 1 avocado slice. Repeat the procedure for the remaining 4 tacos.

Nutrition Facts

Serves: 5
Serving Size: 1 taco

Amount per serving
Calories   **230**

Calories from fat 90

Total fat 10.0 g

  Saturated fat 2.4 g

  Trans fat 0.0 g

Cholesterol 10 mg

Sodium 400 mg

Potassium 670 mg

Total carbohydrate 31 g

  Dietary fiber 14 g

  Sugars 5 g

Protein 14 g

Phosphorus 245 mg

Choices/Exchanges: 1 1/2 Starch, 2 Nonstarchy Vegetable, 1 Lean Protein, 1 Fat

VEGETABLE STEW WITH WHOLE-WHEAT DUMPLINGS

WHAT'S BETTER DURING THE FALL THAN A WARM, TASTY STEW? THIS BUDGET-FRIENDLY RECIPE IS FAIRLY EASY.

- ⏱ 20 minutes
- 🍲 50 minutes
- 🍽 8 servings
- 🍴 1 1/2 cups stew and 1 dumpling

Recipe Cost: $10.40

STEW

1	tablespoon olive oil
1	fennel bulb, diced
1	onion, diced
2	stalks celery, diced
4	cups butternut squash, peeled and diced
1	teaspoon ground sage
4	cups fat-free low-sodium chicken broth
4	cups water
1/4	teaspoon salt
1	teaspoon salt-free all-purpose seasoning (such as Spike or Mrs. Dash)
1/2	teaspoon ground black pepper
2	bay leaves
4	cups chopped kale (1 bunch, stemmed)

DUMPLINGS

1	cup whole-wheat flour
1/2	cup all-purpose flour
1	tablespoon baking powder
1/2	teaspoon salt
1/4	teaspoon ground black pepper
1	teaspoon herbes de Provence (or dried sage)
1	large egg
1/2	cup fat-free plain Greek yogurt
1/2	cup water

1. Add oil to a large soup pot over medium-high heat.
2. Add fennel, onion, and celery to oil and sauté until onions turn clear (about 4–5 minutes). Add squash, sage, chicken broth, water, salt, no-salt seasoning, pepper, and bay leaves. Bring to a boil; then reduce to a simmer.
3. Simmer stew 20 minutes. Then add kale and simmer 10 more minutes.
4. While stew is simmering, whisk together dumpling ingredients to form a stiff batter. Set aside.
5. After stew has simmered with kale 10 minutes, remove bay leaves.
6. Use a 1/4 cup measure to scoop dumplings on top of stew to make 8 dumplings. Do not stir once dumplings have been added to the top of the stew. Cover, reduce heat, and simmer 10 minutes until dumplings are cooked through and puffed.

CHEF TIP: *Serve with a green salad with low-fat honey mustard dressing.*

Nutrition Facts

Serves: 8
Serving Size: 1 1/2 cups stew and 1 dumpling

Amount per serving
Calories **180**

Calories from fat 25	
Total fat 3.0 g	
Saturated fat 0.6 g	
Trans fat 0.0 g	
Cholesterol 25 mg	
Sodium 470 mg	
Potassium 710 mg	
Total carbohydrate 31 g	
Dietary fiber 6 g	
Sugars 4 g	
Protein 9 g	
Phosphorus 345 mg	

Choices/Exchanges: 1 1/2 Starch, 1 Nonstarchy Vegetable, 1/2 Fat

THIS BUDGET-FRIENDLY RECIPE COMES TOGETHER QUICKLY FOR A WEEKNIGHT DINNER, WITH THE FLAVORS OF FALL COMING FROM THE APPLES, ONION, AND CABBAGE.

CHICKEN SAUSAGE AND CABBAGE SKILLET

- ⏱ 10 minutes
- 🍳 20 minutes
- 🍽 4 servings
- 🥄 1 2/3 cups

Recipe Cost: $7.65

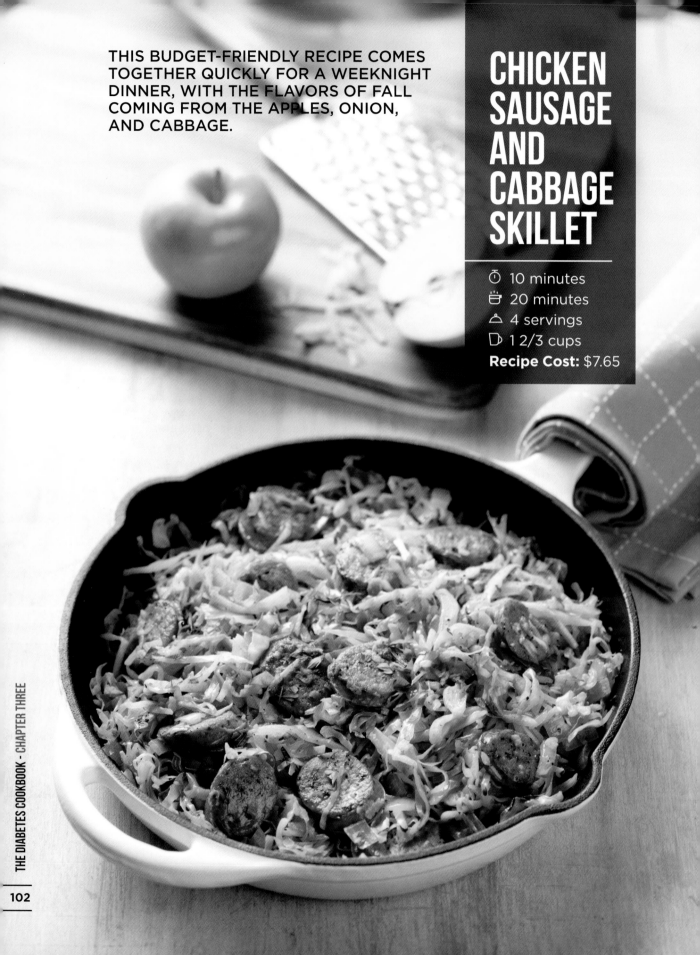

Nonstick cooking spray
1 teaspoon olive oil
3 links fully cooked roasted garlic chicken sausage (about 3 ounces each), sliced
2 small Granny Smith apples, peeled and grated (use large hole on grater)
1 onion, diced
8 cups shredded cabbage (1 small head)
1 tablespoon honey or 2 packets artificial sweetener
1/4 cup white wine
1 tablespoon white wine vinegar
1 teaspoon salt-free all-purpose seasoning (such as Spike or Mrs. Dash)
1/2 teaspoon ground black pepper

1. Spray a large sauté pan with cooking spray and then add oil and heat over medium-high heat.
2. Sauté sausage until it begins to brown. Remove from pan and set aside.
3. Add apples, onion, and cabbage to the pan and sauté 8–10 minutes or until cabbage is soft and beginning to lightly brown.
4. Return sausage to the pan and add remaining ingredients. Sauté until all the liquid is reduced.

CHEF TIP: *If you don't want to use white wine, use 2 tablespoons white wine vinegar and omit the additional white wine vinegar from the ingredient list.*

MAKE IT GLUTEN-FREE: *Confirm that all ingredients, including chicken sausage, are gluten-free.*

Nutrition Facts

Serves: 4
Serving Size: 1 2/3 cups

Amount per serving
Calories 220

Calories from fat 60

Total fat 7.0 g

Saturated fat 1.7 g

Trans fat 0.0 g

Cholesterol 50 mg

Sodium 390 mg

Potassium 530 mg

Total carbohydrate 27 g

Dietary fiber 5 g

Sugars 19 g

Protein 14 g

Phosphorus 180 mg

Choices/Exchanges: 1/2 Starch, 1/2 Carbohydrate, 2 Nonstarchy Vegetable, 1 Lean Protein, 1 Fat

BRAISED CHICKEN THIGHS WITH MUSHROOMS

- ⏱ 15 minutes
- 🍲 40 minutes
- 🍽 4 servings
- 🍴 1 chicken thigh with 1/4 cup mushrooms

Recipe Cost: $7.90

LC

HEALTHY EATING CAN BE DONE ON A BUDGET, AND THIS DINNER PROVES IT! CHICKEN THIGHS ARE LESS EXPENSIVE THAN CHICKEN BREASTS AND CAN BE A NICE CHANGE. THIS RECIPE MAKES A TASTY, LOW-CARB, BUDGET-FRIENDLY MEAL.

1	tablespoon olive oil
1	pound boneless skinless chicken thighs
1	teaspoon trans fat–free margarine
1/2	onion, finely diced
1	(8-ounce) package sliced mushrooms
3	tablespoons balsamic vinegar
1 1/2	cups fat-free low-sodium chicken broth

1. Heat oil in a large Dutch oven over medium-high heat.
2. Add chicken thighs and sauté 3 minutes per side. Remove from pan and set aside.
3. Add margarine to the Dutch oven and melt. Once margarine is melted, add onion and sauté 2 minutes. Add mushrooms and sauté 3–5 minutes, stirring frequently, until liquid is released.

4. Add balsamic vinegar to the Dutch oven and cook with mushrooms 1 minute. Add chicken thighs back to pan and spoon mushrooms on top of chicken. Pour chicken broth into pan.
5. Bring the chicken broth to a boil. Reduce the heat to medium-low; cover the Dutch oven with a heavy, tight-fitting lid; and simmer 25 minutes.

CHEF TIP: *Heat up your favorite frozen vegetable medley and serve alongside the braised chicken. You could also add 1/3 cup brown rice to the meal.*

MAKE IT GLUTEN-FREE: *Use gluten-free chicken broth and confirm all other ingredients are gluten-free.*

Nutrition Facts

Serves: 4

Serving Size: 1 chicken thigh with 1/4 cup mushrooms

Amount per serving	
Calories	**210**
Calories from fat 100	
Total fat 11.0 g	
Saturated fat 2.4 g	
Trans fat 0.0 g	
Cholesterol 105 mg	
Sodium 130 mg	
Potassium 510 mg	
Total carbohydrate 6 g	
Dietary fiber 1 g	
Sugars 4 g	
Protein 22 g	
Phosphorus 250 mg	

Choices/Exchanges: 1 Nonstarchy Vegetable, 3 Lean Protein, 1 Fat

CHICKEN PICCATA

TRY THIS LIGHTER VERSION OF THE TRADITIONAL ITALIAN FAVORITE.

- ⏱ 20 minutes
- 🍲 15 minutes
- 🍽 4 servings
- 🍴 1 chicken breast and 1 tablespoon sauce

Recipe Cost: $6.80

CHICKEN

	Nonstick cooking spray
2	large boneless skinless chicken breasts (about 10 ounces each)
1/4	teaspoon salt
1/2	teaspoon ground black pepper
1/4	cup whole-wheat flour
1	egg
1	teaspoon lemon juice
1/2	cup bread crumbs
1	teaspoon Italian seasoning

SAUCE

1	teaspoon olive oil plus cooking spray
2	tablespoons capers, drained and rinsed
1	tablespoon lemon juice
1/2	cup fat-free low-sodium chicken broth
1/4	cup chopped fresh parsley

1. Preheat oven to 475°F. Coat a baking sheet with cooking spray and set aside.
2. Slice the chicken breasts in half lengthwise and then use a mallet to pound to 1/4-inch thickness. Season each chicken breast with salt and black pepper.
3. Set up three wide bowls or flat-bottom containers. Fill the first bowl with the whole-wheat flour, the second bowl with the egg and lemon juice, and the third bowl with the bread crumbs and Italian seasoning. Whisk the egg and lemon juice together. Combine the bread crumbs and Italian seasoning and mix well.
4. Dredge a chicken breast in the flour and shake off the excess. Then dip the chicken breast in the egg, and then coat it in the bread crumb mixture. Place the chicken breast on the baking sheet. Repeat this process for the remaining three chicken breasts.
5. Spray the top of each chicken breast with cooking spray and bake 8 minutes. Turn the chicken breasts over and bake 5 more minutes. Ensure that the chicken is cooked to an internal temperature of 165°F.
6. While the chicken is baking, heat the oil and a generous amount of cooking spray in a small nonstick skillet over medium heat. Add the capers and sauté 2–3 minutes.

7. Add the lemon juice and cook until the juice is completely reduced. Add the chicken broth and simmer until reduced by half. Stir in the parsley.
8. Remove the chicken from the oven and serve with 1 tablespoon of sauce drizzled over the chicken.

CHEF TIP: *Serve the chicken on a bed of baby spinach.*

Nutrition Facts

Serves: 4

Serving Size: 1 chicken breast and 1 tablespoon sauce

Amount per serving

Calories 280

Calories from fat 70	
Total fat 8.0 g	
Saturated fat 1.9 g	
Trans fat 0.0 g	
Cholesterol 130 mg	
Sodium 470 mg	
Potassium 380 mg	
Total carbohydrate 17 g	
Dietary fiber 2 g	
Sugars 1 g	
Protein 35 g	
Phosphorus 305 mg	

Choices/Exchanges: 1 Starch, 5 Lean Protein

THIS CHOWDER IS FULL OF CHUNKY GOODNESS, INCLUDING SWEET CORN AND JUICY CHICKEN, AND IT IS HEARTY ENOUGH TO BE A MAIN DISH. JALAPEÑO PEPPERS GIVE IT A TOUCH OF SPICY HEAT.

JALAPEÑO CHICKEN AND CORN CHOWDER

- ⏱ 25 minutes
- 🍲 30 minutes
- 🍽 8 servings
- 🥣 1 1/4 cups

Recipe Cost: $8.60

1	tablespoon olive oil
1	medium yellow onion, peeled and chopped
2	medium carrots, peeled and chopped
2	stalks celery, chopped
2	medium jalapeño peppers, seeded and chopped
2	cloves garlic, peeled and smashed
4	ears sweet corn, kernels cut off the cob (or 4 cups frozen kernels, thawed and drained)
1	tablespoon salt-free all-purpose seasoning (such as Spike or Mrs. Dash)
1/2	teaspoon ground black pepper
4	cups fat-free low-sodium chicken broth
2	cups cooked chicken breast, chopped
1	cup fat-free plain Greek yogurt

1. Heat the oil in a large soup pot over medium heat.

2. Add the onion, carrot, celery, jalapeño pepper, garlic, and corn and sauté 5–7 minutes.

3. Add the no-salt seasoning, black pepper, and chicken broth. Bring to a boil; then reduce the heat and simmer, covered, 20 minutes.

4. Remove the pot from the heat and purée about half the soup, using an immersion blender or an upright blender. If using an upright blender, purée in batches and be sure not to overfill the blender. Return the purée to the pot.

5. Add the chicken and heat through. Remove the pot from the heat.

6. Stir in the yogurt and serve. Do not boil the soup once the yogurt is added.

CHEF TIP: *For a crunchy garnish, serve this soup with a few baked tortilla chips, crushed and sprinkled on top.*

Nutrition Facts

Serves: 8
Serving Size: 1 1/4 cups

Amount per serving

Calories	**180**

Calories from fat 30	
Total fat 3.5 g	
Saturated fat 0.7 g	
Trans fat 0.0 g	
Cholesterol 30 mg	
Sodium 130 mg	
Potassium 550 mg	
Total carbohydrate 21 g	
Dietary fiber 3 g	
Sugars 6 g	
Protein 18 g	
Phosphorus 225 mg	

Choices/Exchanges: 1 Starch, 1 Nonstarchy Vegetable, 2 Lean Protein

CILANTRO LIME ROASTED CHICKEN

⏱ 5 minutes
🍲 50 minutes
🍽 6 servings
🍴 1/2 breast, 1 thigh, or 1 drumstick and 1 wing

Recipe Cost: $9.90

CILANTRO AND LIME MAKE A FRESH AND ZESTY FLAVOR COMBINATION IN THIS CHICKEN DISH.

Nonstick cooking spray
1 (2 1/2-pound) whole chicken, cut into 8 pieces
2 tablespoons chopped fresh cilantro
Juice and zest of 1 lime
1 tablespoon honey or 2 packets artificial sweetener
2 cloves garlic, minced
1/2 teaspoon ground black pepper
1/2 teaspoon salt

1. Preheat oven to 375°F. Coat a baking dish with cooking spray.
2. Remove the skin from the chicken and arrange the chicken pieces in a single layer in the baking pan.
3. In a small bowl, whisk together the cilantro, lime zest, lime juice, honey, garlic, pepper, and salt. Pour the mixture evenly over the chicken and bake 45–50 minutes or until the internal temperature of the largest piece of chicken is 165°F.

CHEF TIP: *Serve with frozen tricolor pepper mixture, steamed.*

Nutrition Facts

Serves: 6

Serving Size: 1/2 breast, 1 thigh, or 1 drumstick and 1 wing

Amount per serving

Calories 130

Calories from fat 40

Total fat 4.5 g

   Saturated fat 1.2 g

   Trans fat 0.0 g

Cholesterol 55 mg

Sodium 250 mg

Potassium 160 mg

Total carbohydrate 4 g

   Dietary fiber 0 g

   Sugars 3 g

Protein 18 g

Phosphorus 120 mg

Choices/Exchanges: 3 Lean Protein

HONEY MUSTARD CHICKEN THIGHS WITH WILD RICE AND BROCCOLI

HONEY DIJON MUSTARD MAKES THESE CHICKEN THIGHS SWEET AND TANGY. ADD A SIDE OF NONSTARCHY VEGETABLES AND DINNER IS DONE!

GF

- ⏱ 5 minutes
- 🍲 40 minutes
- 🍽 4 servings
- 🍽 1 chicken thigh, 1/2 cup cooked wild rice, and 1 cup broccoli

Recipe Cost: $6.35

Nonstick cooking spray
1/4 cup honey Dijon mustard
2 cloves garlic, minced
1/4 teaspoon ground black pepper
1 pound boneless skinless chicken thighs
3/4 teaspoon dried thyme
2 cups cooked wild rice (prepare according to directions on the package)
4 cups steamed broccoli

1. Preheat oven to 375°F. Spray baking dish with cooking spray.
2. In a small bowl, combine mustard, garlic, and pepper.
3. Spread about 1 1/2 tablespoons mustard mixture evenly on top of each chicken thigh.
4. Arrange chicken in the prepared baking dish. Bake 40 minutes or until mustard mixture has formed a crust and is slightly hardened.
5. Remove from oven and sprinkle thyme on top of each thigh. Serve each chicken thigh over 1/2 cup wild rice and 1 cup steamed broccoli.

DIETITIAN TIP: *Whole grains such as oats, wild rice, whole-wheat bread, and quinoa provide more fiber, vitamins, and minerals than refined grains. Portion control is still important when including these healthier carbohydrates in your meal plan. Broccoli Amandine (page 255) would be a great side dish with this meal.*

Nutrition Facts

Serves: 4

Serving Size: 1 chicken thigh, 1/2 cup cooked wild rice, and 1 cup broccoli

Amount per serving

Calories	**280**

Calories from fat 70

Total fat 8.0 g
Saturated fat 1.9 g
Trans fat 0.0 g
Cholesterol 105 mg
Sodium 300 mg
Potassium 610 mg
Total carbohydrate 30 g
Dietary fiber 5 g
Sugars 6 g
Protein 25 g
Phosphorus 320 mg

Choices/Exchanges: 1 Starch, 1/2 Carbohydrate, 2 Nonstarchy Vegetable, 3 Lean Protein

CHICKEN CHILI

⏱ 10 minutes
🍲 25 minutes
🍽 4 servings
🥛 1 1/4 cups
Recipe Cost: $7.50

GF

THIS CHILI IS PERFECT FOR A FALL DINNER, AND IT'S FULL OF VITAMIN C, PROTEIN, AND FIBER. FEEL FREE TO EXPERIMENT WITH DIFFERENT BEANS SUCH AS BLACK OR GREAT NORTHERN.

Nonstick cooking spray
8   ounces boneless skinless chicken breast, diced
1   green bell pepper, diced
1   small onion, diced
1   clove garlic, minced
2   (14.5-ounce) cans diced tomatoes
1   (16-ounce) can navy beans, rinsed and drained
1/4   teaspoon ground black pepper
2   teaspoons chili powder
1/2   teaspoon cumin

1. Spray a large soup pot with cooking spray. Add chicken and sauté over medium heat 7 minutes or until done. Remove from pot.
2. Add green pepper and onion to pot and sauté over medium-high heat 3 minutes or until onion is clear. Add garlic and sauté 30 more seconds.
3. Add remaining ingredients along with cooked chicken and bring to a boil. Reduce heat and simmer 20 minutes.

Nutrition Facts

Serves: 4
Serving Size: 1 1/4 cups

Amount per serving	
Calories	**210**

Calories from fat 20	
Total fat 2.5 g	
Saturated fat 0.6 g	
Trans fat 0.0 g	
Cholesterol 30 mg	
Sodium 470 mg	
Potassium 860 mg	
Total carbohydrate 30 g	
Dietary fiber 10 g	
Sugars 7 g	
Protein 19 g	
Phosphorus 235 mg	

Choices/Exchanges: 1 Starch, 3 Nonstarchy Vegetable, 1 Lean Protein

SUMMER CHICKEN SPRING ROLLS

WITH NO COOKING NEEDED, THESE ROLLS ARE A GREAT ADDITION TO ANY SUMMER MENU.

⏱ 20 minutes
△ 4 servings
▭ 2 rolls
Recipe Cost: $9.65

SPRING ROLLS

1	cup shredded cabbage
1 1/2	cups shredded cooked chicken
1/2	cup shredded carrots
1/2	cup peeled, seeded, and diced cucumber
1/4	cup chopped fresh cilantro
1/2	cup thinly sliced shiitake mushrooms
1	green onion, chopped
8	medium spring roll skins (about 8 5/8 inches diameter or 1/2 ounce)

DIPPING SAUCE

2	tablespoons reduced-sodium soy sauce
3	tablespoons rice wine vinegar
2	tablespoons hot water
1	tablespoon olive oil
1	teaspoon ground ginger

1. In a medium bowl combine cabbage, chicken, carrot, cucumber, cilantro, mushrooms, and green onion.

2. In a small bowl, whisk together dipping sauce ingredients.

3. Before using, soak spring roll skins in water 10–15 seconds, then shake off excess water. Place about 1/4 cup chicken-vegetable mixture at the bottom of a spring roll skin. Fold over the spring roll edge nearest to you to cover the filling. Fold in the side edges tightly. Roll away from you to seal. Repeat procedure for remaining spring rolls.

4. Serve spring rolls with dipping sauce.

DIETITIAN TIP: *You can make this dish gluten-free by using gluten-free soy sauce. You could also try these spring rolls with shrimp in place of chicken.*

Nutrition Facts

Serves: 4
Serving Size: 2 rolls

Amount per serving
Calories 250

Calories from fat 70	
Total fat 8.0 g	
Saturated fat 1.7 g	
Trans fat 0.0 g	
Cholesterol 45 mg	
Sodium 420 mg	
Potassium 300 mg	
Total carbohydrate 26 g	
Dietary fiber 2 g	
Sugars 2 g	
Protein 18 g	
Phosphorus 160 mg	

Choices/Exchanges: 1 1/2 Starch, 1 Nonstarchy Vegetable, 2 Lean Protein, 1/2 Fat

CHICKEN SAUSAGE HASH

⏱ 15 minutes
🍲 15 minutes
🍽 4 servings
🍽 1 1/2 cups
Recipe Cost: $7.50

GF

YOU CAN FEED A FAMILY OF FOUR FOR UNDER $10 WITH THIS RECIPE. MAKE IT THE NIGHT BEFORE TO SAVE TIME.

Nonstick cooking spray
1   tablespoon olive oil
1   onion, diced
1   cup mushrooms, sliced
1   medium red bell pepper, seeded and diced
1/2   teaspoon dried thyme
1/4   teaspoon crushed red pepper flakes
1/4   teaspoon ground black pepper
1   clove garlic, minced
3   links gluten-free apple chicken sausage, diced
1/4   cup water
1   pound (2 large or 4 small) cooked sweet potatoes, roasted whole, peeled, and diced

1. Spray a large sauté pan with cooking spray, add olive oil and heat over medium-high.
2. Sauté the onion, mushrooms, and red bell pepper 6–7 minutes or until they start to caramelize.
3. Add the thyme, crushed red pepper flakes, black pepper, and garlic. Mix well and sauté 1–2 more minutes.
4. Stir in the chicken sausage and water and sauté 3–4 more minutes, scraping the bottom of the pan to mix in any brown bits on the bottom.
5. Add cooked sweet potatoes and gently stir them into the hash. Heat them through and serve.

CHEF TIP: *Serve with a mixed green salad tossed with a light balsamic vinaigrette. This would increase the cost of the meal to $9.95.*

Nutrition Facts

Serves: 4
Serving Size: 1 1/2 cups

Amount per serving
Calories   **230**

Calories from fat 70

Total fat 8.0 g

   Saturated fat 2.0 g

   Trans fat 0.0 g

Cholesterol 35 mg

Sodium 290 mg

Potassium 930 mg

Total carbohydrate 29 g

   Dietary fiber 4 g

   Sugars 13 g

Protein 11 g

Phosphorus 200 mg

Choices/Exchanges: 1 1/2 Starch, 1 Nonstarchy Vegetable, 1 Lean Protein, 1 Fat

GRILLED CHICKEN SAUSAGE WITH ZUCCHINI AND PEPPERS

LC

- ⏱ 10 minutes
- ⏲ 10 minutes
- 🍽 4 servings
- 🍴 1 sausage link and 1/2 cup zucchini-pepper mixture

Recipe Cost: $7.50

NEED A QUICK WEEKNIGHT DINNER AND DON'T FEEL LIKE HEATING UP THE HOUSE? THIS FOUR-INGREDIENT BUDGET-FRIENDLY DISH, COOKED ON THE GRILL, IS FULL OF FLAVOR AND LOW IN CARBS. IF DESIRED, SERVE IT WITH A SIDE OF WILD RICE OR QUINOA.

Nonstick cooking spray
2 large zucchini, sliced into rounds
1 red bell pepper, sliced in 1-inch strips
4 sun-dried tomato chicken sausage links (already cooked; shop for precooked sausages with the lowest fat and sodium content that you can find, such as Al Fresco)

1. Preheat a grill to medium-high. Spray grill rack with cooking spray. Place the zucchini and pepper on the grill or place in a veggie basket and grill 8–10 minutes, until tender. **2.** While the vegetables are cooking, place the chicken sausage on the grill and heat through 4–5 minutes, turning frequently.

MAKE IT GLUTEN-FREE: *Confirm that the sausage and all other ingredients are gluten-free.*

Nutrition Facts

Serves: 4

Serving Size: 1 sausage link and 1/2 cup zucchini-pepper mixture

Amount per serving

Calories 180

Calories from fat 70	
Total fat 8.0 g	
Saturated fat 2.1 g	
Trans fat 0.0 g	
Cholesterol 65 mg	
Sodium 470 mg	
Potassium 710 mg	
Total carbohydrate 9 g	
Dietary fiber 2 g	
Sugars 8 g	
Protein 17 g	
Phosphorus 235 mg	

Choices/Exchanges: 2 Nonstarchy Vegetable, 2 Lean Protein, 1/2 Fat

THIS FRITTATA IS A GREAT WAY
TO GET MORE VEGGIES INTO
YOUR DAY. HAVE IT FOR BRUNCH
OR DINNER!

SUMMER VEGETABLE FRITTATA

- ⏱ 20 minutes
- 🍲 25 minutes
- △ 4 servings
- ⌓ 2 wedges

Recipe Cost: $7.70

GF
LC
VG

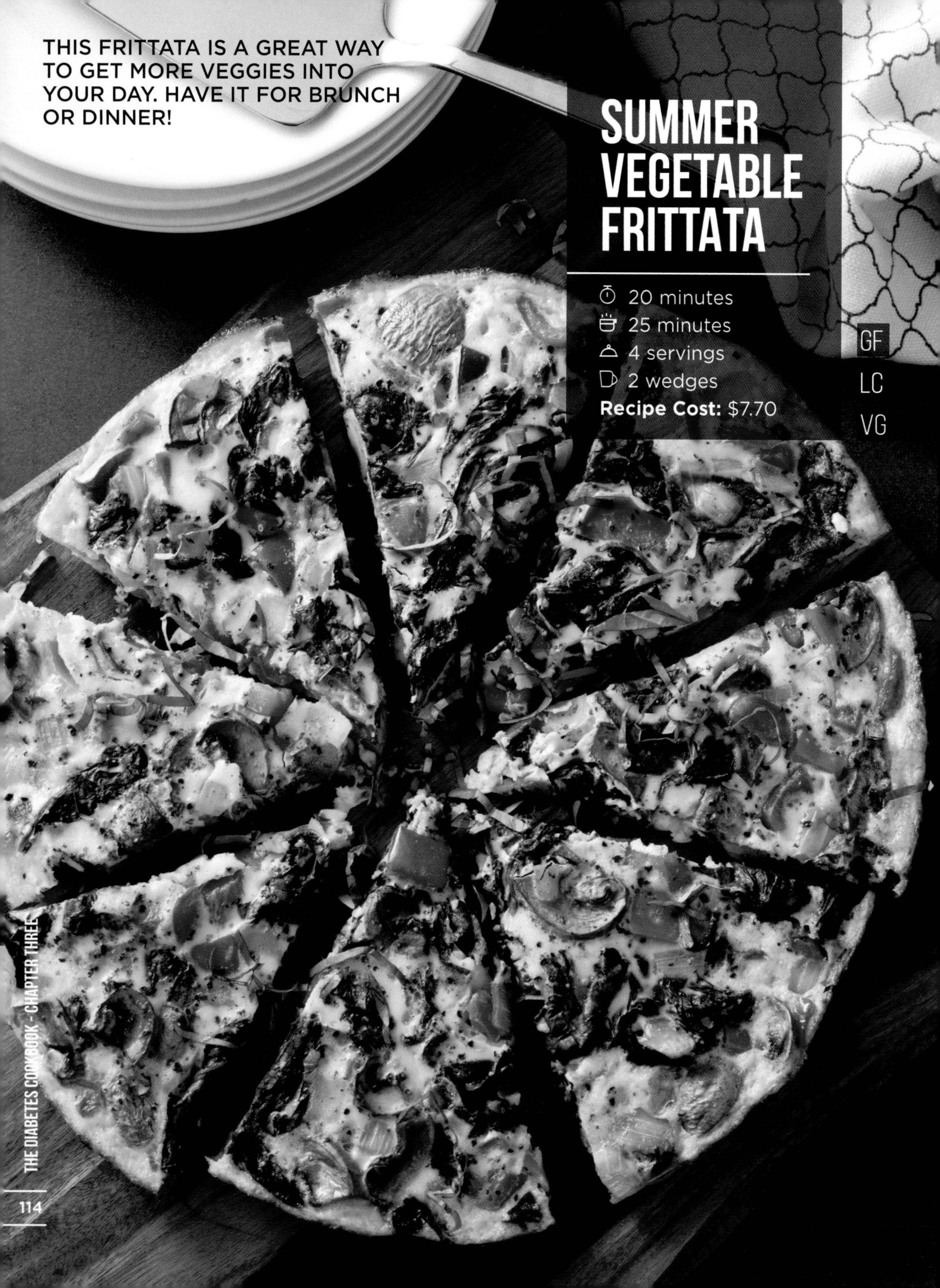

1	tablespoon olive oil
8	ounces mushrooms, diced
1	medium red bell pepper, seeded and diced
1	small onion, diced
3	cups fresh spinach
2	eggs
5	egg whites
1/4	cup skim milk
1/2	teaspoon salt
1/2	teaspoon ground black pepper
1/4	teaspoon cayenne pepper
1	tablespoon chopped fresh basil

1. Preheat oven to 350°F.

2. Add olive oil to an oven-safe, nonstick sauté pan and place over medium high heat.

3. Add mushrooms and sauté until all the liquid from the mushrooms is evaporated.

4. Add bell pepper, onion, and spinach and sauté until vegetables are softened and liquid is evaporated.

5. Whisk eggs, egg whites, milk, salt, pepper, cayenne pepper, and basil in a medium bowl. Pour over vegetables and stir until eggs start to set.

6. Smooth the top of the frittata with a spatula, and put in oven to bake 20 minutes or until eggs are set.

7. Slide the frittata out of the pan onto a plate and slice into 8 pie wedges.

CHEF TIP: *Serve this frittata with a green salad with light balsamic vinaigrette.*

Nutrition Facts

Serves: 4
Serving Size: 2 wedges

Amount per serving
Calories 130

Calories from fat 50	
Total fat 6.0 g	
Saturated fat 1.3 g	
Trans fat 0.0 g	
Cholesterol 95 mg	
Sodium 420 mg	
Potassium 550 mg	
Total carbohydrate 9 g	
Dietary fiber 2 g	
Sugars 5 g	
Protein 11 g	
Phosphorus 150 mg	

Choices/Exchanges: 2 Nonstarchy Vegetable, 1 Lean Protein, 1 Fat

MISO GLAZED COD

○ 15 minutes
🍲 5 minutes
△ 4 servings
▭ 1 fish fillet and
   3/4 cup stir-fry
Recipe Cost: $10.50

LC

BROILING THE FISH FILLETS AND STIR-FRYING THE VEGETABLES MAKE THIS SAVORY 20-MINUTE MEAL COME TOGETHER IN A FLASH. SERVE WITH BROWN RICE OR ANOTHER WHOLE GRAIN IF DESIRED.

Nonstick cooking spray
1 pound white fish, such as cod, sea bass, or orange roughy
1 tablespoon toasted sesame oil, divided
1 tablespoon powdered instant miso soup mix (powder only)
1/4 teaspoon ground black pepper
4 cups shredded napa cabbage
2 cloves garlic, grated or minced
2 cups snow peas, sliced
1 tablespoon Asian-style hot sauce (sambal oelek)

1. Place a rack in the middle of the oven. Preheat oven to broil. Coat a baking sheet with cooking spray.
2. Cut the fish into 4 (4-ounce) portions and arrange on the prepared baking sheet.
3. In a small bowl, mix together 1 1/2 teaspoons of sesame oil, the miso soup mix powder, and black pepper to form a paste. Brush the top of each of fish fillet with the glaze (coating will be very thin). Spray each fillet with cooking spray and place baking sheet on middle rack of the oven. Broil 6 minutes.
4. While the fish is broiling, add the remaining 1 1/2 teaspoons sesame oil and more cooking spray to a wok or large sauté pan over high heat. Stir-fry the cabbage, garlic, snow peas, and hot sauce 4 minutes, until just wilted but still slightly crunchy.
5. Remove fish from baking sheet and serve on top of 3/4 cup of the stir-fried vegetables.

CHEF TIP: *Have leftover napa cabbage? It's sweeter and more tender than regular green cabbage. Enjoy it raw and shredded in a salad or on a burger or sandwich.*

Nutrition Facts

Serves: 4
**Serving Size: 1 fish fillet and
3/4 cup stir-fry**

Amount per serving
Calories 170

Calories from fat 40	
Total fat 4.5 g	
Saturated fat 0.7 g	
Trans fat 0.0 g	
Cholesterol 50 mg	
Sodium 230 mg	
Potassium 510 mg	
Total carbohydrate 8 g	
Dietary fiber 2 g	
Sugars 4 g	
Protein 24 g	
Phosphorus 175 mg	

Choices/Exchanges: 2 Nonstarchy Vegetable, 3 Lean Protein

GRILLED FLANK STEAK QUESADILLA

SERVE THIS QUESADILLA WITH A SIDE SALAD LIGHTLY TOSSED WITH A LOW-FAT CILANTRO VINAIGRETTE.

⏱ 35 minutes
🍲 10 minutes
🍽 4 servings
🍴 1 quesadilla

Recipe Cost: $10.10

Juice and zest of 4 limes (about 1/2 cup lime juice, 2 tablespoons lime zest)
2   tablespoons chopped fresh cilantro
2   cloves garlic, minced
1/2 pound flank steak
1/2 teaspoon ground black pepper
1   large red bell pepper, seeded and sliced
Nonstick cooking spray
1/2 cup shredded reduced-fat mozzarella cheese
8   (6-inch) low-carb high-fiber whole-wheat tortillas

1. Prepare an indoor or outdoor grill.
2. Combine lime zest, lime juice, cilantro, garlic, and flank steak in a resealable plastic bag or bowl. Let marinate in the refrigerator 30 minutes.
3. Remove steak from marinade and discard remaining marinade. Season steak with pepper on both sides and grill over medium-high heat 5–7 minutes on each side. Set aside to rest.
4. While steak is grilling, coat the red bell pepper slices with cooking spray and grill on each side 4–5 minutes. When done grilling, dice the pepper and set aside.
5. After meat has finished resting, thinly slice the meat against the grain, then chop to mince the meat. Stir the minced meat and peppers together.
6. Add the cheese to the meat mixture and stir to incorporate.
7. Heat a nonstick pan over medium heat. Spray with cooking spray and place one tortilla in the pan.

Top with 1/4 of the meat mixture and then place another tortilla on top of that.
8. Sauté the quesadilla 2 minutes on each side.
9. Repeat the process for the remaining 3 quesadillas.

Nutrition Facts

Serves: 4
Serving Size: 1 quesadilla

Amount per serving	
Calories	**200**

Calories from fat 70	
Total fat 8.0 g	
Saturated fat 2.5 g	
Trans fat 0.0 g	
Cholesterol 40 mg	
Sodium 460 mg	
Potassium 290 mg	
Total carbohydrate 22 g	
Dietary fiber 13 g	
Sugars 2 g	
Protein 23 g	
Phosphorus 225 mg	

Choices/Exchanges: 1 Starch, 1 Nonstarchy Vegetable, 2 Lean Protein, 1/2 Fat

PARMESAN LEMON CRUSTED FLOUNDER WITH GREEN BEANS AMANDINE

⏱ 10 minutes

🍳 20 minutes

△ 4 servings

🍽 1 piece fish and 1 cup green beans

Recipe Cost: $10.15

FEEL FREE TO SUBSTITUTE ANY WHITE FISH FOR THE FLOUNDER IN THIS RECIPE.

Nonstick cooking spray

8 cups water

1/2 cup panko bread crumbs

Zest and juice of 1 lemon (juice divided)

1/4 cup grated parmesan cheese

2 teaspoons olive oil

3 cloves garlic, minced or grated, divided

4 (4-ounce) frozen flounder fillets (do not thaw)

1 egg white

1 pound fresh green beans, trimmed and cut in half

1 tablespoon trans fat–free margarine

1/4 cup slivered almonds

1. Preheat oven to 375°F. Coat a baking sheet with cooking spray and set it aside. Add 8 cups of water to a large soup pot over high heat and bring to a boil.

2. In a small bowl, combine the panko bread crumbs, lemon zest, grated parmesan cheese, olive oil, and half of the garlic. Mix until the panko is coated with the olive oil.

3. Lay the fish fillets on the prepared baking sheet and brush the top of each fillet with egg whites. Coat the top of each fillet with 2 tablespoons of panko mixture and press it into the fish. Drizzle with 2 tablespoons lemon juice. Spray the top of each fish with cooking spray.

4. Bake 20 minutes.

5. While the fish is baking, par-cook (blanch) the green beans 2 minutes. Drain and set aside.

6. Add the margarine to a nonstick sauté pan over medium heat. Add reamaining garlic, almonds, and green beans and sauté 4–5 minutes.

7. Drizzle with remaining 2 tablespoons lemon juice and sauté 2 more minutes.

8. Serve 1 fish fillet with 1 cup green beans.

Nutrition Facts

Serves: 4

Serving Size: 1 piece fish and 1 cup green beans

Amount per serving

Calories 290

Calories from fat 110	
Total fat 12.0 g	
Saturated fat 2.5 g	
Trans fat 0.0 g	
Cholesterol 65 mg	
Sodium 210 mg	
Potassium 560 mg	
Total carbohydrate 18 g	
Dietary fiber 4 g	
Sugars 3 g	
Protein 28 g	
Phosphorus 370 mg	

Choices/Exchanges: 1/2 Starch, 2 Nonstarchy Vegetable, 3 Lean Protein, 1 Fat

PASTITSIO (GREEK LASAGNA)

- ⏱ 30 minutes
- 🍲 60 minutes
- 🍽 12 servings
- ▯ 1 slice

Recipe Cost: $9.90

THIS VERSION OF PASTITSIO IS A GREAT FAMILY MEAL THAT PAIRS WELL WITH A GREEN SALAD TOPPED WITH A LITTLE FETA CHEESE AND LIGHT GREEK SALAD DRESSING.

Nonstick cooking spray
1 medium onion, diced
20 ounces lean ground turkey
2 1/2 teaspoons ground cinnamon
1 teaspoon ground oregano
1/2 teaspoon salt
1/2 teaspoon ground black pepper
2 (15-ounce) cans low-sodium tomato sauce
1 tablespoon chopped fresh parsley
16 ounces brown rice or quinoa penne pasta (or whole-wheat penne pasta)
1 tablespoon olive oil
2 tablespoons whole-wheat flour
2 cups skim milk
1/8 teaspoon ground nutmeg
1/3 cup freshly grated parmesan cheese
1 egg

1. Preheat oven to 350°F. Coat a 9-by-13-inch baking pan with cooking spray. Set aside.

2. Spray a large nonstick sauté pan with cooking spray. Sauté onion 4–5 minutes or until translucent. Add ground turkey and sauté 8–10 minutes, or until turkey is cooked through.
3. Add cinnamon, oregano, salt, pepper, and tomato sauce. Stir to combine and bring to a simmer 5–7 minutes or until it starts to thicken.
4. Stir in parsley and set aside.
5. Cook pasta according to directions on the package, omitting salt. Drain and immediately add to turkey mixture. Pour the pasta and turkey mixture into the baking pan and press down so it is evenly spread in the pan.
6. Add the olive oil to a small saucepan over medium heat. Stir in flour and cook 1–2 minutes, taking care not to brown it. Stir constantly.
7. Slowly whisk in the skim milk and bring to a boil, whisking constantly. Whisk in the nutmeg and parmesan cheese.
8. In a small bowl, whisk the egg and then slowly whisk in the hot milk mixture to temper the egg. Add the rest of the milk mixture to the egg and then pour over the top of the pasta, spreading to coat it completely.
9. Bake on the middle rack of the oven 30 minutes or until bubbly and top is golden brown.

Nutrition Facts

Serves: 12
Serving Size: 1 slice

Amount per serving

Calories 280

Calories from fat 60

Total fat 7.0 g	
Saturated fat 1.9 g	
Trans fat 0.1 g	
Cholesterol 55 mg	
Sodium 190 mg	
Potassium 530 mg	
Total carbohydrate 37 g	
Dietary fiber 4 g	
Sugars 6 g	
Protein 16 g	
Phosphorus 310 mg	

Choices/Exchanges: 2 Starch, 1 Nonstarchy Vegetable, 2 Lean Protein, 1/2 Fat

KALE AND SAUSAGE SAUTÉ

ENJOY THIS SIMPLE DISH OF GREENS, BEANS, AND CHICKEN SAUSAGE. IT CAN BE PREPARED IN JUST 10 MINUTES!

- 10 minutes
- 15 minutes
- 6 servings
- 1 cup

Recipe Cost: $9.90

1 tablespoon olive oil
3 links Italian-style chicken sausage (about 3 ounces each), diced
1 onion, diced
1 (10-ounce) bag chopped kale
1/2 cup fat-free low-sodium chicken broth
1 (15.5-ounce) can cannellini (white kidney) beans, drained and rinsed
1/4 teaspoon crushed red pepper flakes
1/4 teaspoon salt
1/2 teaspoon ground black pepper

1. Heat olive oil in a large sauté pan over medium heat.
2. Add diced sausage and onion and sauté until onion begins to turn golden brown.
3. Add the kale and chicken broth and sauté until kale softens.
4. Add remaining ingredients and sauté 3-4 more minutes until beans are heated through.

SERVING SUGGESTION: *You can try serving this dish over cauliflower rice for a double veggie meal. Cauliflower rice can be found in the freezer section of your local grocery store.*

It's a great low-carb substitute for regular rice.

Nutrition Facts

Serves: 6
Serving Size: 1 cup

Amount per serving	
Calories	**170**
Calories from fat 50	
Total fat 6.0 g	
Saturated fat 1.4 g	
Trans fat 0.0 g	
Cholesterol 35 mg	
Sodium 410 mg	
Potassium 560 mg	
Total carbohydrate 17 g	
Dietary fiber 5 g	
Sugars 2 g	
Protein 14 g	
Phosphorus 195 mg	

Choices/Exchanges: 1/2 Starch, 1 Nonstarchy Vegetable, 2 Lean Protein, 1/2 Fat

STUFFED PEPPERS

⏱ 20 minutes
🍲 1 1/4 hours
🍽 6 servings
🍴 1 stuffed pepper
Recipe Cost: $7.60

GF

MAKE THIS DISH THE NIGHT BEFORE AND KEEP IT IN THE REFRIGERATOR. JUST HEAT THE PEPPERS IN THE OVEN OR IN THE MICROWAVE FOR DINNER IN NO TIME.

1	cup red or brown lentils
2	cups water
1	tablespoon grated ginger
2	cloves garlic, minced
1	teaspoon turmeric
1	pound lean ground chicken
1	tablespoon chopped fresh cilantro
1/2	teaspoon salt
1/2	teaspoon ground black pepper
1/4	teaspoon cayenne pepper
6	small bell peppers (any color or assorted colors)
1/2	cup fat-free, gluten-free, low-sodium chicken broth

1. Preheat oven to 350°F.
2. Add lentils, water, ginger, garlic, and turmeric to a medium saucepan. Bring to a boil; then reduce to a simmer. Simmer partially covered 20 minutes. Set aside to cool.
3. While lentils are cooking, mix ground chicken, cilantro, salt, black pepper, and cayenne pepper in a medium bowl and set aside.

4. Cut the tops off the bell peppers and cut out the seed pods. Save the tops and set them aside. Clean out the inside of the peppers, removing the ribs and seeds, and set the peppers cut side up in a baking dish. (Note: If the peppers won't sit upright, trim a little bit off the bottom of the peppers to even them out so they will sit up straight. Be careful not to cut a hole in the bottom so the mixture inside does not fall out.)
5. Once the lentils have cooled, stir them into the chicken mixture and mix well.
6. Fill each pepper with the chicken and lentil mixture, but do not pack the mixture in tightly. Just gently fill to the top.
7. Once filled, place the tops on back on the peppers, then pour the chicken broth into the bottom of the pan.
8. Bake 1 hour or until the internal temperature of the chicken mixture is 165°F.

CHEF TIP: *Serve with a steamer bag of broccoli florets. Adding a vegetable side increases the cost of this meal to $9.95—still less than $10 for 6 servings!*

Nutrition Facts

Serves: 6
Serving Size: 1 stuffed pepper

Amount per serving
Calories   **230**

Calories from fat 40

Total fat 4.5 g

   Saturated fat 1.5 g

   Trans fat 0.0 g

Cholesterol 55 mg

Sodium 290 mg

Potassium 930 mg

Total carbohydrate 23 g

   Dietary fiber 9 g

   Sugars 4 g

Protein 25 g

Phosphorus 325 mg

Choices/Exchanges: 1 Starch, 1 Nonstarchy Vegetable, 3 Lean Protein

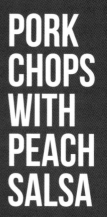

PORK CHOPS WITH PEACH SALSA

- ⏱ 20 minutes
- 🍳 8 minutes
- 🍽 4 servings
- 🍴 1 pork chop and 1/4 cup salsa

Recipe Cost: $9.05

GF
LC

TAKE ADVANTAGE OF SEASONAL PRODUCE BY PAIRING A MOUTHWATERING SALSA WITH PORK CHOPS, OR EVEN CHICKEN.

PORK CHOPS

1	pound (4 pork chops) boneless pork loin chops
1/4	teaspoon ground black pepper
1/2	teaspoon garlic powder
1	teaspoon dried oregano

PEACH SALSA

2	peaches, peeled, pitted, and diced
1/2	green bell pepper, finely diced
1/3	cup finely diced red onion
1	tablespoon rice wine vinegar
1	teaspoon olive oil
1	teaspoon chopped fresh cilantro
1	packet sugar substitute

1. Prepare an indoor or outdoor grill. Season pork chops with pepper, garlic powder, and oregano. Grill pork chops over medium heat 3–4 minutes per side or until done.
2. In a small bowl, mix together salsa ingredients.
3. Top each cooked pork chop with about 1/4 cup salsa mixture and serve.

Nutrition Facts

Serves: 4
Serving Size: 1 pork chop and 1/4 cup salsa

Amount per serving
Calories **210**

Calories from fat 80	
Total fat 9.0 g	
Saturated fat 2.7 g	
Trans fat 0.0 g	
Cholesterol 60 mg	
Sodium 50 mg	
Potassium 510 mg	
Total carbohydrate 10 g	
Dietary fiber 2 g	
Sugars 8 g	
Protein 22 g	
Phosphorus 200 mg	

Choices/Exchanges: 1/2 Fruit, 3 Lean Protein, 1/2 Fat

ASIAN PORK CHOPS

- ⏱ 25 minutes
- 🍲 17 minutes
- 🍽 4 servings
- 🍴 1 pork chop and 1/2 cup broccoli
- **Recipe Cost:** $10.00

LC

REGULAR SOY SAUCE CONTAINS WHEAT AND GLUTEN, SO IF YOU NEED TO FOLLOW A GLUTEN-FREE DIET, MAKE SURE YOU PURCHASE GLUTEN-FREE SOY SAUCE.

VEGETABLE SIDE

2	cups broccoli florets

MARINADE

2	tablespoons plus 1 teaspoon reduced-sodium soy sauce
3	tablespoons rice wine vinegar
2	tablespoons water
1	tablespoon olive oil
1/4	teaspoon crushed red pepper
1	clove garlic, minced

PORK

4	pork loin boneless chops (each 1/2 inch thick, about 1 pound total)
2	teaspoons olive oil
2	tablespoons chopped fresh cilantro

1. Steam the broccoli 5 minutes, until tender.
2. In a medium bowl, combine the marinade ingredients. Add the pork chops and marinate in the refrigerator 20 minutes or longer.

3. Add 2 teaspoons olive oil to a large sauté pan over medium-high heat.
4. Sauté the pork chops about 5 minutes per side or until done. (Reserve marinade for later.)
5. Place the marinade in a small saucepan. Bring it to a boil, reduce heat, and simmer about 2 minutes. Place the pork chops on a serving platter and pour the cooked marinade over them.
6. Top the pork chops with chopped cilantro and serve with the steamed broccoli.

CHEF TIP: *For an affordable starchy side, add 1/3 cup cooked brown rice to your pork chops and broccoli.*

MAKE IT GLUTEN-FREE: *Confirm that all ingredients are gluten-free.*

Nutrition Facts

Serves: 4
Serving Size: 1 pork chop and 1/2 cup broccoli

Amount per serving	
Calories	**230**

Calories from fat 120	
Total fat 13.0 g	
Saturated fat 3.4 g	
Trans fat 0.0 g	
Cholesterol 60 mg	
Sodium 390 mg	
Potassium 470 mg	
Total carbohydrate 5 g	
Dietary fiber 2 g	
Sugars 1 g	
Protein 23 g	
Phosphorus 220 mg	

Choices/Exchanges: 1 Nonstarchy Vegetable, 3 Lean Protein, 1 1/2 Fat

SALMON BURGERS

- 🕐 15 minutes
- 🍽 15 minutes
- 🍲 6 servings
- 🍔 1 burger

Recipe Cost: $10.30

LC

THESE BURGERS ARE A GOOD WAY TO SPICE UP YOUR MENU! THEY ARE PACKED WITH HEART-HEALTHY SALMON, PLUS SOME VEGGIES. TO KEEP THE CARBOHYDRATE COUNT LOW, THESE ARE SERVED OVER BIBB LETTUCE INSTEAD OF ON A BUN.

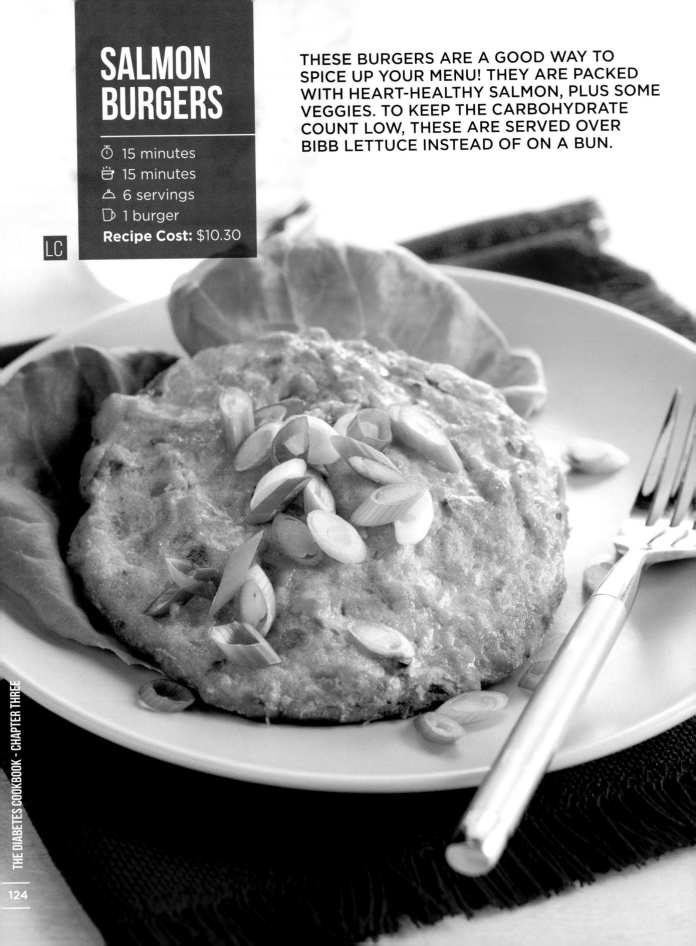

Nonstick cooking spray
1/2 small onion, chopped
1 clove garlic, chopped
1 red bell pepper, seeded and chopped
1 tablespoon Thai red curry paste
1 pound skinless salmon, cut into chunks
1 egg
1/4 cup fresh cilantro
6 iceberg or bibb lettuce leaves
2 scallions, thinly sliced

1. Preheat oven to 475°F. Coat a baking sheet with cooking spray and set aside.
2. Place the onion, garlic, bell pepper, and Thai curry paste in a large food processor and blend until smooth.
3. Add the salmon and purée until smooth. Add the egg and cilantro and purée until incorporated.
4. Scoop the mixture in 1/2-cup portions onto the baking sheet, and press lightly to form a patty. Repeat to make 6 patties.
5. Spray the top of each patty with cooking spray and bake 15 minutes.
6. Serve each salmon burger on a lettuce leaf, and top each with 1 tablespoon sliced scallions.

CHEF TIP: *Serve these burgers with a green salad that has been drizzled with a light sesame ginger vinaigrette.*

Nutrition Facts

Serves: 6
Serving Size: 1 burger

Amount per serving
Calories 150

Calories from fat 60

Total fat 7.0 g

Saturated fat 1.5 g

Trans fat 0.0 g

Cholesterol 70 mg

Sodium 160 mg

Potassium 390 mg

Total carbohydrate 4 g

Dietary fiber 1 g

Sugars 2 g

Protein 17 g

Phosphorus 225 mg

Choices/Exchanges: 1 Nonstarchy Vegetable, 2 Lean Protein, 1/2 Fat

GRILLED SHRIMP TACOS

⏱ 15 minutes
🍲 10 minutes
🍽 4 servings
🌮 1 taco
Recipe Cost: $9.30

HERE'S A LIGHT AND TASTY SUMMER TACO RECIPE THAT'S GREAT FOR A FAMILY DINNER OR THE NEXT TIME YOU HAVE GUESTS.

YOGURT SAUCE

1/4	cup fat-free plain Greek yogurt
2	tablespoons light mayonnaise
1/2	teaspoon chili powder

SHRIMP TACO

12	ounces peeled and deveined shrimp
4	long bamboo skewers, soaked in warm water
4	(6-inch) high-fiber tortillas
1	cup shredded lettuce
1/2	cup salsa verde

MARINADE

1	tablespoon olive oil
2	cloves garlic, minced or grated
	Juice of 1 lime
1/4	teaspoon ground black pepper

1. Preheat an indoor or outdoor grill.
2. In a small bowl, whisk together the yogurt, mayonnaise, and chili powder. Cover and keep in the refrigerator until needed.
3. Skewer 3 ounces of shrimp on each skewer.
4. In a small bowl, whisk together olive oil, garlic, lime juice, and pepper. Brush the shrimp with the marinade and grill 3–4 minutes on each side until the shrimp are pink and just firm. Continue to brush with the marinade while grilling, using all the marinade.
5. Heat the tortillas briefly on the grill. Remove the shrimp from one skewer and place in a tortilla. Top the shrimp with 1/4 cup shredded lettuce, a heaping tablespoon of the reserved yogurt sauce, and 2 tablespoons of salsa verde. Repeat for the remaining three tacos.

CHEF TIP: *Serve this dish with a green salad tossed with cilantro lime vinaigrette.*

Nutrition Facts

Serves: 4
Serving Size: 1 taco

Amount per serving

Calories 210

Calories from fat 50

Total fat 6.0 g	
Saturated fat 0.8 g	
Trans fat 0.0 g	
Cholesterol 145 mg	
Sodium 340 mg	
Potassium 380 mg	
Total carbohydrate 17 g	
Dietary fiber 2 g	
Sugars 2 g	
Protein 22 g	
Phosphorus 300 mg	

Choices/Exchanges: 1 Starch, 3 Lean Protein

GRILLED STEAK SALAD

- ⏱ 15 minutes
- ⏲ 12 minutes
- 🍽 4 servings
- 🍴 2 ounces steak, 2 cups salad, and 3 1/2 tablespoons dressing
- **Recipe Cost:** $10.30

LC

SERVE THIS SALAD WITH STEAMED BROCCOLI AND CAULIFLOWER FOR A REAL SUMMER TREAT!

STEAK SALAD

9	ounces sirloin steak
1/2	teaspoon salt-free all-purpose seasoning (such as Spike or Mrs. Dash)
8	cups mesclun salad mix
1/4	red onion, thinly sliced
1	cup cherry tomatoes, sliced in half lengthwise

DRESSING FOR GRILLED STEAK SALAD

1/4	cup light mayonnaise
1/4	cup fat-free plain Greek yogurt
1/4	cup low-fat buttermilk
1	clove garlic, pressed or grated
2	tablespoons crumbled blue cheese
1/4	teaspoon ground black pepper

1. Heat an indoor or outdoor grill. Season both sides of the steak with the salt-free seasoning.
2. Grill the steak 5–6 minutes per side or until cooked to medium well (145°F internal temperature). Cover loosely with foil, and set aside to rest.
3. In a large bowl, toss together salad mix, red onion, and cherry tomatoes. Divide evenly among 4 large plates.
4. Thinly slice steak and top each salad with 2 ounces of steak.

5. In a small bowl, whisk together the mayonnaise, Greek yogurt, buttermilk, garlic, blue cheese, and pepper.
6. Top the steak with 3 1/2 tablespoons of salad dressing.

Nutrition Facts

Serves: 4

Serving Size: 2 ounces steak, 2 cups salad, and 3 1/2 tablespoons dressing

Amount per serving

Calories 170

Calories from fat 60	
Total fat 7.0 g	
Saturated fat 2.1 g	
Trans fat 0.1 g	
Cholesterol 30 mg	
Sodium 260 mg	
Potassium 510 mg	
Total carbohydrate 8 g	
Dietary fiber 1 g	
Sugars 4 g	
Protein 17 g	
Phosphorus 185 mg	

Choices/Exchanges: 1 Nonstarchy Vegetable, 2 Lean Protein, 1 Fat

YOGURT CURRY MARINATED TILAPIA

⏱ 10 minutes
🍲 30 minutes
🍽 4 servings
🍴 1 fillet

GF

Recipe Cost: $7.65

HERE'S AN EASY, BUDGET-FRIENDLY MEAL TO TRY FOR DINNER THIS WEEK. IT'S SIMPLE TO MAKE AND FULL OF SWEET AND SPICY FLAVOR.

Nonstick cooking spray
4 (4-ounce) tilapia fillets
1 medium onion, halved and thinly sliced
1 medium yellow or orange bell pepper, seeded and thinly sliced
1 cup fat-free plain Greek yogurt
1 cup unsweetened coconut milk beverage
2 tablespoons sweet curry powder
1/2 teaspoon cayenne pepper
1 teaspoon paprika
1 teaspoon garlic powder
1/2 teaspoon salt
1/4 teaspoon ground black pepper

1. Preheat oven to 375°F. Coat an 8-by-11-inch baking pan with nonstick cooking spray.
2. Lay the 4 tilapia fillets side by side in the pan.
3. Top the fillets with the sliced onion and bell pepper.
4. In a medium bowl, whisk together all the remaining ingredients and pour over the fish and vegetables.
5. Bake 30 minutes. Let the fish rest 15 minutes before serving. Vegetables should be slightly crisp and fish should be cooked through but tender.

CHEF TIP: *Serve this dish over cooked brown rice. You could also add a side of steamed broccoli.*

Nutrition Facts

Serves: 4
Serving Size: 1 fillet

Amount per serving

Calories 190

Calories from fat 40

Total fat 4.5 g

Saturated fat 2.2 g

Trans fat 0.0 g

Cholesterol 50 mg

Sodium 370 mg

Potassium 630 mg

Total carbohydrate 11 g

Dietary fiber 2 g

Sugars 5 g

Protein 30 g

Phosphorus 290 mg

Choices/Exchanges: 2 Nonstarchy Vegetable, 3 Lean Protein

SLOPPY JANES

⏱ 10 minutes
🍲 20 minutes
🍽 8 servings
🥄 1 sandwich

Recipe Cost: $9.75

SLOPPY JOES GET A MAKEOVER WITH LEAN GROUND TURKEY INSTEAD OF BEEF, PLUS PLENTY OF ZING FROM GARLIC, ONION, PEPPER, TOMATOES, AND HOT SAUCE.

Nonstick cooking spray
1 medium onion, diced
1 medium red bell pepper, seeded and diced
1 clove garlic, minced
1 pound lean ground turkey
1 tablespoon tomato paste
2 tablespoons Dijon mustard
1 tablespoon hot sauce
2 cups no-salt-added canned crushed tomatoes
1 tablespoon honey or 2 packets artificial sweetener
1/2 teaspoon ground black pepper
8 whole-wheat hamburger buns

1. Spray a nonstick sauté pan with nonstick cooking spray and place over medium-high heat.
2. Add onion, red bell pepper, and garlic. Sauté 5 minutes, stirring frequently.
3. Add turkey and sauté 5–7 minutes, stirring frequently until turkey is just cooked through.
4. Add tomato paste, mustard, hot sauce, tomatoes, honey, and black pepper. Bring to a simmer 5 minutes, stirring frequently.
5. Toast the hamburger buns. Fill each bun with 1/2 cup turkey mixture to make 8 sandwiches.

CHEF TIP: *This recipe freezes well. Portion into freezer-safe containers and freeze up to 6 months.*

Nutrition Facts

Serves: 8
Serving Size: 1 sandwich

Amount per serving

Calories 250

Calories from fat 60	
Total fat 7.0 g	
Saturated fat 1.6 g	
Trans fat 0.1 g	
Cholesterol 45 mg	
Sodium 390 mg	
Potassium 510 mg	
Total carbohydrate 31 g	
Dietary fiber 5 g	
Sugars 10 g	
Protein 16 g	
Phosphorus 240 mg	

Choices/Exchanges: 1 1/2 Starch, 1 Nonstarchy Vegetable, 2 Lean Protein, 1/2 Fat

ROASTED TURKEY AND VEGETABLES

SERVE THIS DISH WITH ROASTED SWEET POTATOES. IT'S A GREAT OPTION FOR THE HOLIDAYS IF YOU DON'T WANT TO COOK THE ENTIRE BIRD!

- ⏱ 15 minutes
- 🍲 60 minutes
- 🍽 6 servings
- 🥄 4 ounces turkey and 1/2 cup vegetables

Recipe Cost: $11.85

LC

Nonstick cooking spray
2   stalks celery, chopped
3   small or 2 medium carrots, peeled and chopped
1   onion, chopped
1/2   head cabbage, chopped
5   sprigs fresh thyme
1   cup fat-free low-sodium chicken broth
2 1/2   pounds bone-in turkey breast half
1   teaspoon olive oil
1   tablespoon salt-free all-purpose seasoning (such as Spike or Mrs. Dash)
1/2   teaspoon ground black pepper

1. Preheat oven to 375°F. Coat a baking dish with nonstick cooking spray.
2. Toss all the vegetables and thyme together in a bowl and place in the bottom of the baking dish. Pour the chicken broth over the vegetables.
3. Remove the skin from the turkey breast. Place it breast side up on top of the vegetables. Drizzle the turkey and vegetables with the olive oil and sprinkle them with seasoning and ground black pepper.
4. Roast the turkey and vegetables in the oven 1 hour or until the internal temperature of the turkey is 165°F.

5. When the dish comes out of the oven, set the turkey aside on a cutting board to rest. Remove the thyme stems and stir the vegetables.
6. Slice the turkey and serve with the vegetables.

Nutrition Facts

Serves: 6

Serving Size: 4 ounces turkey and 1/2 cup vegetables

Amount per serving

Calories   **210**

Calories from fat 25

Total fat 3.0 g

   Saturated fat 0.8 g

   Trans fat 0.0 g

Cholesterol 90 mg

Sodium 170 mg

Potassium 610 mg

Total carbohydrate 10 g

   Dietary fiber 3 g

   Sugars 5 g

Protein 35 g

Phosphorus 305 mg

Choices/Exchanges: 2 Nonstarchy Vegetable, 4 Lean Protein

HERB GARLIC MEAT LOAF

⏱ 10 minutes
🍲 35 minutes
🍽 6 servings
🍴 1 slice

Recipe Cost: $8.15

THIS SAVORY, BUDGET-FRIENDLY MEAT LOAF IS JUST AS GOOD AS CLASSIC MEAT LOAF. OUR DIABETES-FRIENDLY VERSION IS MADE WITH LEAN GROUND TURKEY AND IS SEASONED WITH FRESH HERBS AND GARLIC.

Nonstick cooking spray
1   slice whole-wheat bread
1/4   cup egg substitute
20   ounces lean ground turkey
2   cloves garlic, minced
1   tablespoon chopped fresh oregano
1   tablespoon chopped fresh basil
1/2   cup ketchup, divided
1/4   teaspoon salt
1/2   teaspoon ground black pepper
2   tablespoons balsamic vinegar

1. Preheat oven to 375°F. Coat a loaf pan with cooking spray. Set aside.
2. In a medium bowl, tear the slice of bread into pea-size pieces. Add egg substitute and mix well.
3. Add turkey, garlic, oregano, basil, 1/4 cup ketchup, salt, and pepper. Mix well.
4. Press the turkey mixture into the loaf pan tightly, and bake 20 minutes.
5. While meat loaf is baking, whisk together balsamic vinegar, 1 tablespoon hot sauce (optional), and remaining 1/4 cup ketchup.
6. After the meat loaf has baked 20 minutes, pour the ketchup and balsamic glaze over the meat loaf. Return the meat loaf to the oven and bake an additional 15 minutes or until the internal temperature of the meat loaf is 165°F.

7. Let the meat loaf rest 10 minutes before slicing.

CHEF TIP: *Serve with oven-roasted sweet potatoes.*

Nutrition Facts

Serves: 6
Serving Size: 1 slice

Amount per serving

Calories 190

Calories from fat 60

Total fat 7.0 g

Saturated fat 2.1 g

Trans fat 0.1 g

Cholesterol 75 mg

Sodium 430 mg

Potassium 330 mg

Total carbohydrate 9 g

Dietary fiber 0 g

Sugars 6 g

Protein 20 g

Phosphorus 205 mg

Choices/Exchanges:
1/2 Carbohydrate, 3 Lean Protein, 1/2 Fat

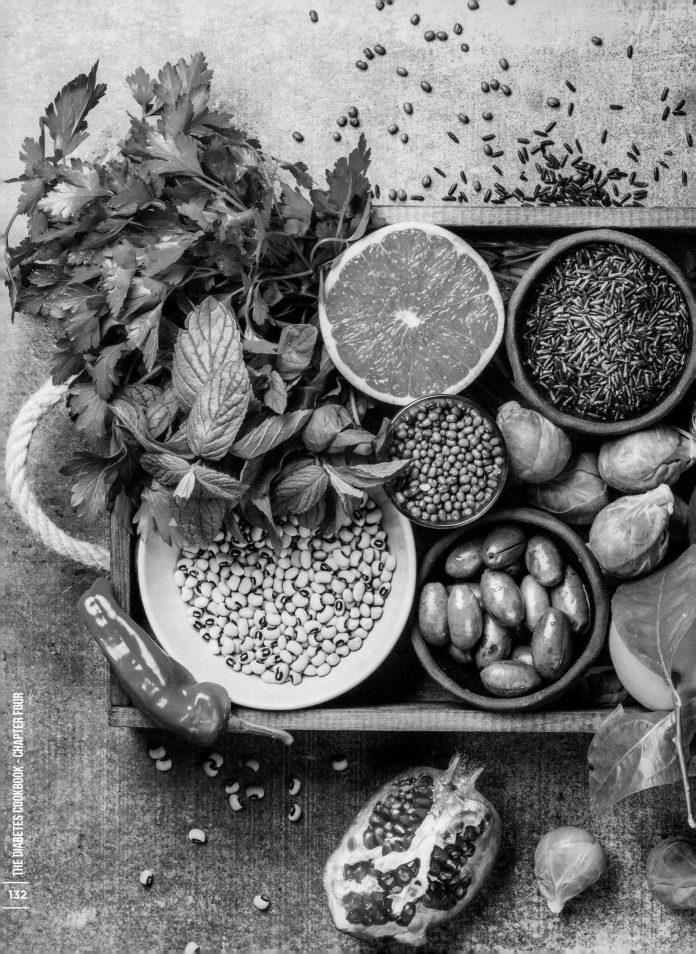

CHAPTER FOUR
SLOW-COOKER RECIPES

THERE IS NOTHING BETTER THAN COMING HOME TO A HEALTHY, HOME-COOKED MEAL AFTER A LONG DAY. THESE SLOW-COOKER MEALS WILL BECOME SOME OF YOUR FAVORITES!

SLOW-COOKER CHICKEN TACO SOUP

SERVE THIS SOUP WITH SOME BAKED TORTILLA CHIPS AND GUACAMOLE.

- 10 minutes
- 6–8 hours
- 8 servings
- 1 1/4 cups

2	pounds (3 large) boneless skinless chicken breasts
1	tablespoon chili powder
2	tablespoons dried parsley
2	teaspoons cumin
1/4	teaspoon cayenne pepper
1/4	teaspoon salt
1/2	teaspoon ground black pepper
1	onion, chopped
1	red bell pepper, seeded and chopped
1	(14.5-ounce) can no-salt-added diced tomatoes
1	(10-ounce) can diced tomatoes with green chilies
1	(15.5-ounce) can black beans, drained and rinsed
1	(8-ounce) can tomato sauce
2	cups fat-free low-sodium chicken broth

1. Place the chicken breasts in the slow cooker. Add the remaining ingredients, stir to incorporate, and cook on high 6 hours (or on low 8 hours).
2. Before serving, shred the chicken meat using two forks.

Nutrition Facts

Serves: 8
Serving Size: 1 1/4 cups

Amount per serving
Calories 210

Calories from fat 20	
Total fat 2.0 g	
Saturated fat 0.5 g	
Trans fat 0.0 g	
Cholesterol 65 mg	
Sodium 490 mg	
Potassium 800 mg	
Total carbohydrate 16 g	
Dietary fiber 5 g	
Sugars 5 g	
Protein 32 g	
Phosphorus 320 mg	

Choices/Exchanges: 1/2 Starch, 2 Nonstarchy Vegetable, 3 Lean Protein

SLOW-COOKER ARROZ CON POLLO WITH CAULIFLOWER RICE

THIS SLOW-COOKER MEAL IS PERFECT FOR WEEKNIGHTS AND MAKES GREAT LEFTOVERS FOR LUNCH.

○ 10 minutes
🍲 6 hours
🍽 6 servings
🥣 1 2/3 cups

2	pounds boneless skinless chicken breasts
1/2	teaspoon salt
1/2	teaspoon ground black pepper
1	medium yellow onion, diced
1	yellow or orange bell pepper, seeded and diced
3	cloves garlic, minced
2	cups fat-free low-sodium chicken broth
2	(14.5-ounce) cans no-salt-added diced tomatoes, with juice
1	tablespoon ground turmeric
1	tablespoon sweet paprika
2	cups frozen green peas
1	(12-ounce) bag frozen cauliflower rice, cooked according to package directions

1. Place chicken in the slow cooker. Season with salt and pepper.
2. Top chicken with remaining ingredients except peas and cauliflower rice.
3. Cook on high 6 hours.
4. In the last 10 minutes of cooking, stir in the peas.

5. Cut chicken into large chunks before serving. Serve over cauliflower rice.

Nutrition Facts

Serves: 6
Serving Size: 1 2/3 cups

Amount per serving
Calories 270

Calories from fat 20

Total fat 2.5 g

Saturated fat 0.7 g

Trans fat 0.0 g

Cholesterol 90 mg

Sodium 440 mg

Potassium 1080 mg

Total carbohydrate 20 g

Dietary fiber 6 g

Sugars 8 g

Protein 42 g

Phosphorus 425 mg

Choices/Exchanges: 1/2 Starch, 3 Nonstarchy Vegetable, 4 Lean Protein

SLOW-COOKER BREAKFAST CASSEROLE

THIS SLOW-COOKER CASSEROLE IS GREAT TO MAKE AT THE HOLIDAYS WHEN YOU HAVE A CROWD TO FEED!

- ⏱ 15 minutes
- 🍲 4 hours
- 🍽 9 servings
- 🍴 About 1 cup

1	pound lean turkey breakfast sausage
	Nonstick cooking spray
4	cups frozen shredded hash browns
2	scallions, white and green parts, minced
3/4	cup shredded low-fat cheddar cheese
1	large red or yellow bell pepper, finely diced
1	small onion, finely diced
8	eggs
1	cup skim milk
1	teaspoon salt-free all-purpose seasoning (such as Spike or Mrs. Dash)
1/2	teaspoon ground black pepper

1. Cook turkey breakfast sausage. Then set aside to cool slightly.
2. Coat the inside of the slow cooker with cooking spray. Add hash browns, scallions, cheese, bell pepper, onion, and cooked sausage. Stir to combine.
3. In a medium bowl, whisk together eggs, milk, salt-free seasoning, and pepper. Pour over the hash brown mixture and mix again to incorporate.
4. Cook on high 4 hours.

Nutrition Facts

Serves: 9
Serving Size: About 1 cup

Amount per serving

Calories 220

Calories from fat 100

Total fat 11.0 g

Saturated fat 4.0 g

Trans fat 0.0 g

Cholesterol 210 mg

Sodium 490 mg

Potassium 420 mg

Total carbohydrate 12 g

Dietary fiber 2 g

Sugars 3 g

Protein 19 g

Phosphorus 280 mg

Choices/Exchanges: 1 Starch, 2 Lean Protein, 1 Fat

SLOW-COOKER BEEF STEW

⏱ 20 minutes
🍲 8 hours
🍽 5 servings
🥣 1 cup

SEARING THE BEEF ON THE STOVETOP ADDS A FEW MINUTES TO YOUR SLOW-COOKER ROUTINE, BUT IT'S WELL WORTH THE PAYOFF IN FLAVOR. SERVE THIS STEW WITH A SIDE OF STEAMED GREEN BEANS FOR A BALANCED WEEKNIGHT MEAL THAT MAKES YOUR KITCHEN SMELL INVITING ALL DAY LONG.

3	tablespoons flour
1	pound lean beef stew meat (such as round), visible fat trimmed and cut into 1-inch cubes
1	tablespoon olive oil
3	cups fat-free low-sodium beef broth
1	cup water
6	large carrots, chopped
8	ounces mushrooms, sliced
1	large sweet potato, peeled and cubed
1	onion, diced
1/2	teaspoon dried thyme
1/2	teaspoon ground black pepper

1. Place the flour in a large resealable plastic bag. Add beef and toss to coat.
2. Add oil to a pan over high heat. Add beef and sauté 6–8 minutes, turning frequently until evenly browned.
3. Transfer beef and all remaining ingredients to a large slow cooker.
4. Cover and cook in slow cooker on low 8 hours.

DIETITIAN TIP: *Sirloin and round cuts of meat are leaner versions. A slow cooker is the perfect way to transform this lean cut of meat into a tender stew.*

MAKE IT GLUTEN-FREE: *Use gluten-free flour and ensure the beef broth is gluten-free.*

Nutrition Facts

Serves: 5
Serving Size: 1 cup

Amount per serving
Calories   **260**

Calories from fat 60

Total fat 7.0 g

    Saturated fat 2.1 g

    Trans fat 0.2 g

Cholesterol 50 mg

Sodium 220 mg

Potassium 930 mg

Total carbohydrate 27 g

    Dietary fiber 5 g

    Sugars 9 g

Protein 22 g

Phosphorus 275 mg

Choices/Exchanges: 1 Starch, 2 Nonstarchy Vegetable, 2 Lean Protein, 1 Fat

SLOW-COOKER CHICKEN AND SWEET POTATOES

○ 20 minutes
⊟ 5–6 hours
△ 4 servings
▷ 1 chicken thigh and 2–3 sweet potato rounds (about 1/2 sweet potato)

GF

NO TIME TO COOK? MAKE THIS SLOW-COOKER CHICKEN FOR DINNER. THE SWEET POTATOES, DIJON MUSTARD, AND BROWN SUGAR MAKE FOR A UNIQUE AND DELICIOUS TASTE.

4	4-ounce boneless skinless chicken thighs
1	onion, chopped
2	large sweet potatoes (about 1 pound total), peeled and sliced into large rounds
1 1/2	cups fat-free, gluten-free, low-sodium chicken broth
3	tablespoons low-calorie brown sugar blend (such as Truvia or Splenda)
1/4	teaspoon dried thyme
2	tablespoons Dijon mustard
1	bay leaf
4	cups steamed broccoli and cauliflower mix

1. Place chicken in the slow cooker. Add onion and sweet potatoes on top of the chicken.
2. Add remaining ingredients, except broccoli and cauliflower mix, and cook on low 5–6 hours or until chicken is done.
3. Remove bay leaf and serve with broccoli and cauliflower.

Nutrition Facts

Serves: 4
Serving Size: 1 chicken thigh and 2–3 sweet potato rounds (about 1/2 sweet potato)

Amount per serving
Calories   **280**

Calories from fat 45

Total fat 5.0 g

  Saturated fat 1.2 g

  Trans fat 0.0 g

Cholesterol 95 mg

Sodium 380 mg

Potassium 750 mg

Total carbohydrate 29 g

  Dietary fiber 5 g

  Sugars 11 g

Protein 28 g

Phosphorus 290 mg

Choices/Exchanges: 1 Starch, 2 Nonstarchy Vegetable, 3 Lean Protein

SLOW-COOKER MOO SHU CHICKEN

HERE'S A SUPER SIMPLE SLOW-COOKER RECIPE THAT COOKS WHILE YOU'RE OUT AND IS READY FOR YOU WHEN IT'S DINNERTIME!

- ⏱ 10 minutes
- 🍲 4–6 hours
- 🍽 4 servings
- 🥡 1 1/2 cups and 1 lettuce leaf

1 (12-ounce) bag broccoli slaw
3 carrots, shredded
1 pound boneless skinless chicken breasts, thinly sliced
3 tablespoons hoisin sauce
1/4 cup water
3 cloves garlic, minced
1 teaspoon reduced-sodium soy sauce
1 tablespoon cornstarch
4 large lettuce leaves

1. Layer the slaw mix and carrots in the bottom of the slow cooker. Top with the chicken.
2. In a small bowl, mix the hoisin sauce, water, garlic, soy sauce, and cornstarch. Pour over the chicken mixture and cook on high 4–6 hours.
3. Serve 1 1/2 cups of mixture in each lettuce leaf.

Nutrition Facts

Serves: 4
Serving Size: 1 1/2 cups and 1 lettuce leaf

Amount per serving	
Calories	**210**

Calories from fat 20	
Total fat 2.5 g	
Saturated fat 0.5 g	
Trans fat 0.0 g	
Cholesterol 65 mg	
Sodium 380 mg	
Potassium 750 mg	
Total carbohydrate 18 g	
Dietary fiber 4 g	
Sugars 8 g	
Protein 29 g	
Phosphorus 305 mg	

Choices/Exchanges:
1/2 Carbohydrate, 2 Nonstarchy Vegetable, 3 Lean Protein

SLOW-COOKER BARBECUE PULLED CHICKEN

USING A SLOW COOKER ALLOWS YOU TO HAVE DINNER READY WHEN YOU GET HOME FROM A BUSY DAY. IF YOU CAN FIND SMOKED PAPRIKA, USE IT IN PLACE OF THE REGULAR PAPRIKA TO ENHANCE THE SMOKY BARBECUE FLAVOR OF THE CHICKEN.

- ⏱ 15 minutes
- 🍲 5–6 hours
- 🍽 8 servings
- 🍴 Heaping 1/2 cup

LC

1	tablespoon paprika
1	teaspoon chili powder
1	teaspoon ground black pepper
1	teaspoon garlic powder
1/4	teaspoon salt
1	whole chicken, cut into 8 pieces, skin removed
1	medium onion, diced
1	cup reduced-carb or reduced-sugar barbecue sauce
8	large lettuce leaves
2	cups shredded cabbage

1. Combine paprika, chili powder, pepper, garlic powder, and salt in a bowl. Add chicken pieces and toss to completely coat chicken.

2. Add chicken and onion to a slow cooker and cook on low 5–6 hours.

3. Remove chicken from slow cooker and set on a cutting board or in a bowl to rest 15 minutes. Take any remaining liquid and onions from slow cooker and mix with the barbecue sauce; set aside.

4. Shred chicken with a fork. Discard bones.

5. Mix pulled chicken with barbecue sauce and onion mixture.

6. To serve, add a heaping 1/2 cup of chicken to a lettuce leaf and top with 1/4 cup shredded cabbage.

Nutrition Facts

Serves: 8
Serving Size: Heaping 1/2 cup

Amount per serving

Calories 160

Calories from fat 50

Total fat 6.0 g

　Saturated fat 1.6 g

　Trans fat 0.0 g

Cholesterol 45 mg

Sodium 450 mg

Potassium 280 mg

Total carbohydrate 9 g

　Dietary fiber 1 g

　Sugars 4 g

Protein 16 g

Phosphorus 130 mg

Choices/Exchanges:
1/2 Carbohydrate, 1 Nonstarchy Vegetable, 2 Lean Protein, 1/2 Fat

SLOW-COOKER CHICKEN FAJITA BURRITOS

THIS CHICKEN DISH IS FULL OF FLAVOR AND HIGH IN FIBER WITH A LOT OF VEGGIES AND BEANS.

- ⏱ 10 minutes
- 🍲 6 hours
- 🍽 8 servings
- 🍴 1 burrito

1	pound boneless skinless chicken strips
1	green bell pepper, sliced
1	red bell pepper, sliced
1	medium onion, sliced
1	tablespoon chili powder
1	teaspoon cumin
1	teaspoon garlic powder
1/2	cup salsa fresca (no added salt)
1/3	cup water
1	(15-ounce) can no-salt-added black beans, rinsed and drained
8	large (burrito-size) whole-wheat low-carb tortillas
1	cup 50% lower-fat shredded cheddar cheese (such as Cabot)

1. Place chicken breast strips in the slow cooker. Top with remaining ingredients except for tortillas and cheese.
2. Cover and cook on low 6 hours or until done. Shred chicken with a fork if needed.
3. Scoop 1/2 cup chicken and bean mixture onto each tortilla and top with 2 tablespoons cheese. Fold into a burrito.

MAKE IT GLUTEN-FREE: *Use gluten-free tortillas and confirm all other ingredients are gluten-free.*

Nutrition Facts

Serves: 8
Serving Size: 1 burrito

Amount per serving
Calories   **260**

Calories from fat 60	
Total fat 7.0 g	
Saturated fat 2.1 g	
Trans fat 0.0 g	
Cholesterol 40 mg	
Sodium 500 mg	
Potassium 490 mg	
Total carbohydrate 33 g	
Dietary fiber 16 g	
Sugars 4 g	
Protein 29 g	
Phosphorus 395 mg	

Choices/Exchanges: 1 1/2 Starch, 1 Nonstarchy Vegetable, 3 Lean Protein

SLOW-COOKER PULLED PORK WITH PINEAPPLE BARBECUE SAUCE

COOKING AT HOME DOES NOT GET ANY EASIER THAN THIS THREE-STEP RECIPE FOR TENDER BARBECUE PULLED PORK. SET THE SLOW COOKER AND ENJOY THE TANTALIZING AROMA.

⏱ 5 minutes
🍲 8 hours
🍽 8 servings
🥄 1/2 cup

1   (2-pound) pork tenderloin
1 1/3 cups sugar-free traditional or honey-mustard barbecue sauce
1   cup canned, crushed, no-sugar-added pineapple with juice
2   cloves garlic, minced
1   small onion, diced

1. Add all ingredients to a slow cooker.
2. Cook on high 8 hours.
3. Shred the meat with two forks and serve.

CHEF TIP: *Serve the pulled pork on a salad or on a lower-carb wrap. If desired, serve with extra barbecue sauce.*

Nutrition Facts

Serves: 8
Serving Size: 1/2 cup

Amount per serving
Calories 190

Calories from fat 25

Total fat 3.0 g

    Saturated fat 0.8 g

    Trans fat 0.0 g

Cholesterol 75 mg

Sodium 400 mg

Potassium 630 mg

Total carbohydrate 15 g

    Dietary fiber 1 g

    Sugars 8 g

Protein 25 g

Phosphorus 300 mg

Choices/Exchanges:
1 Carbohydrate, 3 Lean Protein

SLOW-COOKER HAWAIIAN PORK TACOS

⏱ 10 minutes
🍲 8 hours
🍽 11 servings
🥡 1 taco

SLOW-COOKER RECIPES LIKE THESE SPICY-SWEET TACOS ARE GREAT TIME-SAVERS FOR WEEKNIGHT MEALS. IF YOU DON'T USE ALL THE PORK, FREEZE SOME FOR ANOTHER QUICK DINNER!

1	(3 3/4-pound) lean boneless pork shoulder/Boston butt roast
1/2	teaspoon ground black pepper
1/4	teaspoon ground ginger
1	teaspoon cumin
1	medium onion, sliced
2	cloves garlic, minced
8	ounces pineapple juice
1	cup white wine
11	(soft taco–size) high-fiber tortillas, warmed
1	cup shredded lettuce

1. Place pork shoulder/Boston butt roast in a slow cooker. Sprinkle with pepper, ginger, and cumin. Add onion and garlic. Pour pineapple juice and wine over the roast.
2. Cover and cook on high 7–8 hours. Drain liquid and shred the meat with a fork.
3. Scoop about 1/2 cup pork into each tortilla. Top each taco with shredded lettuce and any additional toppings of your choice.

DIETITIAN TIP: *Try topping these tacos with salsa, avocado slices, and reduced-fat shredded cheese for even more flavor!*

MAKE IT GLUTEN-FREE: *This recipe can be made gluten-free by using gluten-free tortillas.*

Nutrition Facts

Serves: 11
Serving Size: 1 taco

Amount per serving
Calories **280**

Calories from fat 70

Total fat 8.0 g

Saturated fat 2.7 g

Trans fat 0.0 g

Cholesterol 95 mg

Sodium 330 mg

Potassium 680 mg

Total carbohydrate 17 g

Dietary fiber 9 g

Sugars 2 g

Protein 40 g

Phosphorus 450 mg

Choices/Exchanges: 1 Starch, 4 Lean Protein

SLOW-COOKER ITALIAN SAUSAGE AND VEGETABLES

GF

- ⏱ 10 minutes
- 🍲 6 hours
- 🍽 5 servings
- 🥤 1 cup

NEED A FLAVORFUL MEAL BUT DON'T HAVE TIME TO COOK? YOUR FAMILY WILL LOVE THIS MOUTHWATERING MEAL, AND IT SMELLS DELICIOUS COOKING ALL DAY IN YOUR KITCHEN. SERVE IT ON A WHOLE-WHEAT BUN OR WITH A SMALL SIDE OF PASTA OR SPAGHETTI SQUASH.

1	(14.5-ounce) can no-salt-added diced tomatoes
1	teaspoon dried oregano
1	teaspoon dried basil
1	clove garlic, minced
2	teaspoons olive oil
4	ready-to-cook gluten-free Italian turkey sausage links (about 3 ounces each)
1	large green bell pepper, sliced
1	medium onion, sliced
16	ounces frozen Italian-style vegetables (unseasoned broccoli, cauliflower, carrots, green beans, and zucchini)

1. In a small bowl, mix together the tomatoes, oregano, basil, and garlic. Set aside.
2. Heat the oil in a medium sauté pan over medium-high heat. Add the sausage and sauté about 2 minutes per side until brown. Remove from the pan.
3. Layer the green pepper slices and onion slices in the slow cooker.
4. Place the sausage links on top of the peppers and onions. Pour frozen Italian vegetables on top of the sausage.
5. Pour the diced tomatoes mixture on top of the sausage.
6. Cover the slow cooker and cook on low 6 hours or until done (cooking times vary based on the slow cooker).

Nutrition Facts

Serves: 5
Serving Size: 1 cup

Amount per serving

Calories 190

Calories from fat 70

Total fat 8.0 g

Saturated fat 1.7 g

Trans fat 0.3 g

Cholesterol 55 mg

Sodium 460 mg

Potassium 650 mg

Total carbohydrate 13 g

Dietary fiber 4 g

Sugars 6 g

Protein 17 g

Phosphorus 200 mg

Choices/Exchanges: 3 Nonstarchy Vegetable, 2 Lean Protein, 1/2 Fat

SLOW-COOKER ROPA VIEJA

GF
LC

⏱ 10 minutes
🍲 6 hours
△ 10 servings
🥛 1/2 cup

ROPA VIEJA LITERALLY MEANS "OLD CLOTHES" AND COMES FROM THE TEXTURE OF THE MEAT WHEN IT IS SHREDDED. THIS DISH IS JUICY AND FLAVORFUL AND IS A GREAT FILLING FOR TACOS OR SERVED WITH VEGETABLES.

2 pounds flank steak
2 red bell peppers, seeded and sliced
1 large red onion, sliced
1 cup fresh cilantro (with stems)
1 (15-ounce) can no-salt-added diced tomatoes
1/2 cup red wine vinegar
4 cloves garlic, minced
1/2 teaspoon salt
1/2 teaspoon ground black pepper
1 teaspoon cumin
1/4 teaspoon crushed red pepper flakes

1. Add all ingredients to the slow cooker, cover, and cook on high 6 hours.
2. When the meat is done, gently remove it from the sauce. Purée the sauce with an immersion blender or in an upright blender.
3. Shred the beef and return it to the sauce.

CHEF TIP: *Serve this dish with a salad, corn tortillas, or cauliflower rice.*

Nutrition Facts

Serves: 10
Serving Size: 1/2 cup

Amount per serving
Calories 170

Calories from fat 60

Total fat 7.0 g

    Saturated fat 2.9 g

    Trans fat 0.0 g

Cholesterol 45 mg

Sodium 200 mg

Potassium 530 mg

Total carbohydrate 6 g

    Dietary fiber 1 g

    Sugars 3 g

Protein 20 g

Phosphorus 205 mg

Choices/Exchanges: 1 Nonstarchy Vegetable, 2 Lean Protein, 1 Fat

SLOW-COOKER FLANK STEAK TACOS

⏱ 10 minutes
🍲 6 hours
🍽 12 servings
🍴 1 taco

GF

PICO DE GALLO IS A FRESH SALSA MADE OF DICED TOMATO, ONION, CILANTRO, AND GREEN OR JALAPEÑO PEPPERS. YOU CAN BUY IT FRESHLY PREPARED IN THE PRODUCE SECTION OF MOST GROCERY STORES. YOU CAN ALSO TOP THESE TASTY TACOS WITH AVOCADO AND CHEESE IF DESIRED. FLANK STEAK IS A LEANER CUT OF RED MEAT.

1 1/4 pounds flank steak
2 teaspoons chili powder
1 teaspoon cumin
1 teaspoon garlic powder
Juice of 1 lime
1/2 cup water
12 (6-inch) corn tortillas
3/4 cup pico de gallo

1. Place the flank steak in a slow cooker. Sprinkle the meat with chili powder, cumin, and garlic powder. Pour the lime juice over the steak. Pour the water over the steak.
2. Cover and cook on low 6 hours or until done. Shred the steak with a fork.
3. Scoop about 1 1/2 ounces steak into each tortilla. Top each taco with 1 tablespoon pico de gallo.

Nutrition Facts

Serves: 12
Serving Size: 1 taco

Amount per serving
Calories 130

Calories from fat 35	
Total fat 4.0 g	
Saturated fat 1.5 g	
Trans fat 0.0 g	
Cholesterol 20 mg	
Sodium 40 mg	
Potassium 240 mg	
Total carbohydrate 13 g	
Dietary fiber 2 g	
Sugars 1 g	
Protein 11 g	
Phosphorus 175 mg	

Choices/Exchanges: 1 Starch, 1 Lean Protein

SLOW-COOKER GARLIC LIME CHICKEN

THIS CHICKEN WOULD BE GREAT SERVED WITH A SIDE OF QUINOA AND BROCCOLI FOR A BALANCED MEAL!

⏱ 10 minutes
🍲 6 hours
🍽 6 servings
🍴 About 3 ounces

GF
LC

Juice of 3 limes
3 cloves garlic, minced
2 tablespoons balsamic vinegar
1 tablespoon olive oil
2 1/4 pounds boneless skinless chicken thighs (about 6)
1/2 teaspoon ground black pepper

1. In a small bowl, whisk together lime juice, garlic, vinegar, and olive oil.
2. Season the chicken with pepper.
3. Put chicken in the slow cooker. Pour lime juice mixture over chicken. Cover and cook on low 6 hours.

Nutrition Facts

Serves: 6
Serving Size: About 3 ounces

Amount per serving
Calories **210**

Calories from fat 110	
Total fat 12.0 g	
Saturated fat 2.9 g	
Trans fat 0.0 g	
Cholesterol 85 mg	
Sodium 75 mg	
Potassium 200 mg	
Total carbohydrate 3 g	
Dietary fiber 0 g	
Sugars 1 g	
Protein 24 g	
Phosphorus 145 mg	

Choices/Exchanges: 3 Lean Protein 1 1/2 Fat

SLOW-COOKER POT ROAST

- ⏱ 10 minutes
- 🍲 7–8 hours
- 🍽 14 servings
- 🍴 3 1/2 ounces roast and 1/4 cup carrots and mushrooms in juice

GF
LC

IT DOESN'T GET ANY EASIER AND TASTIER THAN THIS ROAST! THE SMALL AMOUNT OF RED WINE ADDS A LARGE AMOUNT OF FLAVOR THAT WILL HAVE YOUR MOUTH WATERING. IF DESIRED, YOU CAN OMIT THE RED WINE AND USE BEEF BROTH.

3	pounds boneless lean bottom round roast
1	teaspoon ground black pepper
1	teaspoon dried thyme
1	onion, sliced
2	cloves garlic, minced
2	bay leaves
2	cups baby carrots
8	ounces mushrooms, sliced
1	cup water
1/2	cup red wine, such as Pinot Noir

1. Place roast in slow cooker. Season with pepper and thyme.
2. Place onion, garlic, and bay leaves on top of roast. Place carrots and mushrooms along sides of roast. Pour water and red wine over roast.
3. Cook on high 7–8 hours, until roast is done and able to shred. Remove bay leaves and serve.

Nutrition Facts

Serves: 14

Serving Size: 3 1/2 ounces roast and 1/4 cup carrots and mushrooms in juice

Amount per serving

Calories   **140**

Calories from fat 45

Total fat 5.0 g

  Saturated fat 1.5 g

  Trans fat 0.0 g

Cholesterol 50 mg

Sodium 65 mg

Potassium 430 mg

Total carbohydrate 4 g

  Dietary fiber 1 g

  Sugars 2 g

Protein 19 g

Phosphorus 200 mg

Choices/Exchanges: 3 Lean Protein

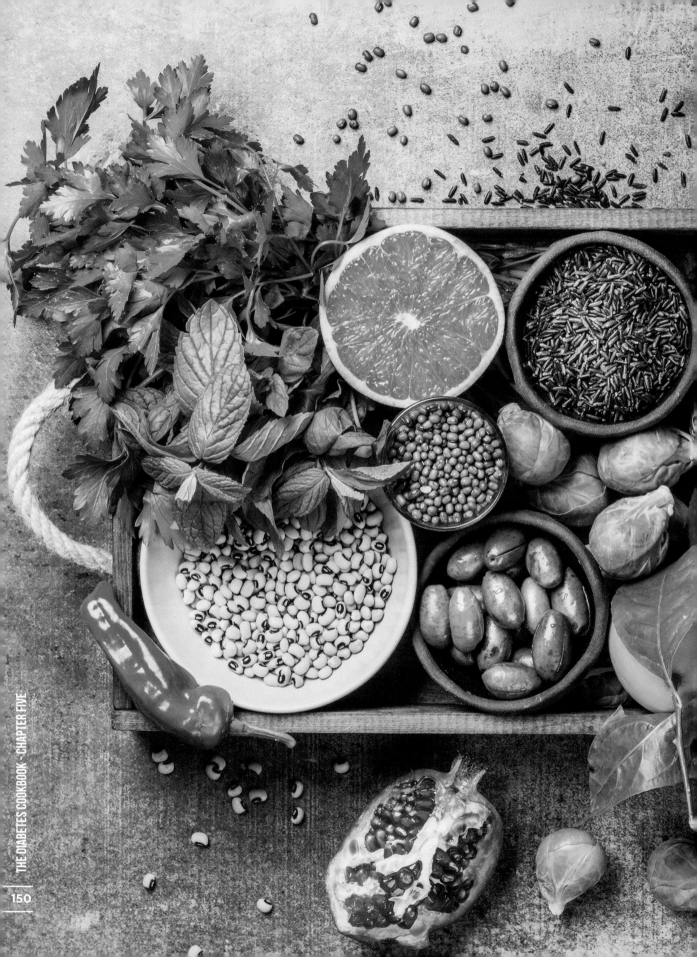

CHAPTER FIVE
KID-FRIENDLY RECIPES

GET YOUR KIDS INVOLVED IN THE KITCHEN AND YOU'LL FIND THAT THEY ARE MORE LIKELY TO EAT THE HEALTHY FOODS THEY HELPED CREATE. THESE RECIPES ARE ONES THE WHOLE FAMILY WILL ENJOY. DON'T TAKE OUR WORD FOR IT; TRY THESE OUT WITH YOUR KIDS TODAY.

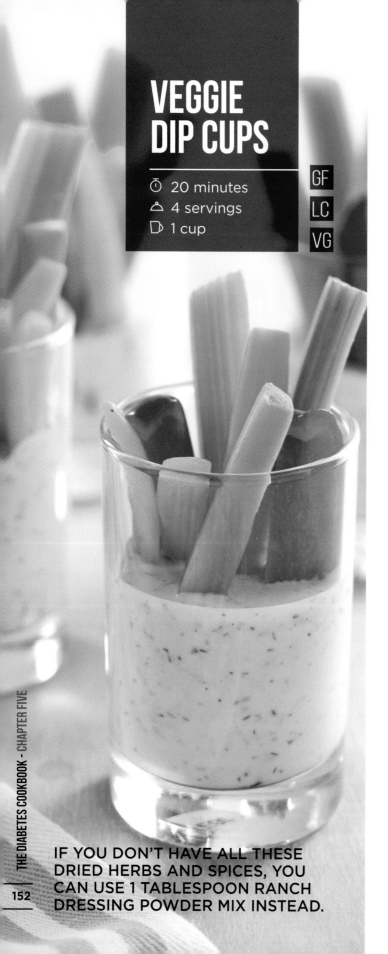

VEGGIE DIP CUPS

- ⏱ 20 minutes
- 🍽 4 servings
- 🥤 1 cup

GF
LC
VG

1/4 cup low-fat buttermilk
1/2 cup fat-free plain Greek yogurt
1/4 cup light mayonnaise
1 tablespoon minced fresh parsley
1/2 teaspoon dried dill
1/2 teaspoon garlic powder
1/2 teaspoon onion powder
1/8 teaspoon salt
1/4 teaspoon ground black pepper
4 cups assorted vegetable sticks for dipping (carrots, cucumbers, celery, bell peppers)

1. In a medium bowl combine buttermilk, yogurt, mayonnaise, parsley, dill, garlic powder, onion powder, salt, and pepper.
2. Pour 1/4 of the dip into a plastic or glass cocktail cup.
3. Arrange 1 cup of assorted vegetable sticks in the cup so all of them are touching the dip.
4. Repeat process for 3 more cups.
5. Feel free to double-dip your veggie sticks out of your own cup!

Nutrition Facts

Serves: 4
Serving Size: 1 cup

Amount per serving
Calories **90**

Calories from fat 35

Total fat 4.0 g

   Saturated fat 0.5 g

   Trans fat 0.0 g

Cholesterol 4 mg

Sodium 260 mg

Potassium 350 mg

Total carbohydrate 10 g

   Dietary fiber 2 g

   Sugars 6 g

Protein 5 g

Phosphorus 90 mg

Choices/Exchanges: 2 Nonstarchy Vegetable, 1 Fat

IF YOU DON'T HAVE ALL THESE DRIED HERBS AND SPICES, YOU CAN USE 1 TABLESPOON RANCH DRESSING POWDER MIX INSTEAD.

KID-FRIENDLY HASH BROWN WAFFLES

⏲ 5 minutes
🍽 10 minutes
🛎 8 servings
🍽 1 waffle

FOR A BELGIAN-STYLE WAFFLE MAKER, USE 1 CUP OF MIXTURE, AND THE SERVING SIZE IS 1/2 WAFFLE.

4   cups frozen shredded hash browns
4   eggs
1/4 cup skim milk
1/2 cup shredded reduced-fat cheddar cheese
1   cup cooked, crumbled gluten-free lean turkey breakfast sausage
1/2 teaspoon salt
1/2 teaspoon ground black pepper
Nonstick cooking spray

1. Preheat a waffle iron to high.
2. In a large bowl, mix the hash browns, eggs, milk, cheese, sausage, salt, and pepper.
3. Coat the top and bottom irons of the heated waffle maker with cooking spray.
4. Scoop 1/2 cup of mixture into each square of a four-square waffle maker (makes four 4-inch-square waffles). Spread the mixture just barely to the edges of the waffle iron. Close the waffle maker and cook 10 minutes or until the waffles stop steaming.
5. Repeat for remaining 4 waffles.

Nutrition Facts

Serves: 8
Serving Size: 1 waffle

Amount per serving
Calories   **130**

Calories from fat 50

Total fat 6.0 g

   Saturated fat 2.2 g

   Trans fat 0.1 g

Cholesterol 110 mg

Sodium 360 mg

Potassium 250 mg

Total carbohydrate 9 g

   Dietary fiber 1 g

   Sugars 1 g

Protein 11 g

Phosphorus 150 mg

Choices/Exchanges: 1/2 Starch, 1 Medium-Fat Protein

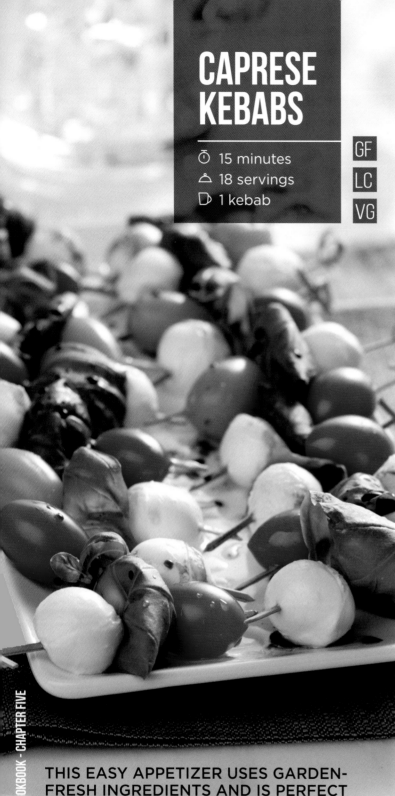

CAPRESE KEBABS

- 🕐 15 minutes
- 🍽 18 servings
- 🍴 1 kebab

GF LC VG

KEBABS

18	grape tomatoes
18	small basil leaves, folded in half
18	fresh mozzarella balls (1/4 ounce each)
18	bamboo mini forks or small skewers

DRESSING

1	tablespoon extra-virgin olive oil
1 1/2	tablespoons balsamic vinegar

1. Place 1 grape tomato, 1 basil leaf, and 1 mozzarella ball on each bamboo fork or skewer. Repeat this process for 18 kebabs. Place the kebabs on a serving platter.

2. In a small bowl, whisk together the dressing ingredients. Right before serving, pour the dressing over the kebabs to coat evenly.

Nutrition Facts

Serves: 18
Serving Size: 1 kebab

Amount per serving	
Calories	**25**

Calories from fat 20	
Total fat 2.0 g	
Saturated fat 1.0 g	
Trans fat 0.0 g	
Cholesterol 5 mg	
Sodium 25 mg	
Potassium 30 mg	
Total carbohydrate 1 g	
Dietary fiber 0 g	
Sugars 0 g	
Protein 1 g	
Phosphorus 30 mg	

Choices/Exchanges: 1/2 Fat

THIS EASY APPETIZER USES GARDEN-FRESH INGREDIENTS AND IS PERFECT FOR SUMMER. THE KEBABS ARE PACKED WITH FLAVOR AND LOW IN CARBOHYDRATES. THEY ALSO LOOK BEAUTIFUL ON A SERVING PLATTER AND ARE SURE TO IMPRESS GUESTS!

BROWN RICE BALLS

GF

⏱ 10 minutes
🍽 8 servings
▷ 2 balls

FUN TO MAKE AND DELICIOUS TO SERVE, THESE BROWN RICE BALLS ARE A GREAT WAY TO GET DIFFERENT VEGETABLES INTO YOUR KID'S DIET IN A FUN AND EASY WAY.

2 cups cooked brown rice, cooled
1/2 cup minced carrot
1/2 cup minced bell pepper (any color)
1/2 cup gluten-free turkey lunch meat, minced
1/2 cup shredded reduced-fat cheddar cheese
1/4 cup light Italian salad dressing
1/2 cup chopped pecans
Sandwich bags

1. In a large bowl, mix all the ingredients together.
2. Place 1/4 cup of the mixture into a sandwich bag and press the mixture into one corner of the bag. Squeeze the mixture in the corner of the bag to make a ball.
3. Eat the rice ball right out of the bag.

NOTE: *If you have a nut allergy, you can omit the pecans and this will still be delicious.*

Nutrition Facts

Serves: 8
Serving Size: 2 balls

Amount per serving
Calories 150

Calories from fat 70

Total fat 8.0 g

Saturated fat 1.5 g

Trans fat 0.0 g

Cholesterol 10 mg

Sodium 220 mg

Potassium 150 mg

Total carbohydrate 16 g

Dietary fiber 2 g

Sugars 2 g

Protein 6 g

Phosphorus 135 mg

Choices/Exchanges: 1 Starch, 1 1/2 Fat

FISH NUGGETS

⏱ 15 minutes
🍲 12 minutes
🍽 5 servings
🍴 4 nuggets

THESE NUGGETS CAN BE SERVED WITH A SIDE OF TARTAR SAUCE IF DESIRED. BROCCOLI AND SWEET POTATO FRIES WOULD BALANCE THIS MEAL PERFECTLY!

Nonstick cooking spray
1/2 cup all-purpose flour
1 egg
1 egg white
Dash hot sauce
2/3 cup whole-wheat panko bread crumbs
1/2 teaspoon garlic powder
1/4 teaspoon ground black pepper
10 ounces cod or haddock fillets, cut into 1-inch pieces

1. Preheat oven to 400°F. Spray a baking sheet with cooking spray.
2. Place flour in a shallow baking dish.
3. In another shallow baking dish, whisk together egg, egg white, and hot sauce.
4. In a separate shallow dish, mix together bread crumbs, garlic powder, and pepper.
5. Dip each fish nugget in flour, then egg mixture, and then dredge in bread crumb mixture. Coat well and place on a baking sheet. Spray nuggets with cooking spray.
6. Bake 12–15 minutes; turn fish pieces over halfway through cooking time (or cook at 400°F in a convection oven if available).

Nutrition Facts

Serves: 5
Serving Size: 4 nuggets

Amount per serving
Calories 130

Calories from fat 15

Total fat 1.5 g
  Saturated fat 0.5 g
  Trans fat 0.0 g
Cholesterol 60 mg
Sodium 75 mg
Potassium 170 mg
Total carbohydrate 14 g
  Dietary fiber 1 g
  Sugars 1 g
Protein 15 g
Phosphorus 110 mg

Choices/Exchanges: 1 Starch, 1 Lean Protein

CHEESY CAULIFLOWER TOTS

⏱ 20 minutes
🍲 25 minutes
🍽 7 servings
🍴 5 tots

LC
VG

SERVE THESE AS A SIDE WITH DINNER. THE TASTE IS SO SIMILAR TO TRADITIONAL TATER TOTS, YOUR FAMILY MAY NOT REALIZE THAT THEY ARE EATING CAULIFLOWER!

Nonstick cooking spray
1   head cauliflower
     (about 1 1/2 pounds), trimmed
1   egg
1   egg white
1/2 cup shredded reduced-fat cheddar cheese
1/3 cup whole-wheat bread crumbs
2   scallions, white and green parts, minced
1/8 teaspoon salt
1/4 teaspoon ground black pepper

1. Preheat oven to 400°F. Coat one large or two small baking sheets with cooking spray. Set aside.
2. Steam the cauliflower 10–12 minutes or until soft. Set aside to cool. Once cool, mince the cauliflower.
3. Stir the remaining ingredients into the minced cauliflower, and let the mixture rest 10 minutes.
4. After resting, stir the mixture again. Scoop cauliflower mixture with a tablespoon measure onto the prepared baking sheet. Form the mixture into the shape of a tater tot. Repeat to make 35 tots.

5. Spray the top of each tot with cooking spray. Bake 15 minutes. Turn the tots and bake an additional 10 minutes or until golden brown.

Nutrition Facts

Serves: 7
Serving Size: 5 tots

Amount per serving
Calories 80

Calories from fat 25	
Total fat 3.0 g	
Saturated fat 1.4 g	
Trans fat 0.0 g	
Cholesterol 30 mg	
Sodium 160 mg	
Potassium 340 mg	
Total carbohydrate 9 g	
Dietary fiber 3 g	
Sugars 2 g	
Protein 6 g	
Phosphorus 115 mg	

Choices/Exchanges: 1 Nonstarchy Vegetable, 1 Fat

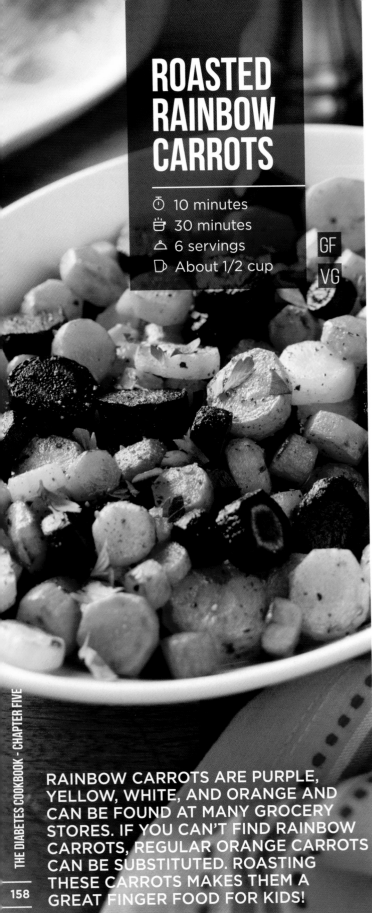

ROASTED RAINBOW CARROTS

- ⏱ 10 minutes
- 🍲 30 minutes
- 🍽 6 servings
- 🥄 About 1/2 cup

GF
VG

Nonstick cooking spray
1   (2-pound) package rainbow carrots
3   tablespoons olive oil
1/4 teaspoon ground black pepper

1. Preheat oven to 425°F. Spray a baking sheet with cooking spray.
2. Peel and cut carrots into equal-size rounds and wedges, about 1/2 inch in size.
3. Place carrots on a baking sheet. Pour olive oil over carrots and mix well. Sprinkle with pepper.
4. Bake 30 minutes until soft and crinkly.

Nutrition Facts

Serves: 6
Serving Size: About 1/2 cup

Amount per serving	
Calories	**110**

Calories from fat 60	
Total fat 7.0 g	
Saturated fat 1.0 g	
Trans fat 0.0 g	
Cholesterol 0 mg	
Sodium 95 mg	
Potassium 430 mg	
Total carbohydrate 13 g	
Dietary fiber 4 g	
Sugars 6 g	
Protein 1 g	
Phosphorus 45 mg	

Choices/Exchanges: 2 Nonstarchy Vegetable, 1 1/2 Fat

RAINBOW CARROTS ARE PURPLE, YELLOW, WHITE, AND ORANGE AND CAN BE FOUND AT MANY GROCERY STORES. IF YOU CAN'T FIND RAINBOW CARROTS, REGULAR ORANGE CARROTS CAN BE SUBSTITUTED. ROASTING THESE CARROTS MAKES THEM A GREAT FINGER FOOD FOR KIDS!

POWER SNACK MIX

⏱ 5 minutes
🍽 6 servings
🥄 1/3 cup

VG

DRIED FRUITS ARE HIGH IN CARBS, BUT USED SPARINGLY THEY CAN ADD A SWEET AND FRUITY TASTE. THIS SNACK MIX WILL APPEAL TO BOTH KIDS AND ADULTS!

1   cup multigrain oat cereal
3   tablespoons mini chocolate chips
3/4 cup almonds
1/3 cup dried cherries

1. In a medium bowl, mix together all ingredients. Portion into 1/3-cup servings.

Nutrition Facts

Serves: 6
Serving Size: 1/3 cup

Amount per serving
Calories   **190**

Calories from fat 110

Total fat 12.0 g

   Saturated fat 2.0 g

   Trans fat 0.0 g

Cholesterol 0 mg

Sodium 20 mg

Potassium 200 mg

Total carbohydrate 19 g

   Dietary fiber 3 g

   Sugars 11 g

Protein 4 g

Phosphorus 150 mg

Choices/Exchanges: 1/2 Fruit, 1 Carbohydrate, 2 Fat

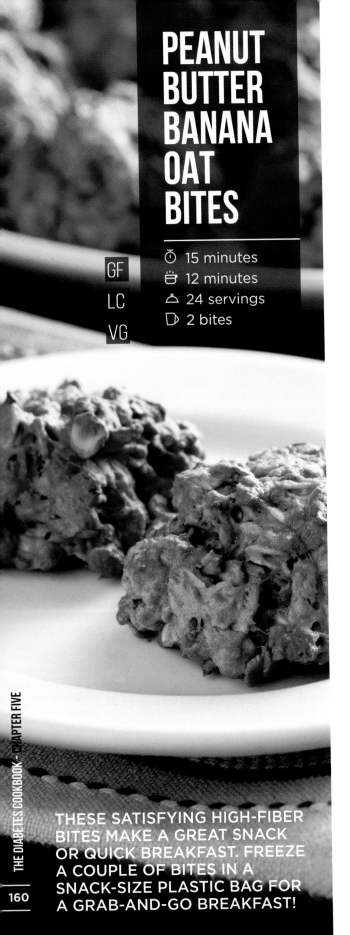

PEANUT BUTTER BANANA OAT BITES

GF
LC
VG

- ⏱ 15 minutes
- 🍳 12 minutes
- △ 24 servings
- ▭ 2 bites

1/2	cup peanut butter, heated in microwave 30 seconds
1	ripe banana, mashed
1	egg
1	teaspoon vanilla extract
2	tablespoons low-calorie brown sugar blend (such as Truvia or Splenda)
2	cups certified gluten-free rolled oats
1	teaspoon baking soda
1/2	teaspoon salt
1/4	cup milled flaxseed

1. Preheat oven to 350°F. Line a baking sheet with parchment paper.
2. In a medium bowl whisk together peanut butter, banana, egg, vanilla, and brown sugar blend.
3. In a small bowl mix together oats, baking soda, and salt. Add flaxseed.
4. Add oat mixture to peanut butter mixture and mix well.
5. Scoop batter in 1-tablespoon balls and place on baking sheet. Bake 10–12 minutes. Cool on wire rack.

Nutrition Facts

Serves: 24
Serving Size: 2 bites

Amount per serving
Calories **70**

Calories from fat 35

Total fat 4.0 g

Saturated fat 0.8 g

Trans fat 0.0 g

Cholesterol 10 mg

Sodium 130 mg

Potassium 90 mg

Total carbohydrate 8 g

Dietary fiber 1 g

Sugars 2 g

Protein 3 g

Phosphorus 60 mg

Choices/Exchanges:
1/2 Carbohydrate, 1 Fat

THESE SATISFYING HIGH-FIBER BITES MAKE A GREAT SNACK OR QUICK BREAKFAST. FREEZE A COUPLE OF BITES IN A SNACK-SIZE PLASTIC BAG FOR A GRAB-AND-GO BREAKFAST!

BLUEBERRY LEMON YOGURT PARFAIT

GF
VG

- 🕐 5 minutes
- 🍴 4 servings
- 🍶 1 parfait

TRY MAKING THIS PARFAIT WITH A VARIETY OF BERRIES, SUCH AS RASPBERRIES, BLACKBERRIES, AND STRAWBERRIES.

3 cups fat-free plain Greek yogurt
Juice and zest of 2 small lemons
1/4 cup stevia
1 tablespoon vanilla extract
2 cups fresh blueberries
1/4 cup sliced almonds

1. In a medium bowl, whisk together yogurt, lemon juice, lemon zest, stevia, and vanilla extract.
2. Add 1/2 cup yogurt to a parfait dish or small bowl. Top with 1/2 cup blueberries, then another 1/4 cup of yogurt. Sprinkle with 1 tablespoon sliced almonds.
3. Repeat with 3 more parfait glasses. Serve immediately or refrigerate.

Nutrition Facts

Serves: 4
Serving Size: 1 parfait

Amount per serving
Calories 190

Calories from fat 35

Total fat 4.0 g

Saturated fat 0.4 g

Trans fat 0.0 g

Cholesterol 10 mg

Sodium 65 mg

Potassium 360 mg

Total carbohydrate 21 g

Dietary fiber 2 g

Sugars 14 g

Protein 19 g

Phosphorus 265 mg

Choices/Exchanges: 1 Fruit, 1/2 Fat-Free Milk, 2 Lean Protein

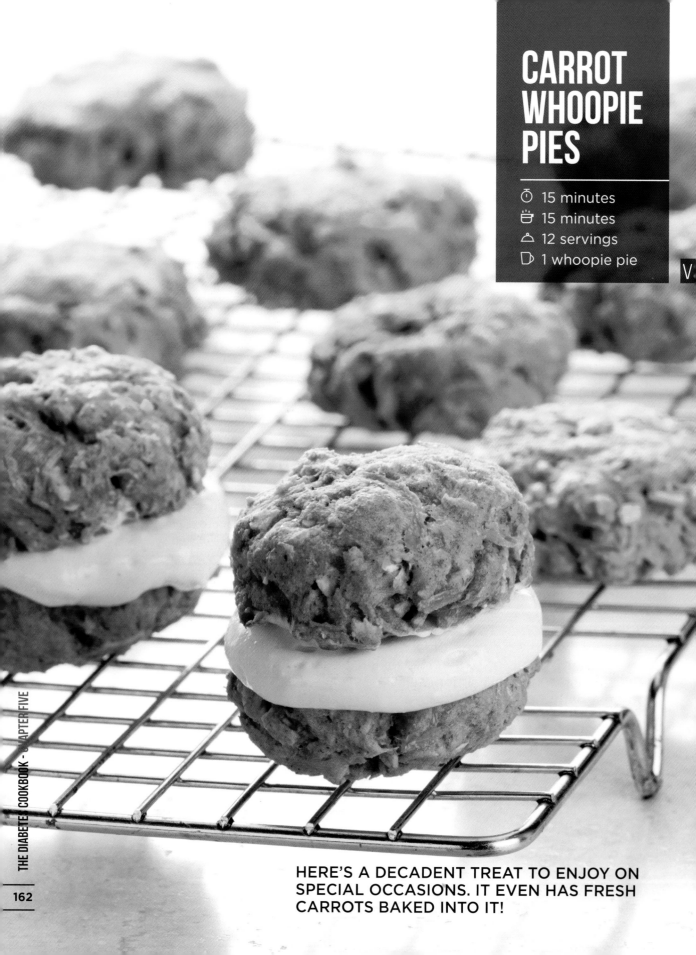

CARROT WHOOPIE PIES

- ⏱ 15 minutes
- 🍲 15 minutes
- 🍽 12 servings
- 🥧 1 whoopie pie

HERE'S A DECADENT TREAT TO ENJOY ON SPECIAL OCCASIONS. IT EVEN HAS FRESH CARROTS BAKED INTO IT!

WHOOPIE PIE

Nonstick cooking spray
1/2 cup low-calorie brown sugar blend (such as Truvia or Splenda)
1/2 cup unsweetened applesauce
1/4 cup olive oil
1/2 cup egg substitute
1   teaspoon vanilla extract
1   cup whole-wheat flour
1   cup old-fashioned rolled oats
2   teaspoons baking powder
1/2 teaspoon baking soda
1   teaspoon ground cinnamon
1/4 teaspoon nutmeg
2   cups shredded carrots

MAPLE CREAM CHEESE FILLING

8   ounces fat-free cream cheese, softened
1   teaspoon vanilla extract
2   tablespoons real maple syrup
2   tablespoons low-calorie granulated sugar substitute (such as Truvia)
1   teaspoon lemon juice

1. Preheat oven to 350°F. Line two baking sheets with parchment paper and coat with cooking spray. Set aside.
2. In a medium bowl, combine the brown sugar blend, applesauce, oil, egg substitute, and vanilla. Mix well and set aside.
3. In a large bowl, combine the flour, oats, baking powder, baking soda, cinnamon, and nutmeg.
4. Make a well in the center of the dry ingredients. Add the sugar (wet) mixture to the dry ingredients all at once and mix well.

5. Stir in the carrots. Scoop mounds of batter the size of a heaping tablespoon onto the baking sheets. Space them about 2 inches apart for a total of 24 cookies (2 sheets of 12).
6. Bake 15 minutes. Set aside to cool.
7. In a small bowl, beat the filling ingredients until smooth and fluffy. Spread a light layer of frosting between two cookies.

CHEF TIP: *You can use maple extract to cut the carbs a little in the filling.*

Nutrition Facts

Serves: 12
Serving Size: 1 whoopie pie

Amount per serving	
Calories	**160**

Calories from fat 45	
Total fat 5.0 g	
Saturated fat 0.7 g	
Trans fat 0.0 g	
Cholesterol 5 mg	
Sodium 270 mg	
Potassium 200 mg	
Total carbohydrate 23 g	
Dietary fiber 3 g	
Sugars 9 g	
Protein 6 g	
Phosphorus 245 mg	

Choices/Exchanges: 1 Starch, 1/2 Carbohydrate, 1 Fat

CHOCOLATE PEANUT BUTTER CHIA SEED PUDDING

⏱ 5 minutes
🍽 3 servings
🥄 1/3 cup

SERVE THIS PUDDING WITH A DOLLOP OF LIGHT WHIPPED CREAM (IF DESIRED) AND A SPRINKLE OF COCOA POWDER FOR A FANCY DESSERT OR SNACK.

2	tablespoons unsweetened cocoa powder
2	tablespoons stevia
1/4	cup powdered peanut butter
1/4	cup chia seeds
1	cup skim milk or unsweetened almond milk
1	teaspoon vanilla extract

1. Mix cocoa powder, stevia, and powdered peanut butter together, and incorporate well so there are no lumps.
2. Stir in the chia seeds and stir well to combine.
3. Whisk in the milk and vanilla. Let sit 5 minutes, then whisk again. Cover and refrigerate for at least 2 hours before serving.

Nutrition Facts

Serves: 3
Serving Size: 1/3 cup

Amount per serving
Calories 150

Calories from fat 60

Total fat 7.0 g

Saturated fat 1.1 g

Trans fat 0.0 g

Cholesterol 0 mg

Sodium 100 mg

Potassium 340 mg

Total carbohydrate 18 g

Dietary fiber 8 g

Sugars 5 g

Protein 10 g

Phosphorus 310 mg

Choices/Exchanges:
1 Carbohydrate, 1 Lean Protein, 1 Fat

OVEN-BAKED CHICKEN TAQUITOS

THIS IS A GREAT HEALTHIER RECIPE TO TRY IN PLACE OF FRIED MEXICAN FOOD. THE TAQUITOS COME OUT PERFECTLY CRISPY!

⏱ 10 minutes
🍲 40 minutes
🍽 4 servings
🍴 2 taquitos

GF

Nonstick cooking spray
1/2 teaspoon cumin
1 teaspoon chili powder
1 teaspoon garlic powder
1/2 teaspoon ground black pepper
8 ounces boneless skinless chicken breasts
1/2 cup shredded 2% Mexican-style cheese blend
1/2 cup fat-free refried beans
8 (6-inch) corn tortillas
1 cup shredded lettuce
1/2 cup prepared guacamole
1 cup diced tomatoes

1. Preheat oven to 400°F. Coat a baking sheet with cooking spray. Set aside.
2. In a small bowl, mix together the cumin, chili powder, garlic powder, and pepper.
3. Lay the chicken breasts on the prepared baking sheet. Sprinkle the chicken with the spice mixture. Roast the chicken in the oven 25 minutes or until the internal temperature is 165°F. Set it aside to cool slightly. Keep the oven on and coat a clean baking sheet with cooking spray.
4. Once the chicken has rested and cooled slightly, shred the chicken meat and place it in a medium bowl. Add the cheese and refried beans and mix well.
5. Place the corn tortillas between two damp paper towels. Microwave on high 30 seconds.

6. Fill each corn tortilla with 1/4 cup chicken filling and roll tightly. Lay seam side down on the prepared baking sheet. Once all the taquitos are on the baking sheet, lightly spray each one with cooking spray.
7. Bake 15 minutes or until the tortillas are crispy.
8. Serve two taquitos topped with 1/4 cup shredded lettuce, 2 tablespoons guacamole, and 1/4 cup diced tomatoes.

Nutrition Facts

Serves: 4
Serving Size: 2 taquitos

Amount per serving
Calories   **320**

Calories from fat 100

Total fat 11.0 g
   Saturated fat 3.1 g
   Trans fat 0.0 g
Cholesterol 40 mg
Sodium 380 mg
Potassium 600 mg
Total carbohydrate 35 g
   Dietary fiber 7 g
   Sugars 2 g
Protein 22 g
Phosphorus 390 mg

Choices/Exchanges: 2 Starch, 1 Nonstarchy Vegetable, 2 Lean Protein, 1 Fat

BARBECUE CHICKEN PIZZA

SERVE THIS PIZZA WITH A BIG GARDEN SALAD DRIZZLED LIGHTLY WITH LOW-FAT RANCH DRESSING. IT'S A QUICK, EASY, AND BUDGET-FRIENDLY MEAL!

- ⏱ 25 minutes
- 🍲 50 minutes
- 🍽 8 servings
- 🍴 1 slice

Nonstick cooking spray
1/2 pound boneless skinless chicken breast
1/4 teaspoon salt
1/4 teaspoon ground black pepper
1/4 cup sugar-free apricot preserves
1/4 cup barbecue sauce
1/2 teaspoon hot sauce
1 (12-inch) prepackaged whole-wheat pizza crust
1/2 medium red onion, thinly sliced
1 cup shredded carrots
1/2 cup reduced-fat shredded Italian-style cheese
1/2 teaspoon dried oregano

1. Preheat oven to 375°F. Spray a baking sheet with cooking spray.
2. Season the chicken with salt and pepper on both sides.
3. Place the chicken on the prepared baking sheet and bake 25 minutes or until the juices run clear. Remove the chicken from the oven and chop into 1/2-inch pieces.
4. In a small saucepan, combine the apricot preserves, barbecue sauce, and hot sauce. Bring to a boil.
5. Spoon the sauce over the pizza crust.

Top the crust with cooked chicken, sliced onion, carrots, and cheese. Sprinkle the pizza with dried oregano.
6. Bake the pizza 20–25 minutes or until the cheese is melted and bubbly.

Nutrition Facts

Serves: 8
Serving Size: 1 slice

Amount per serving
Calories 160

Calories from fat 30

Total fat 3.5 g

Saturated fat 1.4 g

Trans fat 0.0 g

Cholesterol 20 mg

Sodium 400 mg

Potassium 230 mg

Total carbohydrate 23 g

Dietary fiber 4 g

Sugars 5 g

Protein 11 g

Phosphorus 155 mg

Choices/Exchanges: 1 Starch, 1/2 Carbohydrate, 1 Lean Protein

CHICKEN FINGERS

🕐 15 minutes
🍲 30 minutes
🍽 5 servings
🍴 2 chicken strips

GF

DO YOU NEED A HEALTHY DINNER FOR THE ENTIRE FAMILY? THESE BAKED CHICKEN FINGERS ARE COATED IN CORNMEAL, WHICH IS CONSIDERED A WHOLE GRAIN AND MAKES A CRISPY COATING. THE CHICKEN FINGERS TASTE GREAT SERVED OVER SALAD GREENS.

Nonstick cooking spray
1 egg
1 egg white
Dash hot sauce
3/4 cup certified gluten-free cornmeal
1/2 teaspoon garlic powder
1/4 teaspoon ground black pepper
1/4 teaspoon dried thyme
1 pound boneless skinless chicken breast tenderloins, cut into 10 strips

1. Preheat oven to 350°F. Spray a baking sheet with cooking spray.
2. In a shallow baking dish, whisk together the egg, egg white, and hot sauce.
3. In another shallow dish, mix together cornmeal, garlic powder, pepper, and thyme.
4. Dip a chicken breast strip in the egg mixture, and then dredge in the cornmeal mixture. Coat well and place on baking sheet. Repeat procedure for remaining chicken strips.
5. Bake 30 minutes or until done (to an internal temperature of 165°F). Turn chicken pieces over halfway through cooking time.

Nutrition Facts

Serves: 5
Serving Size: 2 chicken strips

Amount per serving
Calories 200

Calories from fat 30

Total fat 3.5 g

Saturated fat 1.0 g

Trans fat 0.0 g

Cholesterol 90 mg

Sodium 75 mg

Potassium 220 mg

Total carbohydrate 17 g

Dietary fiber 1 g

Sugars 0 g

Protein 23 g

Phosphorus 185 mg

Choices/Exchanges: 1 Starch, 3 Lean Protein

CHICKEN CAESAR SALAD LUNCH WRAPS

⏱ 10 minutes
🍽 4 servings
🥡 1 wrap

IF YOU ARE TIRED OF THE SAME BORING SANDWICH FOR LUNCH, TRY THIS RESTAURANT-STYLE WRAP. IT'S PACKED FULL OF FLAVOR, IT'S LOW IN CARBS, AND IT SUPPLIES A SERVING OF VEGGIES. USE COOKED ROTISSERIE CHICKEN FROM THE GROCERY STORE TO SAVE TIME.

1 1/2	cups diced cooked chicken
2	tablespoons light Caesar salad dressing
3	tablespoons freshly grated parmesan cheese
4	cups bagged romaine lettuce salad
4	(10-inch) low-carb whole-wheat tortillas

1. In a medium bowl, mix together all the ingredients except for the tortillas. Toss to coat the salad evenly with the dressing.
2. Spread 1 heaping cup of the chicken salad mixture onto a tortilla. Fold the left and right sides of the wrap in until they touch and roll from the bottom to make a wrap.
3. Repeat procedure for remaining 3 wraps.

MAKE IT GLUTEN-FREE: *Use gluten-free tortillas and confirm the salad dressing is gluten-free.*

Nutrition Facts

Serves: 4
Serving Size: 1 wrap

Amount per serving
Calories 220

Calories from fat 80

Total fat 9.0 g

Saturated fat 1.8 g

Trans fat 0.0 g

Cholesterol 50 mg

Sodium 510 mg

Potassium 280 mg

Total carbohydrate 21 g

Dietary fiber 14 g

Sugars 2 g

Protein 25 g

Phosphorus 260 mg

Choices/Exchanges: 1 1/2 Starch, 2 Lean Protein, 1/2 Fat

CUCUMBER AND TURKEY TEA SANDWICHES

○ 10 minutes
△ 2 servings
▷ 1 sandwich

THIS RECIPE IS SUPER EASY BUT FULL OF CRUNCH, FLAVOR, AND FRESHNESS. IT SERVES TWO BUT IT'S EASY TO INCREASE THE SERVINGS FOR A LUNCHEON OR AFTERNOON GATHERING.

4 teaspoons 1/3-less-fat garden vegetable cream cheese
4 slices whole-wheat bread
1/2 cucumber, peeled and thinly sliced (about 18 slices total)
4 ounces no-salt-added deli-style roasted turkey breast (such as Boar's Head)

1. Spread 2 teaspoons cream cheese on 1 slice of bread. Then top with 6–9 cucumber slices, 2 ounces turkey meat, and another slice of bread. Cut the sandwich diagonally into 4 pieces.
2. Repeat this procedure for the second sandwich.

Nutrition Facts

Serves: 2
Serving Size: 1 sandwich

Amount per serving
Calories   **240**

Calories from fat 40	
Total fat 4.5 g	
Saturated fat 1.9 g	
Trans fat 0.0 g	
Cholesterol 45 mg	
Sodium 370 mg	
Potassium 430 mg	
Total carbohydrate 26 g	
Dietary fiber 4 g	
Sugars 4 g	
Protein 23 g	
Phosphorus 290 mg	

Choices/Exchanges: 2 Starch, 2 Lean Protein

RAINBOW FRUIT PLATTER

A QUICK, EASY, AND COLORFUL RECIPE THAT ANYONE CAN MAKE! TRY IT OUT FOR BREAKFAST, A SNACK, OR EVEN DESSERT.

- ⏱ 30 minutes
- ⌂ 25 servings
- 🍽 1 cup

DIP

1	cup 100-calorie vanilla Greek yogurt
1	tablespoon chia seeds
1/8	teaspoon cinnamon

FRUITS

4	cups whole strawberries, hulled
4	cups cubed cantaloupe
1	pineapple, peeled, cored, and cubed (about 4 cups)
3	cups green grapes
4	cups blueberries
3	cups purple grapes
3	cups blackberries

1. Mix together yogurt and chia seeds. Refrigerate overnight. Mix in cinnamon.

2. On a very large platter, place strawberries in an arc to form the top row of a rainbow pattern.

3. Place cantaloupe cubes as the second row under the strawberries. Continue this process with the pineapple through the blackberries to complete a rainbow. Serve with dip.

DIETITIAN TIP: *Get your kids involved in making this platter. They will love it, and it will teach them that healthy food can be fun, too!*

Nutrition Facts

Serves: 25
Serving Size: 1 cup

Amount per serving
Calories 80

Calories from fat 5	
Total fat 0.5 g	
Saturated fat 0.1 g	
Trans fat 0.0 g	
Cholesterol 0 mg	
Sodium 10 mg	
Potassium 260 mg	
Total carbohydrate 20 g	
Dietary fiber 3 g	
Sugars 15 g	
Protein 2 g	
Phosphorus 40 mg	

Choices/Exchanges: 1 1/2 Fruit

POWER GRANOLA

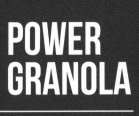

- ⏱ 15 minutes
- ☕ 45 minutes
- △ 22 servings
- ▽ 1/4 cup

THIS GRANOLA IS A GREAT PRE- OR POST-WORKOUT SNACK WITH A GREAT BALANCE OF CARBS AND PROTEIN. IT ALSO MAKES AN EXCELLENT BREAKFAST CEREAL OR CAN BE STIRRED INTO YOUR FAVORITE GREEK YOGURT.

Nonstick cooking spray
1 cup unsalted cashews, chopped
1 cup unsalted raw pumpkin seeds (pepitas)
1 cup unsalted pecans, chopped
1 cup unsalted sunflower seeds
1 cup certified gluten-free old-fashioned oats
1/4 cup natural peanut butter
1/4 cup olive oil
1/4 cup low-calorie brown sugar blend (such as Truvia or Splenda)

1. Preheat oven to 300°F.
2. Line a baking sheet with parchment paper or foil. Coat with cooking spray and set aside.
3. In a bowl, combine cashews, pumpkin seeds, pecans, sunflower seeds, and oats. Set aside.
4. In the microwave, heat peanut butter, oil, and brown sugar blend together. Stir to combine.
5. Pour peanut butter mixture over oat mixture and stir to coat.
6. Spread granola in a packed, single layer onto the prepared baking sheet. Bake 40–45 minutes, stirring every 10 minutes to ensure even browning.
7. Remove from oven and let cool completely. Break up granola and store in an airtight container.

Nutrition Facts

Serves: 22
Serving Size: 1/4 cup

Amount per serving
Calories 200

Calories from fat 150

Total fat 17.0 g
    Saturated fat 2.2 g
    Trans fat 0.0 g
Cholesterol 0 mg
Sodium 0 mg
Potassium 190 mg
Total carbohydrate 8 g
    Dietary fiber 2 g
    Sugars 2 g
Protein 5 g
Phosphorus 210 mg

Choices/Exchanges:
1/2 Carbohydrate, 1 Lean Protein, 2 1/2 Fat

HEALTHY BACK-TO-SCHOOL LUNCH

⏱ 10 minutes
△ 1 serving
▯ 1 lunch

COMING UP WITH IDEAS FOR SCHOOL LUNCHES CAN BE OVERWHELMING. THIS HEALTHY LUNCH IS QUICK, FUN, AND TASTY. YOUR CHILD (AND YOU) WILL LOVE IT! YOU CAN MODIFY PORTION SIZES BASED ON YOUR CHILD'S AGE AND APPETITE. FOR EXAMPLE, AN OLDER CHILD MAY NEED TWO MINI SANDWICHES.

MINI TURKEY SANDWICH

- 1 teaspoon mustard
- 1 whole-grain dinner roll
- 2 ounces no-salt-added deli-style turkey breast
- 1/2 ounce reduced-fat cheddar cheese
- 1 romaine lettuce leaf

CUCUMBER SANDWICH

- 1 teaspoon hummus
- 4 cucumber slices
- 1 teaspoon sunflower seeds

SIDES

- 1/2 cup blueberries and sliced strawberries
- 1 (2-ounce) tube Greek yogurt

1. Spread mustard on the roll. Top it with turkey, cheese, and lettuce to make a sandwich.
2. Spread 1/2 teaspoon hummus on 1 cucumber slice. Top it with 1/2 teaspoon sunflower seeds and top with another cucumber slice to make a sandwich. Repeat the process to make another cucumber sandwich.
3. Assemble all meal components including blueberries and yogurt in separate sections of a divided lunch container.

Nutrition Facts

Serve: 1
Serving Size: 1 lunch

Amount per serving
Calories 310

Calories from fat 80

Total fat 9.0 g

Saturated fat 3.1 g

Trans fat 0.0 g

Cholesterol 55 mg

Sodium 460 mg

Potassium 570 mg

Total carbohydrate 34 g

Dietary fiber 5 g

Sugars 15 g

Protein 30 g

Phosphorus 440 mg

Choices/Exchanges: 1 Starch, 1/2 Fruit, 1/2 Fat-Free Milk, 1 Nonstarchy Vegetable, 3 Lean Protein

HEALTHY HOMEMADE LUNCH IN A PACK

⏱ 10 minutes
🍽 1 serving
🍱 1 lunch

MAKE THIS QUICK AND DELICIOUS HOMEMADE LUNCH-IN-A-PACK FOR YOUR CHILD'S FIRST DAY BACK TO SCHOOL. IT WILL BE A TREAT FOR YOUR KIDS, AND YOU WILL KNOW THEY ARE EATING HEALTHY. YOU COULD ALSO MAKE ONE FOR YOURSELF!

SNACK MIX

1/4	cup chocolate oat cereal
1/4	cup mini pretzels (or pretzel sticks broken into 1-inch pieces)
1	tablespoon unsalted peanuts

LUNCH

2	stalks celery (4 inches each)
2	teaspoons hummus
3	ounces no-salt-added deli-style turkey breast (cut each slice into 4 pieces)
1	slice reduced-fat cheddar cheese, cut into 4 squares
8	multigrain crackers
1	nectarine, pitted and sliced
4	baby carrots

1. In a small bowl, combine all the snack mix ingredients.
2. Spread 1 teaspoon hummus on each celery stalk. Using a compartmentalized plastic container, place the turkey, cheese, crackers, and nectarine in separate sections of the container.
3. Place snack mix, carrots, and celery with hummus in a section of the container or in a separate container, if needed.

Nutrition Facts

Serve: 1
Serving Size: 1 lunch

Amount per serving

Calories	**470**

Calories from fat 130
Total fat 14.0 g
Saturated fat 4.1 g
Trans fat 0.0 g
Cholesterol 65 mg
Sodium 620 mg
Potassium 940 mg
Total carbohydrate 53 g
Dietary fiber 8 g
Sugars 21 g
Protein 35 g
Phosphorus 510 mg

Choices/Exchanges: 2 Starch, 1 Fruit, 1 Nonstarchy Vegetable, 4 Lean Protein, 1 Fat

GRILLED BANANA SPLIT SUNDAES

A NEW SPIN ON A TIMELESS CLASSIC. KEEP THE PEELS ON THE BANANAS FOR A BUILT-IN BAKING DISH AS YOU GRILL THEM—THE HEAT CARAMELIZES THE SUGAR BLEND IN THIS SENSATIONAL DESSERT.

GF
VG

- ⏱ 5 minutes
- 🍲 10 minutes
- 🍽 6 servings
- 🍨 1 sundae

2 teaspoons low-calorie brown sugar blend (such as Truvia or Splenda)
1/2 teaspoon ground cinnamon
2 firm unpeeled bananas, split in 1/2 lengthwise (leave peels on)
2 cups reduced-fat, reduced-calorie strawberry ice cream
6 tablespoons no-sugar-added crushed pineapple, drained
6 tablespoons sugar-free chocolate sauce
6 tablespoons fat-free whipped topping
6 tablespoons pecans, chopped

1. Preheat indoor or outdoor grill to medium heat.
2. In a small bowl, whisk the brown sugar blend and cinnamon together. Sprinkle the cut side of the bananas with the cinnamon mixture.
3. Place the bananas cut side down on the grill and cook until grill marks appear, about 2–3 minutes. Flip the bananas over and cook until the peel just starts to pull away from the banana. Remove the bananas from the grill and remove the peels. Cut each half in thirds, crosswise.
4. Scoop 1/3 cup ice cream into a sundae bowl. Tuck two pieces of banana into the ice cream so they are sticking up. Top the ice cream with 1 tablespoon pineapple, 1 tablespoon chocolate sauce, 1 tablespoon whipped topping, and 1 tablespoon pecans. Repeat for the remaining 5 sundaes.

CHEF TIP: *If you prefer, choose a different flavor of ice cream and use any no-sugar-added canned fruit or fresh fruit instead of the pineapple.*

Nutrition Facts

Serves: 6
Serving Size: 1 sundae

Amount per serving
Calories   **180**

Calories from fat 60	
Total fat 7.0 g	
Saturated fat 1.8 g	
Trans fat 0.0 g	
Cholesterol 10 mg	
Sodium 85 mg	
Potassium 300 mg	
Total carbohydrate 28 g	
Dietary fiber 3 g	
Sugars 9 g	
Protein 3 g	
Phosphorus 80 mg	

Choices/Exchanges: 1 Fruit, 1 Carbohydrate, 1 Fat

NO-BAKE PEANUT BUTTER AND CHOCOLATE BITES

GF
LC
VG

○ 10 minutes
☕ 2 minutes
△ 24 servings
▱ 2 bites

NEED A HEALTHY SNACK FOR YOUR SUMMER ROAD TRIP? THIS SIMPLE TREAT IS MUCH HEALTHIER THAN ANY PROCESSED SNACK THAT YOU MIGHT BUY AT A GAS STATION.

1/3	cup low-calorie granulated sugar blend (such as Domino Light Sugar & Stevia Blend)
1/3	cup skim milk
1/2	cup peanut butter
1	teaspoon vanilla extract
2	cups certified gluten-free rolled oats
3	tablespoons mini chocolate chips

1. In a small saucepan, combine sugar blend with milk over medium heat. Stir well and bring to a boil for 1 1/2 minutes. Stir in peanut butter and vanilla.
2. Remove from heat and add remaining ingredients; stir to incorporate.
3. Scoop oat mixture into 1-tablespoon balls and place on wax paper. Let cool and refrigerate.

Nutrition Facts

Serves: 24
Serving Size: 2 bites

Amount per serving
Calories 80

Calories from fat 30	
Total fat 3.5 g	
Saturated fat 0.7 g	
Trans fat 0.0 g	
Cholesterol 0 mg	
Sodium 20 mg	
Potassium 70 mg	
Total carbohydrate 9 g	
Dietary fiber 1 g	
Sugars 4 g	
Protein 2 g	
Phosphorus 55 mg	

Choices/Exchanges:
1/2 Carbohydrate, 1 Fat

ROASTED PEAR SAUCE

⏱ 10 minutes
🍲 25 minutes
△ 6 servings
🥄 1/2 cup

GF
VG

THERE IS NO REASON TO BUY STORE-BOUGHT APPLESAUCE WHEN YOU CAN MAKE THIS EASY GOURMET PEAR SAUCE AT HOME IN NO TIME.

3   large ripe pears (about 1 1/2 pounds total), cored, and cut in 1-inch pieces
2   teaspoons butter, melted
1   tablespoon honey or 2 packets artificial sweetener
1   tablespoon lemon juice
1/3 cup chopped walnuts, toasted

1. Preheat oven to 350°F.
2. In a large bowl, toss the pears with melted butter. Pour the pears into a baking dish and roast, uncovered, 20–25 minutes or until pears are tender, stirring once or twice. Set the cooked pears aside to cool.
3. Add the pears back to the large bowl; add the honey and lemon juice. Using an immersion blender or upright blender, blend the pear mixture until almost smooth. Stir in the walnuts.

Nutrition Facts

Serves: 6
Serving Size: 1/2 cup

Amount per serving
Calories 120

Calories from fat 50

Total fat 6.0 g

Saturated fat 1.2 g

Trans fat 0.1 g

Cholesterol 6 mg

Sodium 10 mg

Potassium 150 mg

Total carbohydrate 20 g

Dietary fiber 4 g

Sugars 13 g

Protein 1 g

Phosphorus 35 mg

Choices/Exchanges: 1 Fruit, 1/2 Carbohydrate, 1 Fat

RASPBERRY SMOOTHIE POPS

⏱ 5 minutes
Freeze Time: 3 hours
⌂ 4 servings
▷ 1 pop

GF
VG

TRY THESE EASY AND TASTY SMOOTHIE POPS THAT ARE PERFECT ON A HOT SUMMER DAY—A HEALTHY TREAT MADE WITH FRESH INGREDIENTS AND FREE OF FOOD DYES.

1   small banana
1   cup unsweetened frozen raspberries
2   ounces fat-free berry Greek yogurt
1/2 cup skim milk

1. In a blender, mix all ingredients until smooth.
2. Pour smoothie mixture evenly into 4 ice pop molds. Insert ice pop handle. Place upright and freeze until solid, about 3 hours.

DIETITIAN TIP: *Both kids and adults will love these easy smoothie pops.*

Nutrition Facts

Serves: 4
Serving Size: 1 pop

Amount per serving	
Calories	**70**
Calories from fat 5	
Total fat 0.5 g	
Saturated fat 0.2 g	
Trans fat 0.0 g	
Cholesterol 0 mg	
Sodium 20 mg	
Potassium 230 mg	
Total carbohydrate 13 g	
Dietary fiber 3 g	
Sugars 8 g	
Protein 3 g	
Phosphorus 70 mg	

Choices/Exchanges: 1 Fruit

VEGGIE MEATBALLS

⏱ 20 minutes
🍲 45 minutes
🍽 11 servings
🍴 2 meatballs

GF
LC

THIS IS A MEATBALL RECIPE YOUR WHOLE FAMILY WILL LOVE. IT'S ALSO A GREAT WAY TO SNEAK IN SOME EXTRA VEGGIES FOR YOUR KIDS AND YOU.

SAUCE

1/2	cup ketchup
3	tablespoons balsamic vinegar

MEATBALLS

1	pound lean ground turkey
1/2	zucchini, grated
1	carrot, grated
1/2	onion, grated
1	clove garlic, minced
2	teaspoons chili powder
1/4	teaspoon ground black pepper
1/4	teaspoon salt
1	egg, slightly beaten
1/2	cup certified gluten-free rolled oats
3	tablespoons freshly grated parmesan cheese

1. Preheat oven to 350°F.
2. In a small bowl, whisk together sauce ingredients.
3. In a medium bowl, mix together meatball ingredients. Shape into 1-inch balls.
4. Place meatballs on a baking sheet and top evenly with sauce (1 1/2 teaspoons per meatball).
5. Bake 45 minutes or until done.

Nutrition Facts

Serves: 11
Serving Size: 2 meatballs

Amount per serving
Calories 110

Calories from fat 35

Total fat 4.0 g

Saturated fat 1.3 g

Trans fat 0.0 g

Cholesterol 50 mg

Sodium 240 mg

Potassium 220 mg

Total carbohydrate 8 g

Dietary fiber 1 g

Sugars 4 g

Protein 10 g

Phosphorus 125 mg

Choices/Exchanges:
1/2 Carbohydrate, 1 Lean Protein, 1/2 Fat

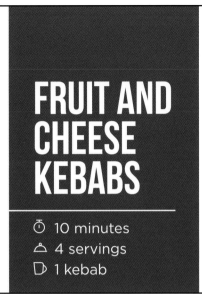

FRUIT AND CHEESE KEBABS

GF
VG

⏱ 10 minutes
🍽 4 servings
🍴 1 kebab

THESE PRETTY KEBABS ARE A GREAT SNACK FOR KIDS AND ADULTS. EXPERIMENT WITH DIFFERENT FRUITS, SUCH AS A MELON OR PINEAPPLE.

8   strawberries, hulled and cut in half
16   grapes
2   kiwis, peeled and sliced
3   light string cheese sticks, each cut into
     4 pieces
4   wooden skewers

1. Skewer strawberries, grapes, kiwi slices, and cheese in random order on a skewer, using 4 strawberry halves, 4 grapes, 2–3 kiwi slices, and 3 pieces cheese per skewer.
2. Repeat the process for the remaining 3 skewers.

Nutrition Facts

Serves: 4
Serving Size: 1 kebab

Amount per serving
Calories   **80**

Calories from fat 20

Total fat 2.0 g

   Saturated fat 0.8 g

   Trans fat 0.0 g

Cholesterol 2 mg

Sodium 115 mg

Potassium 220 mg

Total carbohydrate 12 g

   Dietary fiber 2 g

   Sugars 8 g

Protein 5 g

Phosphorus 120 mg

Choices/Exchanges: 1 Fruit, 1 Lean Protein

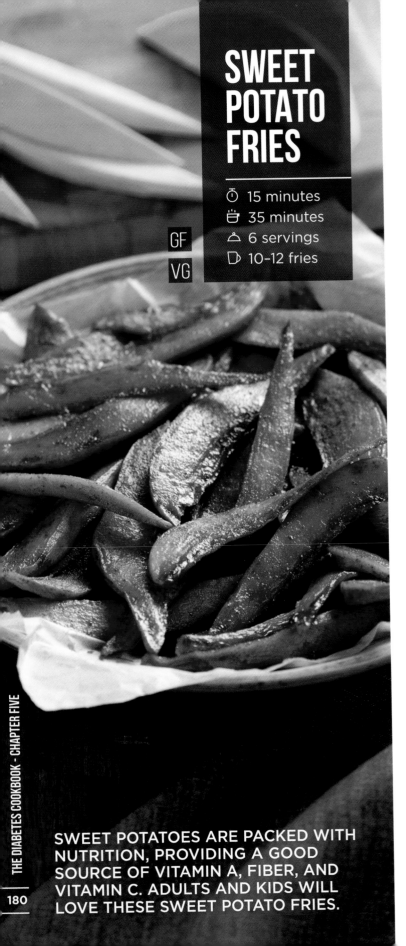

SWEET POTATO FRIES

GF
VG

- ⏱ 15 minutes
- 🍲 35 minutes
- 🍽 6 servings
- 🍟 10–12 fries

Nonstick cooking spray
2   large sweet potatoes (about 2 pounds total), peeled and cut into 1/2-inch wedges
2   tablespoons olive oil
1   teaspoon cinnamon
1/4 cup low-calorie brown sugar blend (such as Truvia)

1. Preheat oven to 400°F. Spray a baking sheet with cooking spray.
2. Place sweet potatoes in a bowl and add oil; toss to coat.
3. Add cinnamon and mix well.
4. Place potatoes on a baking sheet and bake 35 minutes or until potatoes are soft.

Nutrition Facts

Serves: 6
Serving Size: 10–12 fries

Amount per serving
Calories **160**

Calories from fat 40

Total fat 4.5 g

Saturated fat 0.7 g

Trans fat 0.0 g

Cholesterol 0 mg

Sodium 35 mg

Potassium 460 mg

Total carbohydrate 27 g

Dietary fiber 3 g

Sugars 10 g

Protein 2 g

Phosphorus 50 mg

Choices/Exchanges: 1 1/2 Starch, 1/2 Carbohydrate, 1/2 Fat

SWEET POTATOES ARE PACKED WITH NUTRITION, PROVIDING A GOOD SOURCE OF VITAMIN A, FIBER, AND VITAMIN C. ADULTS AND KIDS WILL LOVE THESE SWEET POTATO FRIES.

CHOCOLATE PEANUT BUTTER GRAHAM CRACKER SANDWICHES

THIS RECIPE IS SIMPLE AND IS SURE TO SATISFY YOUR SWEET TOOTH!

⏱ 10 minutes
Freeze Time: 1–2 hours
🔔 14 servings
🍽 1 sandwich

VG

1	(1.4-ounce) package sugar-free instant chocolate pudding mix
1/4	cup peanut butter powder
2	cups skim milk
28	graham cracker sheets (14 rectangles, each 5 inches long), broken into squares

1. In a small bowl, whisk together the pudding mix, peanut butter powder, and milk. Refrigerate 5 minutes.

2. For each sandwich, place 2 tablespoons pudding mixture onto a graham cracker square. Top with another graham cracker square. Repeat for the remaining 13 sandwiches.

3. Place sandwiches on a baking sheet and freeze 1 to 2 hours.

DIETITIAN TIP: *If you like to enjoy dessert from time to time, portion control can help you indulge without overdoing it. Peanut butter powder can be found at some grocery stores, often in the health food section, or in warehouse stores.*

Nutrition Facts

Serves: 14
Serving Size: 1 sandwich

Amount per serving	
Calories	**90**

Calories from fat 15	
Total fat 1.5 g	
Saturated fat 0.3 g	
Trans fat 0.0 g	
Cholesterol 0 mg	
Sodium 190 mg	
Potassium 100 mg	
Total carbohydrate 15 g	
Dietary fiber 1 g	
Sugars 7 g	
Protein 3 g	
Phosphorus 85 mg	

Choices/Exchanges:
1 Carbohydrate, 1/2 Fat

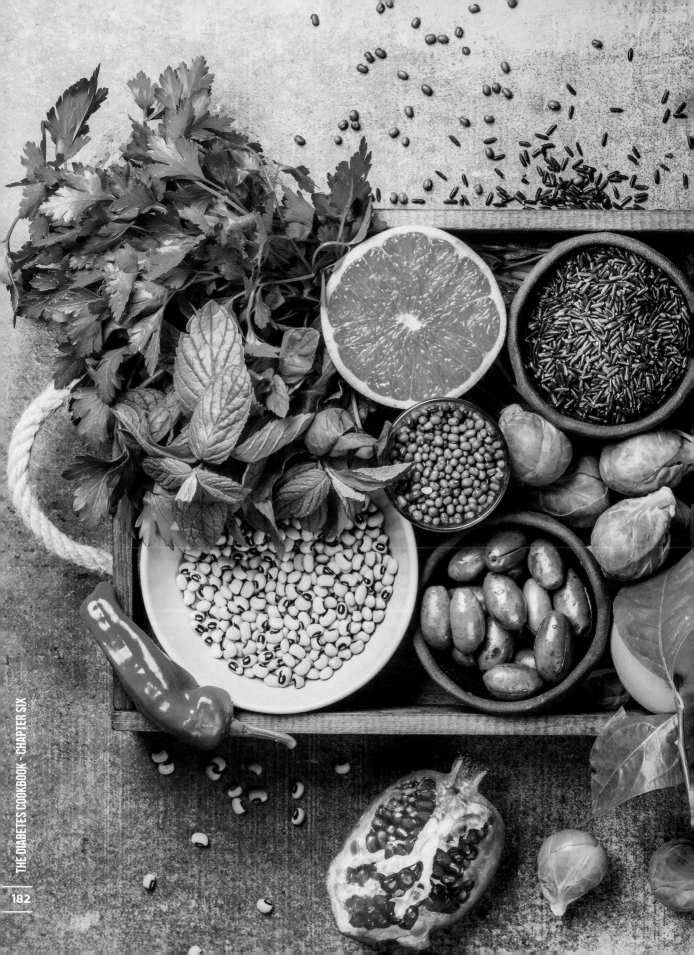

CHAPTER SIX
GLUTEN-FREE RECIPES

GLUTEN-FREE DISHES ARE OFTEN HIGH IN UNHEALTHY CARBS THAT ARE NOT GOOD FOR PEOPLE WITH DIABETES. THESE RECIPES ARE GLUTEN-FREE AND MADE WITH HEALTHY, GLUTEN-FREE GRAINS THAT ARE GOOD FOR PEOPLE WITH DIABETES, CELIAC DISEASE, AND THOSE FOLLOWING A GLUTEN-FREE DIET. OF COURSE, MAKE SURE TO CONFIRM ALL INGREDIENTS YOU USE IN THESE RECIPES ARE GLUTEN-FREE.

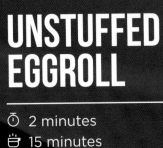

UNSTUFFED EGGROLL

- ⏱ 2 minutes
- 🍲 15 minutes
- 🍽 4 servings
- 🥛 About 1 1/2 cups

GF
LC

THIS DISH IS QUICK, EASY, DELICIOUS, AND CHOCK-FULL OF VEGETABLES WITH THE CONVENIENCE OF USING BAGGED COLESLAW. FOR MORE CRUNCH, ADD SLIVERED ALMONDS.

1	pound lean ground pork
1/2	teaspoon ground black pepper, divided
1	teaspoon garlic powder
1	tablespoon olive oil
1	clove garlic, minced
1	(16-ounce) bag tricolor coleslaw
2	tablespoons lite, gluten-free soy sauce
1	teaspoon ground ginger
3	green onions, sliced

1. Season pork with 1/4 teaspoon pepper and the garlic powder. Sauté pork in a large skillet over medium-high heat until completely cooked. Drain fat if needed. Remove pork from pan and set aside.

2. Heat olive oil in pan and add garlic; sauté 30 seconds. Add coleslaw, soy sauce, ginger, and 1/4 teaspoon pepper. Cook 6 minutes, stirring frequently. Add pork back to pan and top with green onions; heat 1–2 minutes.

3. Serve over brown rice or cauliflower rice if desired.

Nutrition Facts

Serves: 4
Serving Size: About 1 1/2 cups

Amount per serving
Calories **220**

Calories from fat 80

Total fat 9.0 g

 Saturated fat 2.0 g

 Trans fat 0.0 g

Cholesterol 60 mg

Sodium 490 mg

Potassium 680 mg

Total carbohydrate 9 g

 Dietary fiber 4 g

 Sugars 2 g

Protein 25 g

Phosphorus 250 mg

Choices/Exchanges: 2 Nonstarchy Vegetable, 3 Lean Protein, 1 Fat

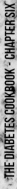

BEEF AND BROCCOLI OVER ZUCCHINI NOODLES

- ⏱ 15 minutes
- 🍲 10 minutes
- 🍽 4 servings
- 🥛 2 cups

GF

IF YOU DON'T HAVE A SPIRALIZER, USE A PEELER TO TRANSFORM ZUCCHINI INTO LONG STRIPS FOR A WIDE NOODLE STYLE.

1 cup fat-free, gluten-free, no-added-salt beef broth
1 tablespoon gluten-free cornstarch
2 tablespoons lite, gluten-free soy sauce
2 cloves garlic, minced
1 tablespoon minced fresh ginger
Nonstick cooking spray
2 teaspoons sesame oil
1 medium onion, sliced
1 pound sirloin beef, sliced
4 heaping cups broccoli florets
2 small zucchini, spiralized into noodles (yields 4 cups)
2 tablespoons toasted sesame seeds

1. In a small bowl, whisk together the broth, cornstarch, soy sauce, garlic, and ginger. Set aside.
2. Spray large sauté pan or wok with cooking spray, add sesame oil, and place over high heat.
3. Add the onion and stir-fry 2 minutes. Add the beef and stir-fry 3 more minutes.
4. Add the broccoli and spiralized zucchini and stir-fry 3 more minutes.
5. Add the broth mixture and bring to a boil, scraping the bottom of the pan to loosen any brown bits. Reduce heat and simmer 2 minutes.
6. Stir in sesame seeds and serve.

DIETITIAN TIP: *You now can find "zucchini noodles" in your grocer's freezer section by the frozen vegetables.*

Nutrition Facts

Serves: 4
Serving Size: 2 cups

Amount per serving
Calories **250**

Calories from fat 80

Total fat 9.0 g

   Saturated fat 2.4 g

   Trans fat 0.1 g

Cholesterol 40 mg

Sodium 500 mg

Potassium 950 mg

Total carbohydrate 15 g

   Dietary fiber 5 g

   Sugars 6 g

Protein 29 g

Phosphorus 330 mg

Choices/Exchanges: 3 Nonstarchy Vegetable, 3 Lean Protein, 1/2 Fat

ASPARAGUS FRITTATA

GF
LC
VG

⏱ 15 minutes
🍲 20 minutes
🍽 6 servings
🍽 1 slice

THIS RECIPE MAKES A GREAT BREAKFAST, BRUNCH, OR QUICK DINNER PACKED WITH PROTEIN AND VEGGIES. IF YOU DON'T LIKE ASPARAGUS, YOU CAN SUBSTITUTE ZUCCHINI OR BROCCOLI.

Nonstick cooking spray
1 bunch (about 12 ounces) thin asparagus, trimmed
1 tablespoon olive oil
1 (16-ounce) container egg substitute
2 tablespoons skim milk
1/2 teaspoon salt
1/4 teaspoon freshly ground black pepper
1/8 teaspoon crushed red pepper flakes
1 teaspoon trans fat–free margarine
1/4 cup shredded reduced-fat mozzarella cheese
1/4 cup freshly grated parmesan cheese

1. Preheat oven to 425°F.
2. Spray a baking sheet with cooking spray. In a small bowl, toss asparagus with olive oil. Place on baking sheet and bake about 12 minutes. Chop cooked asparagus into 1/2-inch pieces. Set aside.
3. In a medium bowl whisk together egg substitute, milk, salt, black pepper, and red pepper flakes. Set aside and preheat broiler.
4. Spray a 9 1/2-inch nonstick ovenproof skillet with cooking spray. Add margarine to skillet and melt over medium heat. Add asparagus to skillet and pour the egg mixture over the asparagus. Cook a few minutes until the eggs start to set.
5. Add the mozzarella and parmesan cheese. Reduce heat to medium-low and cook until the frittata is almost set but the top is still runny, about 2 minutes.

6. Place the skillet under the broiler. Broil until the top is set and golden brown, 2–4 minutes. Let the frittata stand 2 minutes. Using a rubber spatula, loosen the frittata from the skillet and slide the frittata onto a plate. Slice into 6 wedges.

Nutrition Facts

Serves: 6
Serving Size: 1 slice

Amount per serving
Calories **100**

Calories from fat 40

Total fat 4.5 g

Saturated fat 1.5 g

Trans fat 0.0 g

Cholesterol 5 mg

Sodium 430 mg

Potassium 240 mg

Total carbohydrate 4 g

Dietary fiber 1 g

Sugars 2 g

Protein 12 g

Phosphorus 85 mg

Choices/Exchanges: 2 Lean Protein

GLUTEN-FREE BANANA BREAD

⏱ 15 minutes
🍲 35 minutes
🍽 16 servings
☕ 1 slice (1/16 of recipe)

GF
VG

THIS BANANA BREAD MAKES A NICE TREAT, AND IT'S GLUTEN-FREE! INSTEAD OF ONE LARGE LOAF, BAKE IT IN FOUR MINI LOAF PANS FOR SMALLER BREADS THAT CAN BE WRAPPED AND GIVEN AS GIFTS.

Nonstick cooking spray
4 medium very ripe bananas, mashed
2 tablespoons olive oil
1 cup low-fat buttermilk
2 egg whites
1 teaspoon vanilla extract
1/4 cup low-calorie granulated sugar blend (such as Splenda Sugar Blend)
2 cups gluten-free baking mix
3 tablespoons milled flaxseed

1. Preheat oven to 350°F. Spray an 8-by-4-inch loaf pan with cooking spray.
2. In a large bowl, combine bananas, oil, buttermilk, egg whites, vanilla, and sugar blend; mix well.
3. Add gluten-free baking mix and flaxseed and mix until blended. Pour batter into loaf pan. Bake 30–35 minutes or until a toothpick inserted in the center comes out clean.

Nutrition Facts

Serves: 16
Serving Size: 1 slice (1/16 of recipe)

Amount per serving
Calories 140

Calories from fat 25

Total fat 3.0 g	
Saturated fat 0.4 g	
Trans fat 0.0 g	
Cholesterol 0 mg	
Sodium 240 mg	
Potassium 280 mg	
Total carbohydrate 25 g	
Dietary fiber 3 g	
Sugars 9 g	
Protein 4 g	
Phosphorus 70 mg	

Choices/Exchanges: 1 Starch, 1/2 Fruit, 1/2 Fat

GLUTEN-FREE CHOCOLATE ZUCCHINI MUFFINS

⏱ 20 minutes
🍳 20 minutes
△ 14 servings
🍽 1 muffin

GF
VG

TO INCREASE YOUR WHOLE-GRAIN INTAKE, USE A GLUTEN-FREE BAKING MIX THAT LISTS BROWN RICE FLOUR AS THE FIRST INGREDIENT. CERTIFIED GLUTEN-FREE OATS CAN BE SUBSTITUTED FOR QUINOA FLAKES HERE AS WELL.

Nonstick cooking spray
1/4 cup olive oil
1/4 cup low-calorie granulated sugar blend (such as Truvia Baking Blend)
1 teaspoon vanilla extract
1 large zucchini, grated and drained
2 eggs
1 cup all-purpose gluten-free baking mix (such as King Arthur Gluten Free All-Purpose Baking Mix)
1/2 cup quinoa flakes
1/2 cup cocoa powder
1 tablespoon water
2 tablespoons mini chocolate chips

CHEF TIP: *Make sure to squeeze and press any liquid out of the zucchini after grating.*

1. Preheat oven to 350°F. Line muffin tins with muffin papers and spray the papers with cooking spray.
2. In a large bowl, mix together the oil, sugar blend, and vanilla. Add the zucchini and add the eggs one at a time. Mix well.
3. Stir in the baking mix, quinoa flakes, cocoa powder, and water.
4. Spoon the batter into 14 muffin cups. Top each muffin with mini chocolate chips (distribute evenly over all muffins).
5. Bake 20–22 minutes or until a toothpick inserted in the center of a muffin comes out clean.
6. Remove from the oven and let the muffins cool in the pan 10 minutes. Remove the muffins from the pan and cool completely on a wire rack.

Nutrition Facts

Serves: 14
Serving Size: 1 muffin

Amount per serving
Calories 120

Calories from fat 50	
Total fat 6.0 g	
Saturated fat 1.4 g	
Trans fat 0.0 g	
Cholesterol 25 mg	
Sodium 85 mg	
Potassium 170 mg	
Total carbohydrate 16 g	
Dietary fiber 3 g	
Sugars 4 g	
Protein 3 g	
Phosphorus 130 mg	

Choices/Exchanges: 1 Starch, 1 Fat

HIGH-FIBER GLUTEN-FREE BROWNIES

⏱ 15 minutes
🍲 20 minutes
🍽 12 servings
🍴 1 brownie

GF
VG

DON'T BE AFRAID OF THE BLACK BEANS IN THIS RECIPE. YOU CAN'T TASTE THEM, AND THEY ADD A NUTRITION KICK AND FIBER BOOST THAT YOU WON'T FIND IN REGULAR BROWNIES.

Nonstick cooking spray
3/4 cup canned black beans, rinsed and drained
1/4 cup olive oil
2 tablespoons water
1 egg plus 2 egg whites
1/4 cup cocoa powder
1/4 cup plus 1 tablespoon low-calorie granulated sugar blend (such as Truvia Baking Blend)
1 teaspoon instant coffee
1 teaspoon vanilla extract
1/3 cup gluten-free all-purpose baking mix (such as King Arthur Gluten Free All-Purpose Baking Mix)
1/4 cup gluten-free mini chocolate chips

1. Preheat oven to 350°F. Spray a 9-inch square baking pan with cooking spray.
2. In a blender, purée the beans with the oil and water. Add the eggs, cocoa, baking blend, coffee, and vanilla, and blend well.
3. Add the baking mix to the blender and pulse until just incorporated. Stir in mini chocolate chips. Pour into the prepared pan.
4. Bake 18–20 minutes.
5. Let cool at least 15 minutes before cutting and removing from the pan.

Nutrition Facts

Serves: 12
Serving Size: 1 brownie

Amount per serving
Calories 110

Calories from fat 50	
Total fat 6.0 g	
Saturated fat 1.6 g	
Trans fat 0.0 g	
Cholesterol 15 mg	
Sodium 75 mg	
Potassium 125 mg	
Total carbohydrate 12 g	
Dietary fiber 2 g	
Sugars 5 g	
Protein 3 g	
Phosphorus 50 mg	

Choices/Exchanges: 1 Carbohydrate, 1 Fat

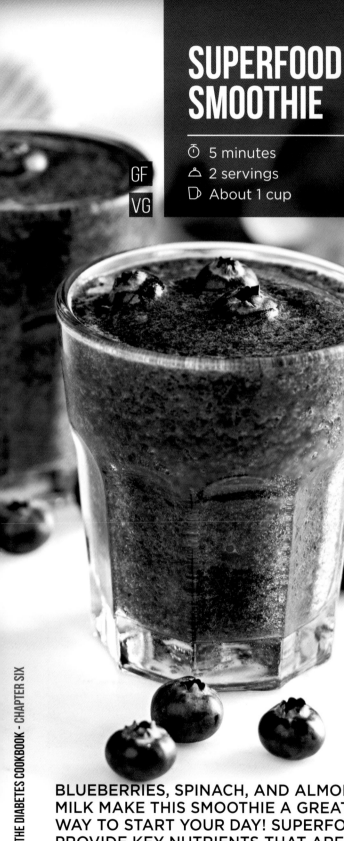

SUPERFOOD SMOOTHIE

GF
VG

- ⏱ 5 minutes
- 🍽 2 servings
- 🥤 About 1 cup

1   cup original almond milk
1   cup frozen blueberries
2   cups baby spinach
1   medium banana

1. Combine all ingredients in a blender and purée until smooth and thick.

Nutrition Facts

Serves: 2
Serving Size: About 1 cup

Amount per serving
Calories 120

Calories from fat 20	
Total fat 2.0 g	
Saturated fat 0.1 g	
Trans fat 0.0 g	
Cholesterol 0 mg	
Sodium 115 mg	
Potassium 510 mg	
Total carbohydrate 25 g	
Dietary fiber 4 g	
Sugars 14 g	
Protein 2 g	
Phosphorus 45 mg	

Choices/Exchanges: 1 1/2 Fruit, 1/2 Fat

BLUEBERRIES, SPINACH, AND ALMOND MILK MAKE THIS SMOOTHIE A GREAT WAY TO START YOUR DAY! SUPERFOODS PROVIDE KEY NUTRIENTS THAT ARE LACKING IN THE TYPICAL WESTERN DIET.

CHICKEN TOSTADAS

THESE CHICKEN TOSTADAS ARE A DELICIOUS DISH THAT WON'T BREAK THE BANK. SAVE TIME BY BUYING A ROTISSERIE CHICKEN.

- ⏱ 10 minutes
- 🍲 5 minutes
- 🍽 4 servings
- 🍴 1 tostada

GF

2	cups shredded cooked chicken breast
3	tablespoons salsa
1	cup canned pinto beans, rinsed and drained
4	tostada shells
4	tablespoons shredded reduced-fat cheddar cheese
1/2	avocado, mashed
1	cup shredded lettuce

1. Preheat oven to 400°F. In a small bowl, mix together the chicken, salsa, and pinto beans.
2. Place the tostada shells on a baking sheet. Top each tostada shell with 1/2 cup chicken mixture and 1 tablespoon cheese. Bake 5 minutes or until the cheese is melted.
3. Remove the tostadas from the oven and top each with a spoonful of mashed avocado and 1/4 cup lettuce.

CHEF TIP: *Heat up some frozen bell peppers and onions by lightly sautéing on the stove. Add some cumin and chili powder to up the flavor of this veggie side dish.*

Nutrition Facts

Serves: 4
Serving Size: 1 tostada

Amount per serving
Calories **310**

Calories from fat 90

Total fat 10.0 g

Saturated fat 2.6 g

Trans fat 0.0 g

Cholesterol 65 mg

Sodium 270 mg

Potassium 550 mg

Total carbohydrate 26 g

Dietary fiber 6 g

Sugars 1 g

Protein 29 g

Phosphorus 310 mg

Choices/Exchanges: 2 Starch, 4 Lean Protein

BROWN RICE AND PINTO BEAN BOWL WITH CHICKEN AND PICO DE GALLO

- ⏱ 10 minutes
- ☕ 10 minutes (includes time to assemble bowl)
- 🍽 6 servings
- 🥣 1 bowl

GF

REFRIED BEANS

- 2 teaspoons olive oil
- 1 medium onion, diced, divided
- 2 cups cooked pinto beans (see Note)
- 1 tablespoon chili powder
- 1 teaspoon cumin
- 1/4 teaspoon ground cayenne pepper
- 1/4 teaspoon ground black pepper
- 1/2 cup water

PICO DE GALLO

- 1 medium tomato, seeded and diced
- 1 medium jalapeño pepper, seeded, deveined, and minced
- 1/4 cup chopped fresh cilantro
- Juice of 1 lime

REMAINING INGREDIENTS

- 2 cups cooked brown rice, warmed (see Note)
- 1/2 teaspoon salt
- 2 cups shredded cooked chicken, warmed
- 1 avocado, peeled, seeded, and sliced
- 1 lime, sliced

1. Add oil to a sauté pan over medium heat. Add half the diced onion, the pinto beans, chili powder, cumin, cayenne pepper, black pepper, and water. Sauté, slightly mashing the beans as you sauté until the liquid is absorbed, about 5 minutes.

2. In a small bowl, mix together the tomato, jalapeño pepper, remaining diced onion, cilantro, and lime juice. Set aside.

3. Season the brown rice with salt.

MAKING YOUR OWN PICO DE GALLO IN THIS RECIPE HELPS YOU AVOID THE SODIUM FOUND IN STORE-BOUGHT SALSAS. THE FRESH FLAVOR IS A BONUS!

4. Divide the brown rice into six salad or soup bowls, top with cooked refried beans, chicken, pico de gallo, sliced avocado, and 1 slice of lime per bowl.

NOTE: *For directions on bulk cooking dry pinto beans, see page 21. For directions on bulk cooking brown rice, see page 21.*

CHEF TIP: *Layer this dish in a jar and take it to work for a fun, appetizing lunch. It can be eaten hot or cold!*

DIETITIAN TIP: *To reduce carbs, substitute cauliflower rice for brown rice here.*

Nutrition Facts

Serves: 6
Serving Size: 1 bowl

Amount per serving
Calories 330

Calories from fat 90	
Total fat 10.0 g	
Saturated fat 2.0 g	
Trans fat 0.0 g	
Cholesterol 40 mg	
Sodium 260 mg	
Potassium 700 mg	
Total carbohydrate 39 g	
Dietary fiber 9 g	
Sugars 3 g	
Protein 22 g	
Phosphorus 280 mg	

Choices/Exchanges: 2 Starch, 1 Nonstarchy Vegetable, 2 Lean Protein, 1 Fat

ASIAN CHICKEN SALAD

GF
LC

⏱ 5 minutes
🍽 4 servings
🥛 2 cups

SALAD

1	(9-ounce) bag romaine lettuce
1	cup shredded cabbage
1	cup shredded carrots
1/4	cup slivered almonds, toasted
1	tablespoon sesame seeds, toasted
2	cups diced cooked chicken breast

DRESSING

2	tablespoons rice vinegar
2	tablespoons lite, gluten-free soy sauce
2	tablespoons extra-virgin olive oil
1	teaspoon toasted sesame seeds
1/4	teaspoon crushed red pepper flakes

1. In a medium bowl mix together all salad ingredients.
2. In a small bowl whisk together dressing ingredients.
3. Pour dressing over salad and toss to coat.

Nutrition Facts

Serves: 4
Serving Size: 2 cups

Amount per serving
Calories 270

Calories from fat 140

Total fat 15.0 g

   Saturated fat 2.2 g

   Trans fat 0.0 g

Cholesterol 60 mg

Sodium 470 mg

Potassium 540 mg

Total carbohydrate 9 g

   Dietary fiber 4 g

   Sugars 3 g

Protein 26 g

Phosphorus 260 mg

Choices/Exchanges: 2 Nonstarchy Vegetable, 3 Lean Protein, 2 Fat

AVOCADO CHICKEN SALAD WRAP

○ 10 minutes
△ 4 servings
▷ 1 wrap

GF

CHECK THE INGREDIENTS IN GLUTEN-FREE TORTILLAS OR WRAPS, AND TRY TO FIND ONES MADE WITH WHOLE GRAINS SUCH AS TEFF OR SORGHUM.

2   cups shredded cooked chicken breast
1/4   cup mashed avocado
2   tablespoons plain hummus
3   stalks celery, diced
1/8   teaspoon ground black pepper
1/4   teaspoon dried thyme
4   gluten-free whole-grain wraps (such as La Tortilla Factory Gluten-Free Wraps)
4   cups field greens

1. In a medium bowl mix together the chicken, avocado, hummus, celery, pepper, and thyme.
2. Spread 1/2 cup chicken salad in the middle of 1 wrap. Top with 1 cup field greens. Fold sides of the wrap in until they touch, and then roll from the bottom to make a wrap.
3. Repeat procedure for remaining 3 wraps.

Nutrition Facts

Serves: 4
Serving Size: 1 wrap

Amount per serving

Calories   **350**

Calories from fat 100	
Total fat 11.0 g	
Saturated fat 2.6 g	
Trans fat 0.0 g	
Cholesterol 60 mg	
Sodium 460 mg	
Potassium 650 mg	
Total carbohydrate 38 g	
Dietary fiber 6 g	
Sugars 3 g	
Protein 25 g	
Phosphorus 430 mg	

Choices/Exchanges: 2 Starch, 1 Nonstarchy Vegetable, 3 Lean Protein, 1 Fat

HERB-STUFFED CHICKEN BREAST WITH BRUSCHETTA SAUCE

THIS LOWER-CARB RECIPE PAIRS WELL WITH A SMALL SERVING OF QUINOA AND A SIDE SALAD.

GF
LC

- ⏱ 15 minutes
- 🍳 45 minutes
- 🍽 6 servings
- 🥄 4 ounces chicken

Nonstick cooking spray

BRUSCHETTA

- 3   roma tomatoes, seeded and diced
- 1/2   small red onion, diced
- 1   tablespoon chopped fresh oregano
- 1   tablespoon red wine vinegar
- 1   tablespoon olive oil

CHICKEN

- 2 1/4   pounds boneless skinless chicken breasts
- 1/2   teaspoon salt
- 1/2   teaspoon ground black pepper
- 1/4   cup chopped fresh basil
- 1/4   cup freshly grated parmesan cheese

1. Preheat oven to 375°F. Coat a baking dish with cooking spray. Set aside.

2. In a small bowl, toss together tomatoes, onion, oregano, vinegar, and olive oil.

3. Butterfly each chicken breast and open. Season both sides of all chicken breasts with salt and pepper.

4. Toss basil and parmesan cheese together in a small bowl, and then divide the mixture evenly among the open chicken breasts. Fold the chicken breasts back in half, and place them in the baking dish.

5. Pour the tomato mixture over the chicken breasts and bake 35–45 minutes (depending on the size of the chicken breasts) or until the internal temperature is 165°F.

Nutrition Facts

Serves: 6

Serving Size: 4 ounces chicken

Amount per serving	
Calories	**230**

Calories from fat 60	
Total fat 7.0 g	
Saturated fat 2.0 g	
Trans fat 0.0 g	
Cholesterol 100 mg	
Sodium 320 mg	
Potassium 400 mg	
Total carbohydrate 2 g	
Dietary fiber 1 g	
Sugars 1 g	
Protein 38 g	
Phosphorus 295 mg	

Choices/Exchanges: 5 Lean Protein

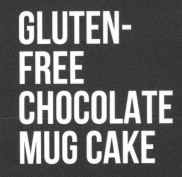

GLUTEN-FREE CHOCOLATE MUG CAKE

⏱ 5 minutes
🍳 1 minute
◁ 1 serving
🥤 1 mug cake

GF
VG

THIS CAKE IS DELICIOUS SERVED WITH RASPBERRIES (IF DESIRED). NO RASPBERRIES? SERVE WITH STRAWBERRIES OR ANOTHER FRUIT. WHEN YOU WANT TO ENJOY A QUICK TREAT, A DESSERT LIKE THIS MUG CAKE WITH FRUIT IS A GOOD PORTION-CONTROLLED CHOICE.

1	tablespoon gluten-free flour
1	tablespoon certified gluten-free oats
1	tablespoon unsweetened cocoa powder
1/8	teaspoon baking powder
1/16	teaspoon salt
4	packets sugar substitute (such as Truvia)
2 1/2	tablespoons skim milk
1 1/2	teaspoons olive oil
1	tablespoon water
1/8	teaspoon vanilla extract
1/2	cup raspberries

1. In a large mug, mix together flour, gluten-free oats, cocoa powder, baking powder, salt, and sugar substitute. Add milk, oil, water, and vanilla. Stir to mix well.
2. Microwave 1 minute to 1 1/2 minutes. Top with fresh raspberries.

DIETITIAN TIP: *You can add 1 teaspoon mini chocolate chips for extra chocolate flavor, but this will increase the carbs and fat a bit.*

Nutrition Facts

Serves: 1
Serving Size: 1 mug cake

Amount per serving
Calories 170

Calories from fat 80

Total fat 9.0 g

   Saturated fat 1.5 g

   Trans fat 0.0 g

Cholesterol 0 mg

Sodium 210 mg

Potassium 290 mg

Total carbohydrate 23 g

   Dietary fiber 7 g

   Sugars 6 g

Protein 5 g

Phosphorus 200 mg

Choices/Exchanges: 1/2 Fruit, 1 Carbohydrate, 1 1/2 Fat

SPINACH, MUSHROOM, EGG, AND HAM CUPS

🕐 15 minutes
⏲ 30 minutes
🍽 8 servings
🍵 1 muffin cup

GF
LC

THESE EGG-AND-HAM CUPS ARE ABSOLUTELY DELICIOUS AND SATISFYING. THEY ARE ALSO MUCH BETTER FOR YOUR BLOOD GLUCOSE THAN A BOWL OF SUGARY CEREAL. AS AN ADDED BONUS, YOU GET SOME VEGGIES IN THIS LOW-CARB BREAKFAST.

Nonstick cooking spray
8 slices (1/2 ounce each) gluten-free lower-in-sodium deli-style smoked ham
2 teaspoons olive oil
1/2 cup diced mushrooms
1 cup chopped baby spinach
5 eggs
1/8 teaspoon fresh ground black pepper
1/3 cup shredded reduced-fat cheddar cheese

1. Preheat oven to 350°F. Spray a muffin tin with cooking spray.
2. Line 8 muffin cups with a slice of ham.
3. Add the oil to a sauté pan and heat over medium-high heat. Add the mushrooms and cook 3 minutes. Add the spinach and cook another 3 minutes. Set the vegetables aside to cool.
4. In a medium bowl, whisk together the eggs, spinach, mushrooms, pepper, and cheese.
5. Carefully fill the 8 muffin cups (lined with ham) with the egg mixture 2/3 full (try not to drip egg mixture under the ham slices).
6. Bake 20–22 minutes, until the eggs are cooked through. Let cool 5 minutes. Use a fork to loosen the edges of the ham-and-egg cups. Use a fork to scoop out each cup.

Nutrition Facts

Serves: 8
Serving Size: 1 muffin cup

Amount per serving
Calories   **80**

Calories from fat 45

Total fat 5.0 g
    Saturated fat 1.8 g
    Trans fat 0.0 g
Cholesterol 125 mg
Sodium 200 mg
Potassium 115 mg
Total carbohydrate 1 g
    Dietary fiber 0 g
    Sugars 1 g
Protein 8 g
Phosphorus 120 mg

Choices/Exchanges: 1 Medium-Fat Protein

SPICY APRICOT-GLAZED PORK WITH SWEET POTATOES AND PEPPERS

- ⏱ 10 minutes
- 🍲 30 minutes
- 🍽 4 servings
- 🍽 3 ounces pork and 2/3 cup vegetables

GF

THIS RECIPE IS HEALTHY, QUICK, AND BUDGET-FRIENDLY. IT MAKES A TASTY MEAL, COMPLETE WITH NONSTARCHY VEGETABLES, STARCHY POTATOES, AND LEAN PORK TENDERLOIN.

PORK

1	pound pork tenderloin
1/4	teaspoon ground black pepper
1/2	teaspoon garlic powder

APRICOT GLAZE

1/2	cup sugar-free apricot preserves
1/4	teaspoon crushed red pepper flakes
1/4	teaspoon dried oregano

VEGETABLES

1	large sweet potato, peeled and cubed
1	large green bell pepper, cut into 1-inch strips

1. Preheat oven to 350°F. Season the pork with black pepper and garlic powder. Place the pork in a baking dish.

2. In a small bowl, mix together the apricot glaze ingredients. Microwave the glaze 1–2 minutes, until the mixture becomes thin and easy to stir. Pour the glaze over the pork tenderloin and coat it evenly.

3. Spread the sweet potato and green pepper around the pork. Bake 30 minutes or until the pork is done (when it reaches an internal temperature of 145°F).

Nutrition Facts

Serves: 4

Serving Size: 3 ounces pork and 2/3 cup vegetables

Amount per serving

Calories 190

Calories from fat 25

Total fat 3.0 g

Saturated fat 1.0 g

Trans fat 0.0 g

Cholesterol 60 mg

Sodium 60 mg

Potassium 680 mg

Total carbohydrate 17 g

Dietary fiber 6 g

Sugars 5 g

Protein 23 g

Phosphorus 235 mg

Choices/Exchanges: 1/2 Starch, 1/2 Carbohydrate, 3 Lean Protein

KALE IS A SUPERFOOD THAT YOU MUST TRY IF YOU HAVEN'T ALREADY. IT'S AN EXCELLENT SOURCE OF ANTIOXIDANT VITAMINS A, C, AND K. IT'S ALSO A GREAT SOURCE OF POTASSIUM AND FIBER WHILE BEING LOW IN CARBOHYDRATES AND CALORIES.

KALE SOUP WITH TURKEY AND BEANS

- ⏱ 20 minutes
- 🍲 30 minutes
- 🍽 7 servings
- 🍵 About 1 cup

GF

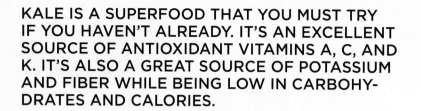

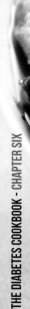

2	teaspoons olive oil
1	yellow onion, diced
1/2	cup diced green bell pepper
1	clove garlic, minced
6	ounces lean ground turkey
32	ounces fat-free, gluten-free, reduced-sodium chicken broth
1/2	cup canned crushed tomatoes
1/2	teaspoon dried basil
1/2	teaspoon dried thyme
1/2	teaspoon dried rosemary
1/8	teaspoon cayenne pepper
1	(15.5-ounce) can black-eyed peas, rinsed and drained
3	cups chopped kale
3	tablespoons freshly grated parmesan cheese

1. Heat the oil in a large soup pot over medium-high heat. Add onion and green pepper, and sauté 3 minutes or until onion is clear. Add the garlic and sauté 30 seconds.
2. Add the turkey and cook about 8 minutes until brown. Add the remaining ingredients except for the parmesan cheese.
3. Bring the soup to a boil; then reduce heat and simmer 15 minutes.
4. Remove the soup from the heat and stir in the parmesan cheese.

Nutrition Facts

Serves: 7
Serving Size: About 1 cup

Amount per serving

Calories 140

Calories from fat 35	
Total fat 4.0 g	
Saturated fat 1.1 g	
Trans fat 0.0 g	
Cholesterol 20 mg	
Sodium 220 mg	
Potassium 460 mg	
Total carbohydrate 14 g	
Dietary fiber 4 g	
Sugars 4 g	
Protein 13 g	
Phosphorus 195 mg	

Choices/Exchanges: 1/2 Starch, 1 Nonstarchy Vegetable, 2 Lean Protein

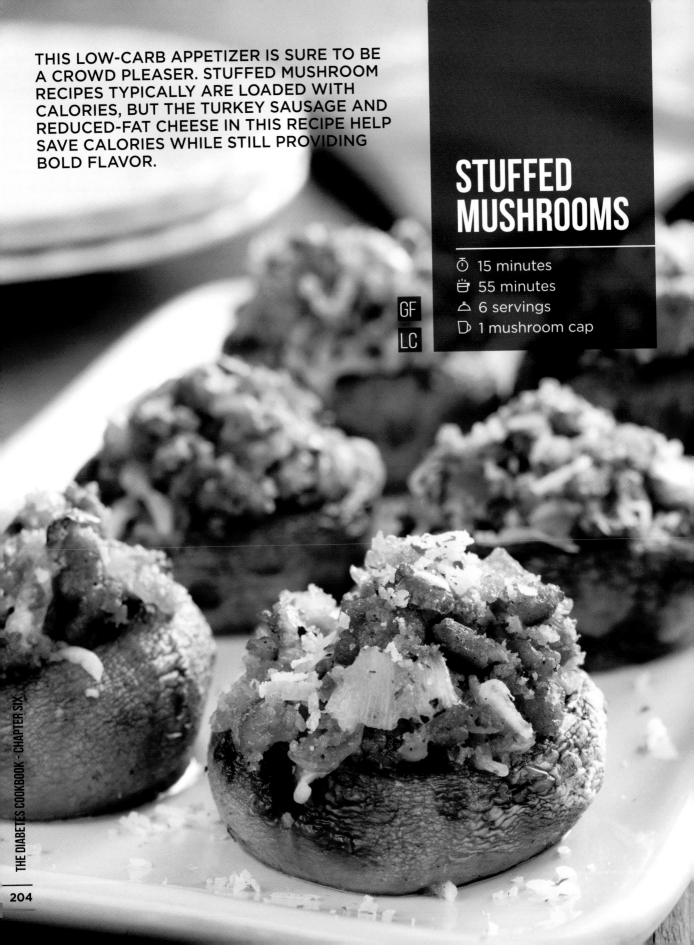

THIS LOW-CARB APPETIZER IS SURE TO BE A CROWD PLEASER. STUFFED MUSHROOM RECIPES TYPICALLY ARE LOADED WITH CALORIES, BUT THE TURKEY SAUSAGE AND REDUCED-FAT CHEESE IN THIS RECIPE HELP SAVE CALORIES WHILE STILL PROVIDING BOLD FLAVOR.

STUFFED MUSHROOMS

GF
LC

- ⏱ 15 minutes
- 🍲 55 minutes
- △ 6 servings
- 🍽 1 mushroom cap

Nonstick cooking spray
6 extra-large white mushrooms (8 ounces)
2 teaspoons olive oil, divided
2 teaspoons balsamic vinegar
1/4 small onion, diced
1/4 small green pepper, diced
2 ounces gluten-free lean turkey breakfast sausage
2 tablespoons gluten-free bread crumbs
1 tablespoon reduced-fat shredded mozzarella cheese
1 tablespoon freshly grated parmesan cheese

1. Preheat oven to 325°F. Coat an 8-inch-by-8-inch square baking dish with cooking spray.
2. Remove the stems from the mushrooms and chop the stems finely. Set aside.
3. Place the mushroom caps in a bowl and toss them with 1 teaspoon olive oil and balsamic vinegar. Set aside the caps.
4. Heat the remaining teaspoon olive oil in a medium skillet over medium heat. Add the onion, green pepper, and mushroom stems, and sauté 3 minutes. Add the sausage and cook another 8–10 minutes, stirring frequently, until the sausage is completely browned.
5. Add the bread crumbs, stirring to combine evenly with all the other ingredients. Stir in the mozzarella cheese and melt.
6. Remove the pan from the heat and stir in the parmesan cheese.

7. Fill each mushroom cap with the sausage mixture (about 1 heaping tablespoon per mushroom cap). Arrange the mushrooms in the baking dish, and bake 40 minutes or until the topping is crispy.

Nutrition Facts

Serves: 6
Serving Size: 1 mushroom cap

Amount per serving
Calories 50

Calories from fat 25

Total fat 3.0 g	
Saturated fat 0.7 g	
Trans fat 0.0 g	
Cholesterol 10 mg	
Sodium 85 mg	
Potassium 160 mg	
Total carbohydrate 3 g	
Dietary fiber 1 g	
Sugars 1 g	
Protein 4 g	
Phosphorus 60 mg	

Choices/Exchanges: 1 Nonstarchy Vegetable, 1/2 Fat

GLUTEN-FREE SCRUMPTIOUS PUMPKIN BREAD

GF
VG

⏱ 10 minutes
🍲 60 minutes
🍽 18 servings
🍴 1 slice

IF YOU DON'T NEED THIS RECIPE TO BE GLUTEN-FREE, YOU COULD USE YELLOW CAKE MIX OR CARROT CAKE MIX IN PLACE OF THE GLUTEN-FREE BREAD MIX. THIS QUICK BREAD IS A FESTIVE AND DELICIOUS HOLIDAY TREAT!

Nonstick cooking spray
1 egg
3 egg whites
1/3 cup skim milk
1 (15-ounce) can pure pumpkin
1/3 cup olive oil
1 (19-ounce) box gluten-free bread mix
1 teaspoon cinnamon
Pinch nutmeg
1/4 cup plus 1 tablespoon mini chocolate chips, divided
1/4 cup plus 1 tablespoon chopped walnuts, divided

1. Preheat oven to 350°F. Spray a large loaf pan with cooking spray.
2. In a large bowl, combine egg, egg whites, milk, pumpkin, and oil. Mix until blended well.
3. Add bread mix, cinnamon, and nutmeg to wet ingredients, and mix well.
4. Stir in 1/4 cup chocolate chips and 1/4 cup walnuts. Pour batter into loaf pan. Sprinkle 1 tablespoon each of chocolate chips and walnuts on top of batter.
5. Bake 50–60 minutes or until toothpick inserted in the center comes out clean.

Nutrition Facts

Serves: 18
Serving Size: 1 slice

Amount per serving
Calories 190

Calories from fat 60

Total fat 7.0 g
    Saturated fat 1.4 g
    Trans fat 0.0 g
Cholesterol 10 mg
Sodium 220 mg
Potassium 115 mg
Total carbohydrate 30 g
    Dietary fiber 1 g
    Sugars 14 g
Protein 2 g
Phosphorus 60 mg

Choices/Exchanges: 2 Carbohydrate, 1 Fat

RAJAS POBLANOS AND SKIRT STEAK TACOS

- ⏱ 30 minutes
- 🍲 20 minutes
- 🍽 4 servings
- 🌮 2 tacos

GF

GREEN OR RED BELL PEPPERS CAN BE USED IN PLACE OF THE POBLANO PEPPERS IN THIS RECIPE.

1	tablespoon olive oil
2	cloves garlic, minced
2	large poblano peppers, seeded and thinly sliced
1	small onion, thinly sliced
1	tablespoon chili powder
1	teaspoon cumin
1/4	teaspoon cayenne pepper
1/2	teaspoon salt
1/4	teaspoon ground black pepper
1/4	cup shredded reduced-fat Mexican-style cheese
1/2	pound skirt steak
8	(6-inch) corn tortillas
2	large tomatoes, diced
4	cups shredded lettuce

1. Preheat an indoor or outdoor grill.

2. Add the oil to a large nonstick sauté pan over medium-high heat. Add the garlic, poblano peppers, onion, chili powder, cumin, cayenne pepper, salt, and pepper. Sauté 8–10 minutes until the vegetables are soft and starting to caramelize.

3. Stir in the cheese and set aside.

4. Season the skirt steak with additional salt and black pepper. Grill on both sides until the steak is medium doneness. Set the steak aside to rest.

5. Once the steak has rested, chop it into small pieces and stir into the pepper and cheese mixture over medium heat until steak has just cooked through.

6. Divide the meat mixture evenly among the 8 tortillas; then top each taco with chopped tomato and shredded lettuce.

Nutrition Facts

Serves: 4
Serving Size: 2 tacos

Amount per serving
Calories 310

Calories from fat 110

Total fat 12.0 g

    Saturated fat 3.3 g

    Trans fat 0.2 g

Cholesterol 40 mg

Sodium 410 mg

Potassium 690 mg

Total carbohydrate 36 g

    Dietary fiber 6 g

    Sugars 6 g

Protein 19 g

Phosphorus 330 mg

Choices/Exchanges: 1 1/2 Starch, 2 Nonstarchy Vegetable, 2 Lean Protein, 1 1/2 Fat

GRILLED STEAK WITH MUSHROOMS

⏱ 5 minutes
🍲 25 minutes
🍽 2 servings
🍴 1 steak with 1 cup mushrooms

GF
LC

THIS PROTEIN-PACKED DISH IS LOW IN SODIUM AND FAT AND MAKES FOR A GREAT HEARTY SUMMER MEAL.

Nonstick cooking spray
2   (4-ounce) fillet steaks (1 1/2 inches thick)
1/4 teaspoon ground black pepper
1   tablespoon trans fat–free margarine
1   pint button mushrooms, sliced

1. Prepare an indoor or outdoor grill and heat to high. Spray grill rack with cooking spray.
2. Sprinkle steaks evenly with salt and pepper.
3. Place steaks on grill with direct high heat and sear 1–2 minutes per side. Reduce heat to medium and cook 18–23 minutes or until done according to your preference (flipping once). Transfer steak to a plate and cover with foil; let rest 5 minutes before serving.
4. In a medium sauté pan, heat margarine over medium-high heat. Add mushrooms and sauté 5–6 minutes until tender.

DIETITIAN TIP: *This steak pairs wonderfully with an arugula salad to make half your plate veggies.*

Nutrition Facts

Serves: 2

Serving Size: 1 steak with 1 cup mushrooms

Amount per serving

Calories 190

Calories from fat 90

Total fat 10.0 g

   Saturated fat 3.1 g

   Trans fat 0.0 g

Cholesterol 60 mg

Sodium 90 mg

Potassium 490 mg

Total carbohydrate 2 g

   Dietary fiber 1 g

   Sugars 1 g

Protein 23 g

Phosphorus 225 mg

Choices/Exchanges: 3 Lean Protein, 1 Fat

SWEET POTATO BURRITO BOWL

⏱ 15 minutes
🍲 60 minutes
🍽 4 servings
🥣 1 bowl

VG
GF

THESE BURRITO BOWLS CAN BE MADE AHEAD OF TIME AND STORED IN A MICROWAVE-SAFE CONTAINER. JUST LEAVE OUT THE LETTUCE, YOGURT, AND TOMATO. WHEN IT'S TIME TO EAT, REHEAT THE BOWL, AND THEN ADD THE COLD TOPPINGS. THIS MAKES A GREAT HOT LUNCH AT THE OFFICE!

Nonstick cooking spray
2 small to medium sweet potatoes (final cooked weight of potatoes is 12 ounces)
1 (12-ounce) bag fozen cauliflower rice
2 teaspoons olive oil
1 small onion, diced small (about 3/4 cup)
2 cloves garlic, minced or grated
1 cup no-salt-added canned black beans, drained and rinsed
1 cup salsa
1/2 cup shredded 2% Mexican-style cheese
2 cups shredded lettuce
1/4 cup fat-free plain Greek yogurt
1 cup diced tomatoes

1. Preheat oven to 400°F. Coat a baking sheet with cooking spray. Scrub and dry the potatoes and place them on the baking sheet. Bake the potatoes 45–60 minutes until very tender.
2. While the potatoes are cooking, cook the cauliflower rice according to directions on the package. Set the cooked rice aside but keep warm.
3. Add the olive oil to a nonstick pan over medium heat. Add the onion and garlic and sauté 5 minutes or until the onion starts to soften.
4. Add the beans and salsa, and simmer to heat the beans through. Set the bean and salsa mixture aside but keep warm.
5. When the potatoes are done cooking, let them cool slightly; then peel and cube.
6. To build 1 burrito bowl, place 1 cup cauliflower rice in a bowl. Top with 1/4 of sweet potatoes. Top with 1/2 cup bean and salsa mixture, then top with 2 tablespoons cheese.
7. To serve, top with 1/2 cup lettuce, 1 tablespoon yogurt, and 1/4 cup tomatoes.
8. Repeat the process for the remaining 3 bowls.

Nutrition Facts

Serves: 4
Serving Size: 1 bowl

Amount per serving
Calories 260

Calories from fat 50

Total fat 6.0 g

Saturated fat 2.3 g

Trans fat 0.0 g

Cholesterol 10 mg

Sodium 530 mg

Potassium 1260 mg

Total carbohydrate 43 g

Dietary fiber 9 g

Sugars 14 g

Protein 14 g

Phosphorus 285 mg

Choices/Exchanges: 2 Starch, 2 Nonstarchy Vegetable, 1 Lean Protein, 1/2 Fat

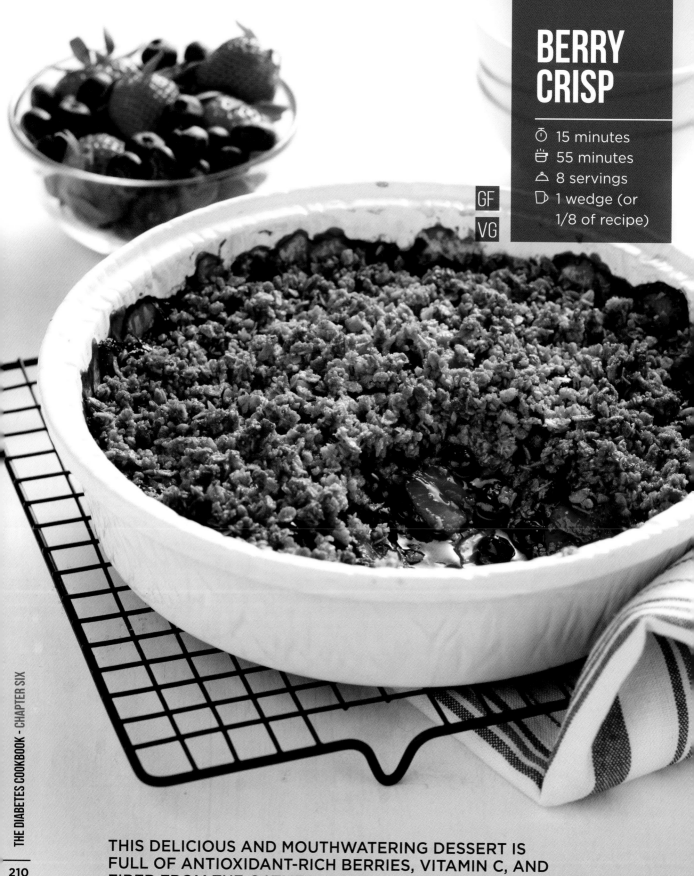

BERRY CRISP

- ⏱ 15 minutes
- 🍲 55 minutes
- △ 8 servings
- 🍽 1 wedge (or 1/8 of recipe)

GF
VG

THIS DELICIOUS AND MOUTHWATERING DESSERT IS FULL OF ANTIOXIDANT-RICH BERRIES, VITAMIN C, AND FIBER FROM THE OATMEAL.

Nonstick cooking spray
1   pound strawberries, sliced
1   pint blueberries
1   teaspoon lemon zest
2   tablespoons lemon juice
2   tablespoons low-calorie granulated
      sugar blend (such as Truvia Baking
      Blend)
1 1/2 tablespoons gluten-free cornstarch
1   teaspoon cinnamon

TOPPING

1   cup certified gluten-free oats
1   tablespoon low-calorie granulated
      sugar blend (such as Truvia Sugar
      Blend)
3   tablespoons low-calorie brown sugar
      blend (such as Truvia or Splenda)
1/2   cup chopped pecans
4   tablespoons trans fat–free margarine,
      diced

1. Preheat oven to 350°F. Spray a 9-inch pie pan with cooking spray.
2. In a medium bowl combine the berries, lemon zest, lemon juice, 2 tablespoons sugar blend, cornstarch, and cinnamon. Mix well and pour into pie pan.
3. In another medium bowl, place all topping ingredients. Use your hands to work the margarine into the dry ingredients until the mixture is crumbly.
4. Sprinkle the topping mixture evenly over the berries. Bake 55 minutes or until the top is brown and the fruit is bubbly. If topping is browning too much during baking, cover with aluminum foil. Serve warm.

Nutrition Facts

Serves: 8
Serving Size: 1 wedge (or 1/8 of recipe)

Amount per serving
Calories 190

Calories from fat 100

Total fat 11.0 g
  Saturated fat 1.8 g
  Trans fat 0.0 g
Cholesterol 0 mg
Sodium 50 mg
Potassium 180 mg
Total carbohydrate 24 g
  Dietary fiber 4 g
  Sugars 11 g
Protein 3 g
Phosphorus 80 mg

Choices/Exchanges: 1/2 Starch, 1/2 Fruit, 1/2 Carbohydrate, 2 Fat

SWEET POTATO SALAD

⏱ 25 minutes
🍲 7 minutes
🍽 12 servings
🍴 1/2 cup

WHO SAYS YOU CAN ONLY USE WHITE POTATOES FOR A POTATO SALAD? THIS DISH WILL BE A WELCOME SURPRISE AT YOUR NEXT SUMMER PICNIC.

SALAD

3	large sweet potatoes (about 13 ounces each)
4	slices turkey bacon

DRESSSING

2	tablespoons extra-virgin olive oil
1	tablespoon apple cider vinegar
1/8	teaspoon ground black pepper
1/2	teaspoon garlic powder
3	stalks celery, diced
2	green onions, sliced

1. Peel and cube sweet potatoes. Place sweet potatoes in a large pot. Cover with water and bring to a boil. Boil until tender, about 5–7 minutes. Drain potatoes, rinse with cold water, and let cool.
2. While potatoes are cooking, cook bacon according to package directions and chop into small pieces.
3. In a small bowl, whisk together olive oil, vinegar, pepper, and garlic powder.
4. Place sweet potatoes in serving bowl, and add celery, green onions, and turkey bacon. Pour dressing over salad and toss until potatoes are coated. Serve cold.

DIETITIAN TIP: *Sweet potatoes have a lower glycemic index than white potatoes.*

Nutrition Facts

Serves: 12
Serving Size: 1/2 cup

Amount per serving
Calories 100

Calories from fat 25

Total fat 3.0 g
Saturated fat 0.6 g
Trans fat 0.0 g
Cholesterol 3 mg
Sodium 95 mg
Potassium 240 mg
Total carbohydrate 15 g
Dietary fiber 2 g
Sugars 5 g
Protein 2 g
Phosphorus 45 mg

Choices/Exchanges: 1 Starch, 1/2 Fat

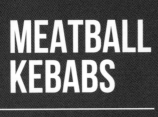

MEATBALL KEBABS

⏱ 20 minutes
🍲 25 minutes
🍽 6 servings
🍴 2 kebabs

GF
LC

THESE MEATBALLS MAKE A FUN FAMILY MEAL. OR SERVE THEM ON A PLATTER AS AN APPETIZER THE NEXT TIME YOU ARE ENTERTAINING.

Nonstick cooking spray
2   egg whites
2   tablespoons grated parmesan cheese
2   cloves garlic, minced
20   ounces lean ground turkey
1/2   teaspoon salt
1/4   teaspoon ground black pepper
12   bamboo skewers
24   grape or cherry tomatoes
8   ounces fresh cremini mushrooms (baby portobello mushrooms), cut in half if needed to make 12 pieces
1   medium onion, quartered, then each quarter cut into thirds (12 onion pieces total)
1/4   cup balsamic vinegar
1   teaspoon olive oil

1. Preheat oven to 375°F. Coat a baking sheet with cooking spray. Set aside.
2. Combine the egg whites, parmesan cheese, garlic, turkey, salt, and pepper. Mix well, and form 24 meatballs. Refrigerate the meatballs for at least 30 minutes.
3. Skewer 2 meatballs, 2 tomatoes, 1 piece of mushroom, and 1 piece of onion alternating on each skewer.
4. In a small bowl, whisk together the vinegar and olive oil.
5. Place the kebabs on the baking sheet and brush the kebabs on all sides with the vinegar and olive oil mixture. Reserve the marinade.
6. Bake the kebabs 10 minutes. Brush all sides with the marinade again and bake an additional 10–15 minutes. The meatballs should be cooked to an internal temperature of at least 165°F.

Nutrition Facts

Serves: 6
Serving Size: 2 kebabs

Amount per serving
Calories **200**

Calories from fat 70

Total fat 8.0 g
    Saturated fat 2.5 g
    Trans fat 0.1 g
Cholesterol 75 mg
Sodium 310 mg
Potassium 520 mg
Total carbohydrate 7 g
    Dietary fiber 1 g
    Sugars 4 g
Protein 22 g
Phosphorus 255 mg

Choices/Exchanges: 1 Nonstarchy Vegetable, 3 Lean Protein, 1/2 Fat

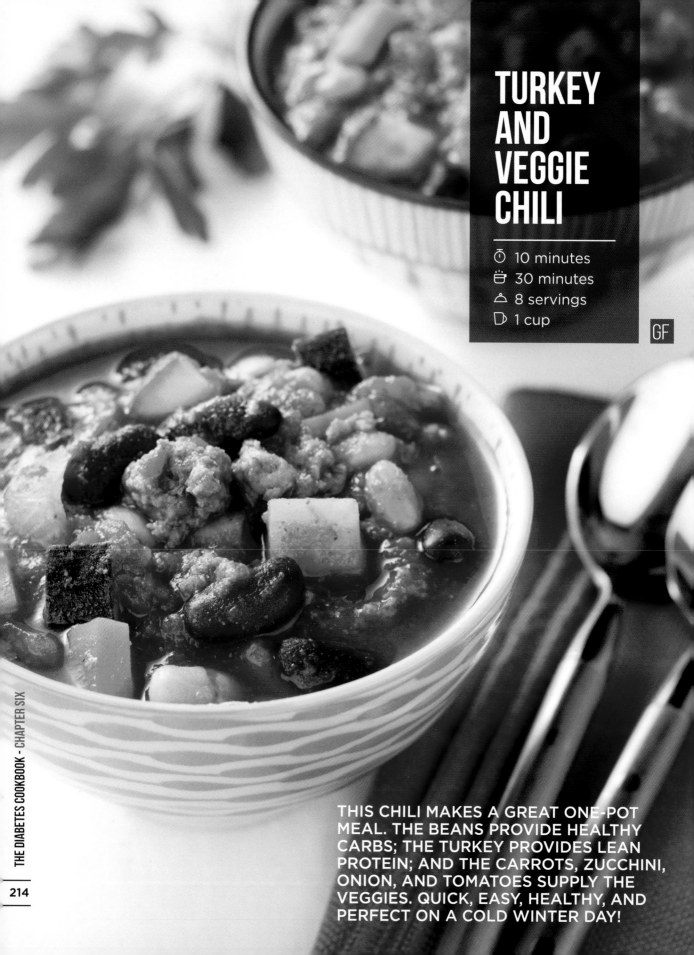

TURKEY AND VEGGIE CHILI

- ⏱ 10 minutes
- 🍲 30 minutes
- 🍽 8 servings
- 🥄 1 cup

GF

THIS CHILI MAKES A GREAT ONE-POT MEAL. THE BEANS PROVIDE HEALTHY CARBS; THE TURKEY PROVIDES LEAN PROTEIN; AND THE CARROTS, ZUCCHINI, ONION, AND TOMATOES SUPPLY THE VEGGIES. QUICK, EASY, HEALTHY, AND PERFECT ON A COLD WINTER DAY!

Nonstick cooking spray
1   small onion, diced
2   medium carrots, diced
1   medium zucchini (6 ounces), diced
1   clove garlic, minced
16   ounces lean ground turkey
1   (14.5-ounce) can no-salt-added diced tomatoes
1   (28-ounce) can no-salt-added crushed tomatoes
1   (15.8-ounce) can gluten-free great northern beans, rinsed and drained
1   (15.25-ounce) can gluten-free no-salt-added kidney beans, rinsed and drained
1/2   teaspoon ground black pepper
1   tablespoon chili powder
1   teaspoon cumin
1   teaspoon garlic powder

1. Spray a large soup pot with cooking spray. Add the onion, carrots, and zucchini, and sauté over medium-high heat 3–4 minutes or until the onion turns clear. Add the garlic and sauté 30 more seconds.
2. Add the ground turkey and cook until brown. Add the remaining ingredients, mix well, and bring the chili to a boil. Reduce the heat and simmer 15–20 minutes.

Nutrition Facts

Serves: 8
Serving Size: 1 cup

Amount per serving
Calories 230

Calories from fat 45	
Total fat 5.0 g	
Saturated fat 1.4 g	
Trans fat 0.1 g	
Cholesterol 45 mg	
Sodium 170 mg	
Potassium 930 mg	
Total carbohydrate 27 g	
Dietary fiber 8 g	
Sugars 8 g	
Protein 20 g	
Phosphorus 280 mg	

Choices/Exchanges: 1 Starch, 2 Nonstarchy Vegetable, 2 Lean Protein

GRILLED ZUCCHINI WITH FETA CHEESE

GF
LC
VG

⏱ 5 minutes
🍳 10 minutes
🍽 6 servings
🍲 1/2 zucchini

GRILLING IS A QUICK AND HEALTHY WAY TO PREPARE VEGGIES. THIS RECIPE IS SIMPLY DELICIOUS AND IS AN EASY SIDE THAT CAN BE ADDED TO ANY MEAL. IF YOU HAVE LEFTOVERS FROM THIS RECIPE, USE THE GRILLED ZUCCHINI IN A BREAKFAST OMELET THE NEXT DAY.

3   medium zucchini, split in half lengthwise (ends trimmed)
1   tablespoon olive oil
1/4 cup crumbled reduced-fat feta cheese

1. Preheat a grill to medium-high.
2. Drizzle the olive oil evenly over the zucchini halves. Grill the zucchini 4–5 minutes per side, until tender.
3. Remove the zucchini from the grill, and sprinkle each piece with feta cheese.

Nutrition Facts

Serves: 6
Serving Size: 1/2 zucchini

Amount per serving
Calories 45

Calories from fat 25

Total fat 3.0 g

   Saturated fat 0.8 g

   Trans fat 0.0 g

Cholesterol 3 mg

Sodium 80 mg

Potassium 260 mg

Total carbohydrate 3 g

   Dietary fiber 1 g

   Sugars 2 g

Protein 2 g

Phosphorus 55 mg

Choices/Exchanges: 1 Nonstarchy Vegetable, 1/2 Fat

ZUCCHINI PIZZA

⏱ 15 minutes
🍲 40 minutes
🍽 3 servings
🍳 2 pieces

GF
LC
VG

THIS RECIPE MAKES A GREAT
VEGETARIAN ENTRÉE OR SIDE DISH.

Nonstick cooking spray
1   cup zucchini, grated
1   egg, beaten
2   ounces shredded reduced-fat mozzarella cheese, divided
3/4 cup no-salt-added tomato sauce
1/2 teaspoon minced garlic
1/4 teaspoon dried oregano
1/2 cup mushrooms, sliced
1/2 cup diced green bell pepper
1/2 cup diced tomato
2   tablespoons freshly grated parmesan cheese

1. Preheat oven to 400°F. Coat an 8-inch square baking dish with cooking spray. Set aside.
2. Place zucchini in a clean kitchen towel or in two layers of paper towel and squeeze as much moisture out of the zucchini as possible.
3. Mix zucchini, egg, and 1/2 ounce of mozzarella cheese. Press tightly into the baking dish. Bake 10 minutes.
4. While zucchini is baking, mix tomato sauce, garlic, and oregano. Set aside.
5. Add cooking spray to a sauté pan over medium heat. Lightly sauté mushrooms, green pepper, and tomato.
6. After zucchini is baked, spread tomato sauce on top of zucchini. Add pizza toppings and top with remaining mozzarella and parmesan cheeses.
7. Bake 25–30 minutes or until cheese is brown and bubbly.

Nutrition Facts

Serves: 3
Serving Size: 2 pieces

Amount per serving

Calories   **130**

Calories from fat 50

Total fat 6.0 g

   Saturated fat 3.1 g

   Trans fat 0.0 g

Cholesterol 75 mg

Sodium 200 mg

Potassium 560 mg

Total carbohydrate 10 g

   Dietary fiber 3 g

   Sugars 6 g

Protein 10 g

Phosphorus 210 mg

Choices/Exchanges: 2 Nonstarchy Vegetable, 1 Medium-Fat Protein

SWEET POTATO SHEPHERD'S PIE

GF

- ⏱ 30 minutes
- 🍳 20 minutes
- 🍽 8 servings
- 🥄 1 1/2 cups

THIS 30-MINUTE MEAL PACKS IN LEAN PROTEIN FROM THE TURKEY, LOTS OF VEGETABLES, AND HEALTHY CARBS FROM THE SWEET POTATOES.

2	large sweet potatoes (about 9 ounces each), peeled and diced

Nonstick cooking spray

1	small onion, diced
2	cloves garlic, minced
1 1/4	pounds lean ground turkey
1	(14.5-ounce) can diced tomatoes
1	(16-ounce) bag frozen mixed vegetables (carrots, corn, peas, and green beans)
1	tablespoon yellow mustard
2	tablespoons gluten-free Worcestershire sauce
1/4	teaspoon ground black pepper
2	teaspoons cornstarch
1	tablespoon cold water
2	tablespoons trans fat–free margarine

1. Place sweet potatoes in steam basket in a medium pot with 2 cups water. Bring to a boil, reduce heat, and simmer. Cover and steam until tender, about 15 minutes.

2. While potatoes are cooking, spray a large sauté pan with cooking spray. Add onion and sauté over medium-high heat 3 minutes or until onion looks clear. Add garlic and sauté 30 seconds. Remove from pan and set aside.

3. Add turkey and cook until brown, about 6–7 minutes. Add onion back to pan and stir to mix.

4. Add diced tomatoes, mixed vegetables, mustard, Worcestershire sauce, and pepper. Bring to a simmer.

5. In a small bowl, mix together cornstarch and water. Add to turkey mixture and stir. Let simmer 5 more minutes.

6. Meanwhile, drain the sweet potatoes. Place sweet potatoes in a medium bowl and mash with a potato masher. Add margarine and whisk until smooth.

7. Preheat broiler. Pour cooked turkey mixture evenly into an 11-by-14-inch pan or medium casserole dish. Spread sweet potatoes evenly on top of turkey mixture.

8. Broil 5 minutes.

Nutrition Facts

Serves: 8
Serving Size: 1 1/2 cups

Amount per serving
Calories 240

Calories from fat 70

Total fat 8.0 g

Saturated fat 2.2 g

Trans fat 0.1 g

Cholesterol 55 mg

Sodium 250 mg

Potassium 550 mg

Total carbohydrate 23 g

Dietary fiber 4 g

Sugars 8 g

Protein 17 g

Phosphorus 205 mg

Choices/Exchanges: 1 Starch, 1 Nonstarchy Vegetable, 2 Lean Protein, 1 Fat

POTATO AND CAULIFLOWER SALAD

GF
VG

- ⏱ 10 minutes
- 🍲 45 minutes
- 🍽 8 servings
- 🥄 1/2 cup

USING VINEGAR-BASED DRESSING IN A POTATO SALAD CUTS DOWN ON THE FAT AND CALORIES FOUND IN A TRADITIONAL POTATO SALAD DRESSING, AND USING CAULIFLOWER IN PLACE OF SOME OF THE POTATOES REDUCES THE CARBS AND INCREASES THE FIBER.

Nonstick cooking spray
4 cups cauliflower florets, roughly chopped
5 red potatoes, cut into 1-inch chunks (4 cups cut)
1/4 cup balsamic vinegar
2 tablespoons olive oil
1 teaspoon Dijon mustard
1 tablespoon honey or 2 packets artificial sweetener
1/4 cup chopped fresh parsley
1/4 cup minced red onion
1 red bell pepper, seeded and diced

1. Preheat oven to 375°F. Coat a baking sheet with cooking spray.
2. Lay cauliflower and potatoes in a single layer on the baking sheet and coat the vegetables with cooking spray. Roast 45 minutes until vegetables are golden brown and tender.
3. In a large bowl, whisk together the vinegar, olive oil, mustard, honey, and parsley.
4. Add onion, bell pepper, and the potatoes and cauliflower right out of the oven. Toss well to coat.
5. Refrigerate salad until cooled (at least 1 hour). Stir again before serving.

Nutrition Facts

Serves: 8
Serving Size: 1/2 cup

Amount per serving
Calories 120

Calories from fat 35

Total fat 4.0 g

Saturated fat 0.6 g

Trans fat 0.0 g

Cholesterol 0 mg

Sodium 40 mg

Potassium 560 mg

Total carbohydrate 20 g

Dietary fiber 3 g

Sugars 6 g

Protein 3 g

Phosphorus 75 mg

Choices/Exchanges: 1 Starch, 1 Nonstarchy Vegetable, 1/2 Fat

EASY HALF-MASHED POTATOES

- ⏱ 15 minutes
- 🍲 20 minutes
- 🍽 11 servings
- 🍶 1/2 cup

LEAVING THE SKIN ON THE POTATOES INCREASES THE FIBER IN THIS RECIPE. BY COMBINING CAULIFLOWER AND POTATOES, YOU GET THE SAME VOLUME AND FEWER CARBS!

1   (24-ounce) bag fingerling potatoes, cut into 1-inch rounds with skin on
1   (16-ounce) bag frozen cauliflower florets
1/3   cup skim milk
5   tablespoons trans fat–free margarine
1/2   teaspoon salt
1/2   teaspoon ground black pepper

1. Place potatoes in a large soup pot. Cover with cold water and bring to a boil. Cook 15 minutes. Add cauliflower to pot, return to a boil, and cook 5 more minutes.
2. Drain potatoes and cauliflower and return them to the pot.
3. Add remaining ingredients and mash mixture with a potato masher. Mix with an electric mixer on low speed about 1 minute.

Nutrition Facts

Serves: 11
Serving Size: 1/2 cup

Amount per serving
Calories **100**

Calories from fat 40	
Total fat 4.5 g	
Saturated fat 1.2 g	
Trans fat 0.0 g	
Cholesterol 0 mg	
Sodium 160 mg	
Potassium 300 mg	
Total carbohydrate 14 g	
Dietary fiber 2 g	
Sugars 1 g	
Protein 2 g	
Phosphorus 45 mg	

Choices/Exchanges: 1 Starch, 1/2 Fat

TWICE-BAKED BUTTERNUT SQUASH

- ○ 10 minutes
- ⏲ 45 minutes
- △ 4 servings
- ▷ 1/4 squash

GF

YOU CAN ALSO MAKE THIS RECIPE WITH SMALL SUGAR PUMPKINS OR ACORN SQUASH INSTEAD OF BUTTERNUT SQUASH.

Nonstick cooking spray
1 (2-pound) butternut squash
1/2 teaspoon salt-free all-purpose seasoning (such as Spike or Mrs. Dash)
1/4 teaspoon ground black pepper
1/4 teaspoon ground nutmeg
1 tablespoon olive oil
2 links gluten-free apple chicken sausage (about 3 ounces each), diced
1/4 cup chopped fresh sage
1/2 cup fat-free, gluten-free, low-sodium chicken broth
1 cup fat-free ricotta cheese
1/4 cup grated parmesan cheese

1. Preheat oven to 425°F. Coat a large baking sheet with cooking spray.
2. Halve the squash lengthwise, scoop out the seeds, and spray with cooking spray. Season the squash with salt-free seasoning, pepper, and nutmeg. Lay the squash cut side up on the baking sheet and roast until just tender, about 45 minutes. Remove the squash from the oven and set aside.
3. While the squash is roasting, add the olive oil to a medium nonstick sauté pan and sauté the sausage and sage until golden brown.
4. Scoop the flesh of the squash into a bowl, keeping the skins intact. Mash the squash flesh with the chicken broth and the ricotta cheese, and then stir in the cooked sausage and sage.
5. Stuff the squash shells with the mashed squash mixture, top with the parmesan cheese, and bake until the cheese is melted and golden brown on top.

6. Cut each squash half in half again before serving.

Nutrition Facts

Serves: 4
Serving Size: 1/4 squash

Amount per serving	
Calories	**240**

Calories from fat 100	
Total fat 11.0 g	
Saturated fat 3.1 g	
Trans fat 0.0 g	
Cholesterol 65 mg	
Sodium 450 mg	
Potassium 530 mg	
Total carbohydrate 20 g	
Dietary fiber 5 g	
Sugars 6 g	
Protein 17 g	
Phosphorus 275 mg	

Choices/Exchanges: 1 Starch, 1/2 Fat-Free Milk, 1 Medium-Fat Protein, 1 Fat

ZUCCHINI LASAGNA SKILLET

- ⏱ 10 minutes
- 🍲 20 minutes
- △ 4 servings
- 🍽 1 cup

GF

THIS IS A GREAT LOW-CARB VERSION OF
TRADITIONAL LASAGNA. YOU CAN ALSO SERVE
THIS DISH OVER WHOLE-GRAIN PASTA.

4 cups water
2 medium zucchini, shaved into strips with a peeler, omitting center seeds
1 teaspoon olive oil
8 ounces lean ground turkey
1 tablespoon Italian seasoning
3 cloves garlic, minced or grated
1/2 (24.5-ounce) jar gluten-free reduced-sodium marinara sauce
1/2 cup skim ricotta cheese
3 tablespoons freshly shredded parmesan cheese

1. Bring the water to a boil in a large saucepan over high heat. Add the zucchini and boil 2 minutes. Drain well and set the cooked zucchini aside in a colander to continue draining.
2. In a large sauté pan, add the olive oil over medium heat. Add the turkey, Italian seasoning, and garlic, and sauté, breaking up the turkey to crumble it. Sauté 5–6 minutes or until the turkey is just cooked through.
3. Add half the jar of marinara sauce and bring to a simmer. Simmer 2 minutes, then stir in the drained zucchini. Continue to simmer 2 more minutes.
4. Stir in both cheeses and stir until melted.

Nutrition Facts

Serves: 4
Serving Size: 1 cup

Amount per serving
Calories 210

Calories from fat 90	
Total fat 10.0 g	
Saturated fat 2.4 g	
Trans fat 0.1 g	
Cholesterol 55 mg	
Sodium 330 mg	
Potassium 590 mg	
Total carbohydrate 11 g	
Dietary fiber 2 g	
Sugars 6 g	
Protein 18 g	
Phosphorus 240 mg	

Choices/Exchange: 2 Nonstarchy Vegetable, 2 Lean Protein, 1 1/2 Fat

GREEN SMOOTHIE BREAKFAST BOWL

GF
VG

⏱ 5 minutes
🍽 2 servings
🥤 About 1 cup

A SMOOTHIE TOPPED WITH SOME CRUNCH MAKES FOR A COMPLETE BREAKFAST IN A BOWL! THE EXTRA INGREDIENTS MAKE THIS THICK FRUIT-AND-VEGGIE BLEND MORE FILLING THAN A DRINKABLE SMOOTHIE.

3/4	cup unsweetened almond milk
4	ounces fat-free plain Greek yogurt
1	cup frozen mixed fruit
2	cups baby spinach
1	medium frozen banana, sliced
1	(1.4-ounce) Maple Glazed Pecan & Sea Salt KIND bar, crumbled

1. Combine all ingredients except KIND bar in a blender. Purée until smooth and thick, stopping to stir mixture a few times. (Add a little more almond milk if needed.)
2. Pour smoothie mixture into 2 bowls. Top each bowl with half of the crumbled KIND bar.

DIETITIAN TIP: *No KIND bar? Top the smoothie with a sprinkle of toasted almonds and unsweetened, shredded coconut.*

Nutrition Facts

Serves: 2
Serving Size: About 1 cup

Amount per serving
Calories **260**

Calories from fat 90	
Total fat 10.0 g	
Saturated fat 0.9 g	
Trans fat 0.0 g	
Cholesterol 10 mg	
Sodium 180 mg	
Potassium 670 mg	
Total carbohydrate 34 g	
Dietary fiber 7 g	
Sugars 19 g	
Protein 11 g	
Phosphorus 170 mg	

Choices/Exchanges: 1 1/2 Fruit, 1 Carbohydrate, 1 Lean Protein, 1 1/2 Fat

GLUTEN-FREE SCRUMPTIOUS PEACH CRISP

GF
VG

- 15 minutes
- 10 servings
- Almost 2/3 cup

2 (16-ounce) bags frozen unsweetened peaches
1 teaspoon cinnamon
1 teaspoon vanilla extract
1 tablespoon honey

TOPPING

1   cup certified gluten-free oats
1/4 cup shredded unsweetened coconut
1/2 teaspoon cinnamon
3   tablespoons trans fat–free margarine
2   tablespoons honey

1. Preheat oven to 350°F. Heat frozen peaches in an oven-safe skillet over medium heat. Cook 10–15 minutes or until soft, stirring frequently. Stir in the cinnamon, vanilla, and honey.
2. While peaches are cooking, combine all topping ingredients in a medium bowl.
3. Sprinkle topping ingredients evenly over peaches (leave some room at edges to see peaches).
4. Bake 25 minutes.

DIETITIAN TIP: *Fresh fruit baked or grilled makes the best natural dessert. This dessert can also be made with blueberries, blackberries, or apples!*

Nutrition Facts

Serves: 10
Serving Size: Almost 2/3 cup

Amount per serving
Calories 130

Calories from fat 40

Total fat 4.5 g

   Saturated fat 2.0 g

   Trans fat 0.0 g

Cholesterol 0 mg

Sodium 30 mg

Potassium 210 mg

Total carbohydrate 21 g

   Dietary fiber 3 g

   Sugars 12 g

Protein 2 g

Phosphorus 60 mg

Choices/Exchanges: 1/2 Starch, 1/2 Fruit, 1/2 Carbohydrate, 1/2 Fat

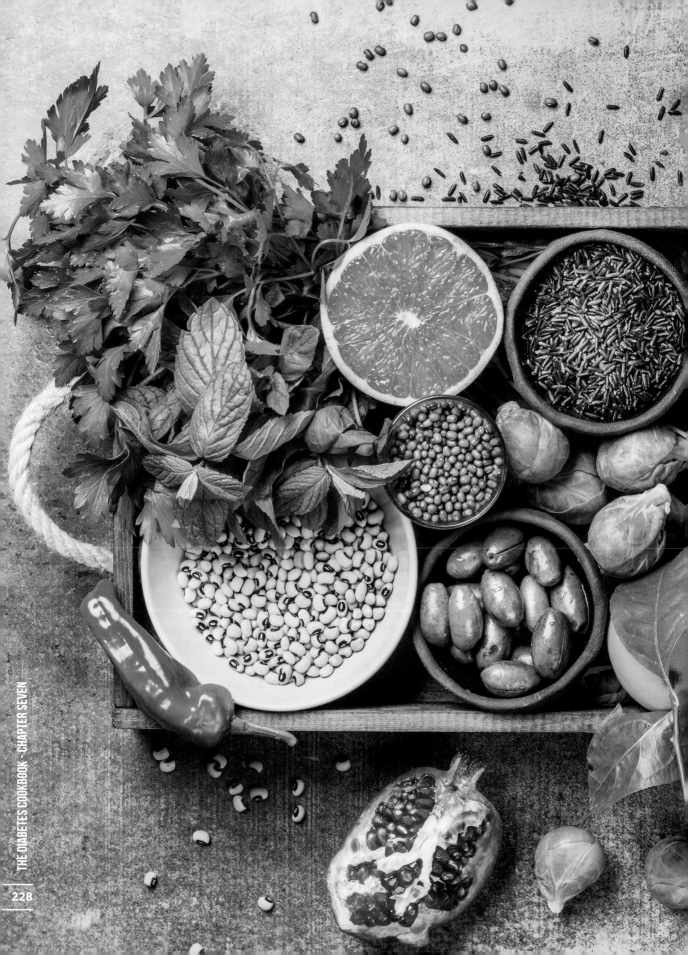

CHAPTER SEVEN

GRAIN-FREE AND DAIRY-FREE RECIPES

ALTHOUGH THERE IS NO IDEAL AMOUNT OF CARBOHYDRATE INTAKE FOR PEOPLE WITH DIABETES, AND THE CARBOHYDRATE AMOUNT SHOULD BE INDIVIDUALIZED FOR EACH PERSON, MONITORING CARBOHYDRATE INTAKE IS A KEY STRATEGY IN ACHIEVING IMPROVED GLYCEMIC CONTROL OR BLOOD SUGAR LEVELS. MANY PEOPLE CHOOSE TO FOLLOW A

LOWER-CARB DIET THAT IS GRAIN-FREE AND DAIRY-FREE DUE TO FOOD ALLERGIES OR INTOLERANCE, OR BECAUSE THEY NOTICE IMPROVEMENTS IN WEIGHT LOSS OR BLOOD SUGAR CONTROL.* RECIPES IN THIS CHAPTER ARE LOWER-CARB, GRAIN-FREE, AND DAIRY-FREE BUT FULL OF HEALTHY FATS, LEAN PROTEINS, AND A LOT OF FREE VEGETABLES. YOU WON'T NOTICE HOW HEALTHY THESE DISHES ARE, BECAUSE THEY TASTE AMAZING!

*As with all eating patterns, you should work with your registered dietitian or certified diabetes educator to find a nutritionally balanced and individualized plan that is best for you.

SWEET AND SPICY NUTS

GF
VG

- ⏱ 5 minutes
- ☕ 8 minutes
- 🍽 8 servings
- 🥄 1/4 cup

FORGET THE POTATO CHIPS! THIS SNACK IS FULL OF PROTEIN AND IT'S SWEET AND SALTY AND FILLING.

1 tablespoon trans fat–free margarine
2 cups unsalted mixed nuts
(1/2 cup each: unsalted cashews, whole almonds, hazelnuts, and pecans)
2 tablespoons honey
1/4 teaspoon ground cayenne pepper
1/2 teaspoon ground black pepper
1/2 teaspoon salt

1. Add margarine to a nonstick skillet over medium heat. Add nuts and sauté 2 minutes.
2. Stir in honey, cayenne pepper, black pepper, and salt.
3. Continue to cook the mixture, stirring constantly, until the nuts are dark golden brown, about 6 minutes.
4. Transfer nuts to a sheet of foil or parchment paper to cool. Break nuts apart and store in an airtight container.

CHEF TIP: *If you like it spicier, add more cayenne pepper.*

Nutrition Facts

Serves: 8
Serving Size: 1/4 cup

Amount per serving
Calories 220

Calories from fat 170

Total fat 19.0 g

Saturated fat 2.2 g

Trans fat 0.0 g

Cholesterol 0 mg

Sodium 160 mg

Potassium 200 mg

Total carbohydrate 11 g

Dietary fiber 2 g

Sugars 6 g

Protein 5 g

Phosphorus 125 mg

Choices/Exchanges:
1 Carbohydrate, 3 1/2 Fat

PALEO 10-MINUTE TACO SALAD

FORGET THE FRIED TORTILLA BOWL AND DIVE INTO THIS LIGHT, FRESH SALAD FOR A GREAT SUMMER LUNCH.

- 🕐 10 minutes
- 🍽 1 serving
- 🍴 1 salad

2	cups shredded iceberg lettuce
1/2	cup grape tomatoes
1/4	cup chopped fresh cilantro
1/2	cup shredded cooked chicken breast meat (such as from a rotisserie chicken)
1/4	cup chopped avocado
1/4	cup fresh no-salt pico de gallo
	Juice of 1 small lime
1	tablespoon extra-virgin olive oil

1. In a salad bowl, gently toss together the lettuce, grape tomatoes, cilantro, chicken, and avocado.

2. Pour the pico de gallo, lime juice, and olive oil over the salad, and toss again gently to coat.

CHEF TIP: *This recipe can be easily doubled or tripled to make enough for a low-carb crowd.*

Nutrition Facts

Serves: 1
Serving Size: 1 salad

Amount per serving
Calories 330

Calories from fat 200

Total fat 22.0 g

    Saturated fat 3.3 g

    Trans fat 0.0 g

Cholesterol 60 mg

Sodium 270 mg

Potassium 900 mg

Total carbohydrate 15 g

    Dietary fiber 6 g

    Sugars 6 g

Protein 23 g

Phosphorus 260 mg

Choices/Exchanges: 1/2 Fruit, 1 Nonstarchy Vegetable, 3 Lean Protein, 3 Fat

ITALIAN STUFFED KALE ROLLS

SERVE THIS HEARTY DISH WITH 1 CUP OF COOKED WHOLE-WHEAT PASTA.

⏱ 20 minutes
🍲 40 minutes
🍽 8 servings
🍴 1 kale roll

GF

Nonstick cooking spray
1 (25-ounce) jar low-sodium tomato basil pasta sauce, divided
20 ounces gluten-free lean sweet Italian turkey sausage
3 tablespoons almond flour
2 tablespoons dried parsley
1 tablespoon garlic powder
1 (8-ounce) can no-salt-added tomato sauce
1/2 teaspoon ground black pepper
8 large curly kale leaves, stems removed

1. Preheat oven to 375°F. Coat a 9-by-13-inch baking dish with cooking spray. Pour 1/4 of the jar of pasta sauce in the baking dish and spread to coat the bottom of the dish.
2. Remove the turkey sausages from their casings; discard the casings, and place the sausages in a medium bowl. Add the almond flour, parsley, garlic powder, tomato sauce, and pepper. Mix together.
3. Fill each kale leaf with 1/3 cup of the meat mixture and roll the leaf around the meat. Place seam side down on top of the sauce in the bottom of the baking dish. Repeat for the remaining 7 rolls.
4. Top with remaining pasta sauce and bake 25 minutes. Turn the rolls over and bake an additional 15 minutes, or until the internal temperature of each roll is 165°F.

Nutrition Facts

Serves: 8
Serving Size: 1 kale roll

Amount per serving
Calories 180

Calories from fat 70

Total fat 8.0 g

　Saturated fat 1.8 g

　Trans fat 0.2 g

Cholesterol 40 mg

Sodium 460 mg

Potassium 730 mg

Total carbohydrate 13 g

　Dietary fiber 3 g

　Sugars 7 g

Protein 15 g

Phosphorus 185 mg

Choices/Exchanges: 1/2 Starch, 1 Nonstarchy Vegetable, 2 Lean Protein, 1/2 Fat

CHIMICHURRI CHICKEN KEBABS

SERVE THESE DELICIOUS KEBABS WITH THE GRILLED VEGGIE KEBABS ON PAGE 384. THESE ARE PERFECT FOR YOUR NEXT SUMMER BARBECUE AND WILL LEAVE YOUR GUESTS SUPER IMPRESSED!

⏱ 2 hours 20 minutes
🍲 15 minutes
△ 8 servings
🍽 1 kebab

GF
LC

SAUCE

1/2	cup chopped fresh Italian parsley
4	cloves garlic, peeled
1/4	teaspoon ground black pepper
1	tablespoon fresh oregano
1/3	cup olive oil
3	tablespoons red wine vinegar

Juice of 2 limes

CHICKEN

2	pounds boneless skinless chicken breast, cut into 1-inch chunks
8	metal skewers

1. Place all the sauce ingredients in a food processor and pulse until blended.
2. Place chicken in a large plastic freezer bag. Pour sauce over chicken and marinate 2 hours or overnight in refrigerator.
3. Preheat the indoor or outdoor grill to medium-high. Skewer chicken on 8 metal skewers. Cook the kebabs, turning after grill marks form, until the chicken is cooked through, 12–15 minutes.

Nutrition Facts

Serves: 8
Serving Size: 1 kebab

Amount per serving
Calories **180**

Calories from fat 80	
Total fat 9.0 g	
Saturated fat 1.6 g	
Trans fat 0.0 g	
Cholesterol 65 mg	
Sodium 60 mg	
Potassium 220 mg	
Total carbohydrate 1 g	
Dietary fiber 0 g	
Sugars 0 g	
Protein 24 g	
Phosphorus 175 mg	

Choices/Exchanges: 3 Lean Protein, 1 Fat

CAULIFLOWER TABBOULEH

⏱ 15 minutes
△ 6 servings
🍽 1 cup

THIS IS A GREAT GRAIN-FREE VERSION OF FLAVORFUL TABBOULEH SALAD.

1 cup packed parsley leaves
1/4 cup packed mint leaves
1 small head cauliflower (about 1 1/2 pounds as purchased), leaves and stem removed
2 roma tomatoes, seeded and diced
2 tablespoons olive oil
3 tablespoons freshly squeezed lemon juice
1/4 teaspoon salt
1/4 teaspoon ground black pepper

1. Mince the parsley and mint leaves (or grind in a food processor) and place in a large bowl.
2. Grate the cauliflower using a box grater and stir together with the parsley and mint.
3. Add the diced tomatoes and stir them into the salad.
4. Drizzle the salad with olive oil and lemon juice, and sprinkle with salt and pepper. Stir to coat.
5. Cover and let the tabbouleh marinate 30 minutes before serving.

Nutrition Facts

Serves: 6
Serving Size: 1 cup

Amount per serving
Calories 70

Calories from fat 45

Total fat 5.0 g
    Saturated fat 0.7 g
    Trans fat 0.0 g
Cholesterol 0 mg
Sodium 130 mg
Potassium 360 mg
Total carbohydrate 6 g
    Dietary fiber 2 g
    Sugars 2 g
Protein 2 g
Phosphorus 45 mg

Choices/Exchanges: 1 Nonstarchy Vegetable, 1 Fat

ROASTED BRUSSELS SPROUTS

⏱ 5 minutes
🍲 45 minutes
△ 5 servings
🍽 6 Brussels sprouts

THESE BRUSSELS SPROUTS ARE LOW IN BOTH CALORIES AND CARBOHYDRATES, WHICH MEANS THEY MAY BE HELPFUL FOR CONTROLLING BLOOD GLUCOSE. ROASTING ENHANCES THEIR FLAVOR.

Nonstick cooking spray
1 pound frozen Brussels sprouts, thawed
2 tablespoons olive oil
1/2 teaspoon ground black pepper
3 slices turkey bacon, cut into 1-inch pieces

1. Preheat oven to 400°F. Spray a baking sheet with cooking spray.
2. Place Brussels sprouts in a bowl and add oil; toss to coat.
3. Add pepper and turkey bacon and mix well.
4. Place Brussels sprouts on a baking sheet and bake 25–30 minutes or until crisp on the outside.

Nutrition Facts

Serves: 5
Serving Size: 6 Brussels sprouts

Amount per serving
Calories 100

Calories from fat 60

Total fat 7.0 g

    Saturated fat 1.1 g

    Trans fat 0.0 g

Cholesterol 5 mg

Sodium 90 mg

Potassium 290 mg

Total carbohydrate 7 g

    Dietary fiber 4 g

    Sugars 2 g

Protein 4 g

Phosphorus 90 mg

Choices/Exchanges: 1 Nonstarchy Vegetable, 1 1/2 Fat

BEEF AND SWEET POTATO STEW

- ⏱ 20 minutes
- 🍽 45 minutes
- 🍲 8 servings
- 🥄 1 cup

GF

YOU CAN SUBSTITUTE BUTTERNUT SQUASH FOR THE SWEET POTATOES IN THIS RECIPE IF YOU'D LIKE. THIS STEW IS EXCELLENT SERVED OVER THE ROOT VEGETABLE CAKES (PAGE 82).

1 tablespoon olive oil
Nonstick cooking spray
1 1/2 pounds lean beef stew meat (chuck or round)
1 onion, diced
2 carrots, sliced into 1/2-inch thick rounds
2 stalks celery, diced
2 1/2 cups fat-free, gluten-free, reduced-sodium beef broth
1/2 cup prunes, diced
1 cup hot water
2 sweet potatoes (about 6 ounces each), peeled and diced into 1-inch chunks
1 1/2 teaspoons ground cinnamon
1 teaspoon ground black pepper
3/4 teaspoon salt
1/4 cup chopped fresh parsley

1. Add olive oil and a generous amount of cooking spray to a large soup pot over high heat. In batches, brown beef on all sides. Do not overcrowd the pan with beef or it will not brown.
2. Remove the beef from the pan and set aside. Add onion, carrots, and celery to the pan and sauté 4–5 minutes.
3. Add the beef broth and scrape the brown bits off the bottom of the pan. Add beef and simmer 1 hour.
4. While the beef is simmering, soak the prunes in hot water for 20 minutes. Drain the prunes, saving the water, and set aside.
5. After the beef has simmered 1 hour, add the drained prunes, sweet potatoes, 1/2 cup of the prune water, cinnamon, pepper, and salt. Bring to a simmer, covered, and simmer 20 minutes or until potatoes are tender.
6. Stir in the parsley and serve.

Nutrition Facts

Serves: 8
Serving Size: 1 cup

Amount per serving
Calories 190

Calories from fat 45

Total fat 5.0 g	
Saturated fat 1.7 g	
Trans fat 0.2 g	
Cholesterol 45 mg	
Sodium 430 mg	
Potassium 540 mg	
Total carbohydrate 18 g	
Dietary fiber 3 g	
Sugars 8 g	
Protein 19 g	
Phosphorus 185 mg	

Choices/Exchanges: 1/2 Starch, 1/2 Fruit, 1 Nonstarchy Vegetable, 2 Lean Protein

THE PEPPERY FLAVOR OF BABY
ARUGULA PAIRS WELL WITH SWEET,
FRESH CITRUS AND CRISPY BACON
IN THIS SIDE SALAD.

ARUGULA SALAD WITH MANDARIN ORANGES

GF

- ⏱ 15 minutes
- 🍽 5 servings
- 🥄 About 1 1/2 cups

SALAD

5	ounces baby arugula
4	cooked bacon slices, chopped
4	medium fresh mandarin oranges (or tangerines or clementines), peeled and segmented

DRESSING

1/4	cup fresh orange juice
1	teaspoon grated orange zest
3	tablespoons extra-virgin olive oil
1/8	teaspoon ground black pepper
1/4	teaspoon dried tarragon

1. In a salad bowl, mix together all salad ingredients.

2. In a small bowl, whisk together dressing ingredients. Pour dressing over salad and toss to coat.

DIETITIAN TIP: *Arugula is a nonstarchy vegetable that's packed with nutrients. Each cup has just 5 calories and 1 gram of carbohydrate along with 10 percent of a day's recommended vitamin A and 25 percent of a day's recommended vitamin K!*

Nutrition Facts

Serves: 5
Serving Size: About 1 1/2 cups

Amount per serving

Calories   **170**

Calories from fat 110

Total fat 12.0 g

   Saturated fat 2.3 g

   Trans fat 0.0 g

Cholesterol 10 mg

Sodium 160 mg

Potassium 320 mg

Total carbohydrate 14 g

   Dietary fiber 2 g

   Sugars 11 g

Protein 5 g

Phosphorus 70 mg

Choices/Exchanges: 1 Fruit, 2 1/2 Fat

CHICKEN AND APRICOT TAGINE

YOU CAN SERVE THIS DISH OVER SPIRALIZED CARROTS, TRI-COLOR QUINOA, OR CAULIFLOWER RICE FOR A FULL MEAL.

- ⏱ 15 minutes
- 🍲 35 minutes
- 🍽 5 servings
- 🍴 1 chicken thigh and 1/3 cup sauce

GF

1/2	teaspoon ground cinnamon
1/2	teaspoon ground ginger
1/2	teaspoon turmeric
1/2	teaspoon ground black pepper
1/2	teaspoon salt
1	tablespoon olive oil
	Nonstick cooking spray
5	(3 1/2-ounce) boneless skinless chicken thighs
1	medium red onion, thinly sliced
4	cloves garlic, minced
1/2	cup dried apricots, quartered
1 1/2	cups fat-free, gluten-free, low-sodium chicken broth
1/4	cup chopped parsley

1. In a small bowl, combine the cinnamon, ginger, turmeric, pepper, and salt.
2. Add oil and a generous amount of cooking spray to a large sauté pan over high heat.
3. Season both sides of the chicken thighs with the spice mixture.
4. Sear the chicken on both sides until golden brown, about 3 minutes per side.
5. Add the onion, garlic, and apricots, and stir in with the chicken thighs. Add the chicken broth and bring to a boil.
6. Reduce heat and simmer 15 minutes or until chicken is cooked through and the internal temperature is at least 165°F.
7. Remove the chicken from the pan and set aside.
8. Bring the sauce to a low boil for 8–10 minutes or until reduced and slightly thickened.
9. Add chicken thighs back into the sauce and stir to coat. Stir in the chopped parsley and serve.

Nutrition Facts

Serves: 5

Serving Size: 1 chicken thigh and 1/3 cup sauce

Amount per serving	
Calories	**200**
Calories from fat 70	
Total fat 8.0 g	
Saturated fat 1.9 g	
Trans fat 0.0 g	
Cholesterol 90 mg	
Sodium 340 mg	
Potassium 500 mg	
Total carbohydrate 14 g	
Dietary fiber 2 g	
Sugars 10 g	
Protein 18 g	
Phosphorus 190 mg	

Choices/Exchanges: 1/2 Fruit, 1 Nonstarchy Vegetable, 2 Lean Protein, 1 Fat

2 large ripe avocados
1/4 cup cocoa powder
3 tablespoons coconut or almond milk
3 tablespoons honey or 3 packets artificial sweetener
1/2 teaspoon vanilla extract
1/2 banana
4 teaspoons dairy-free chocolate chips
1 1/2 cups raspberries

1. Add all the ingredients except chocolate chips and raspberries to a food processor and blend until smooth, scraping the sides of the bowl as needed. Pour mousse into a bowl and refrigerate 1 hour, until cold.
2. Serve 1/3 cup mousse, topped with 1 teaspoon chocolate chips and 1/4 cup raspberries. Repeat for remaining 5 dishes.

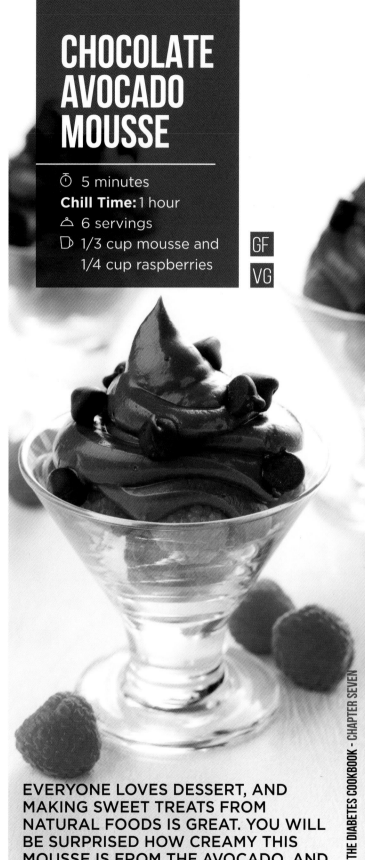

CHOCOLATE AVOCADO MOUSSE

- ⏱ 5 minutes
- **Chill Time:** 1 hour
- 🍽 6 servings
- 🍴 1/3 cup mousse and 1/4 cup raspberries

GF
VG

Nutrition Facts

Serves: 6
Serving Size: 1/3 cup mousse and 1/4 cup raspberries

Amount per serving	
Calories	**180**
Calories from fat 100	
Total fat 11.0 g	
Saturated fat 2.4 g	
Trans fat 0.0 g	
Cholesterol 0 mg	
Sodium 5 mg	
Potassium 440 mg	
Total carbohydrate 24 g	
Dietary fiber 8 g	
Sugars 13 g	
Protein 3 g	
Phosphorus 75 mg	

Choices/Exchanges:
1 1/2 Carbohydrate, 2 Fat

EVERYONE LOVES DESSERT, AND MAKING SWEET TREATS FROM NATURAL FOODS IS GREAT. YOU WILL BE SURPRISED HOW CREAMY THIS MOUSSE IS FROM THE AVOCADO, AND IT'S A NICE DESSERT TO SERVE A GUEST WHO HAS A DAIRY ALLERGY.

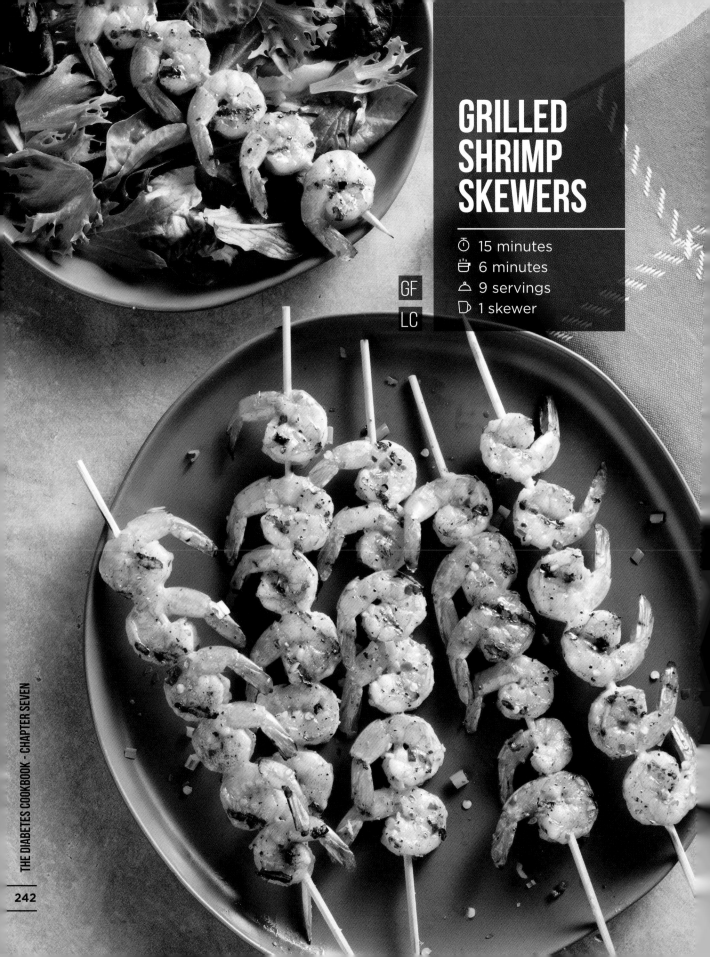

GRILLED SHRIMP SKEWERS

- ⏱ 15 minutes
- 🍲 6 minutes
- 🍽 9 servings
- 🍴 1 skewer

GF
LC

1 1/2   tablespoons olive oil
2   cloves garlic, minced
Juice and zest of 1 medium lemon
1/4   teaspoon crushed red pepper flakes
2   scallions (white and green parts), minced
1/2   teaspoon salt
1/4   teaspoon ground black pepper
1   pound peeled and deveined raw medium shrimp
9   bamboo skewers, soaked in warm water

1. Prepare an indoor or outdoor grill.
2. In a medium bowl, whisk together olive oil, garlic, lemon juice, lemon zest, red pepper flakes, scallions, salt, and black pepper.
3. Add shrimp to bowl and toss to coat evenly. Cover and refrigerate 30 minutes.
4. Divide shrimp evenly among nine skewers. Discard remaining marinade.
5. Grill skewers 2–3 minutes on each side or until shrimp are pink and slightly firm to the touch.

NOTE: *If possible, use fresh (never frozen) shrimp, or shrimp that are free of preservatives (for example, shrimp that have not been treated with salt or STPP [sodium tripolyphosphate]).*

Nutrition Facts

Serves: 9
Serving Size: 1 skewer

Amount per serving
Calories **50**

Calories from fat 5	
Total fat 0.5 g	
Saturated fat 0.1 g	
Trans fat 0.0 g	
Cholesterol 85 mg	
Sodium 75 mg	
Potassium 120 mg	
Total carbohydrate 0 g	
Dietary fiber 0 g	
Sugars 0 g	
Protein 11 g	
Phosphorus 105 mg	

Choices/Exchanges: 1 Lean Protein

QUICK SAUTÉED CABBAGE WITH SESAME SEEDS

GF
LC
VG

⏲ 10 minutes
🍲 4 servings
🥄 1/2 cup

SO MANY PEOPLE SAY THEY LIKE VEGETABLES BUT ADMIT TO NOT EATING ENOUGH. THIS TASTY DISH IS SO EASY AND IS A GREAT WAY TO START EATING MORE VEGETABLES DAILY. BY BUYING BAGGED COLESLAW YOU SAVE ON PREP TIME. ALSO, COCONUT AMINOS CAN BE SUBSTITUTED HERE FOR PEOPLE WHO ARE AVOIDING OR ARE ALLERGIC TO SOY. COCONUT AMINOS IS A SAUCE THAT CAN BE USED IN PLACE OF SOY SAUCE AND CAN BE FOUND AT SPECIALTY GROCERY STORES OR ONLINE.

1 1/2	tablespoons olive oil
1	(14-ounce) bag coleslaw
1 1/2	tablespoons lite, gluten-free soy sauce
1/4	teaspoon ground black pepper
1/4	teaspoon ground ginger
3	tablespoons sesame seeds

1. Heat oil in a large sauté pan over medium heat. Add all ingredients except sesame seeds and cook 9 minutes, stirring frequently.
2. Add sesame seeds and cook 1 additional minute.

Nutrition Facts

Serves: 4
Serving Size: 1/2 cup

Amount per serving
Calories — **120**

Calories from fat 80

Total fat 9.0 g

Saturated fat 1.2 g

Trans fat 0.0 g

Cholesterol 0 mg

Sodium 230 mg

Potassium 290 mg

Total carbohydrate 8 g

Dietary fiber 4 g

Sugars 2 g

Protein 2 g

Phosphorus 75 mg

Choices/Exchanges: 1 Nonstarchy Vegetable, 2 Fat

BEEF AND BRUSSELS SPROUT SKILLET

⏱ 5 minutes
🍲 20 minutes
🍽 5 servings
🥄 1 cup

SOMETIMES THE SIMPLEST INGREDIENTS CREATE THE BEST FLAVORS, AND THIS DISH IS PROOF! MANY PEOPLE PREFER THE FLAVOR OF GRASS-FED BEEF, BUT REGULAR LEAN GROUND BEEF CAN BE USED HERE, TOO. MAKE HALF YOUR PLATE VEGETABLES BY SERVING THIS DISH OVER COOKED CAULIFLOWER RICE—CAULIFLOWER THAT HAS BEEN PROCESSED FINELY TO RESEMBLE RICE—WHICH YOU CAN FIND IN THE FREEZER SECTION OF YOUR LOCAL GROCER.

1	pound 95% lean grass-fed ground beef
2	tablespoons olive oil
2	cloves garlic, minced
1	pound Brussels sprouts, ends trimmed and cut in half
1/4	teaspoon ground black pepper

1. Cook beef in a nonstick pan over medium-high heat about 8–10 minutes, until done. Remove beef from pan and set aside.
2. Heat oil in pan; add garlic and sauté 30 seconds. Add Brussels sprouts and cook 10 minutes, stirring frequently. Add beef back to pan, sprinkle with pepper and cook an additional 1–2 minutes.

Nutrition Facts

Serves: 5
Serving Size: 1 cup

Amount per serving
Calories 200

Calories from fat 100

Total fat 11.0 g
  Saturated fat 3.0 g
  Trans fat 0.1 g
Cholesterol 55 mg
Sodium 70 mg
Potassium 580 mg
Total carbohydrate 7 g
  Dietary fiber 2 g
  Sugars 2 g
Protein 20 g
Phosphorus 215 mg

Choices/Exchanges: 1 Nonstarchy Vegetable, 3 Lean Protein, 1 Fat

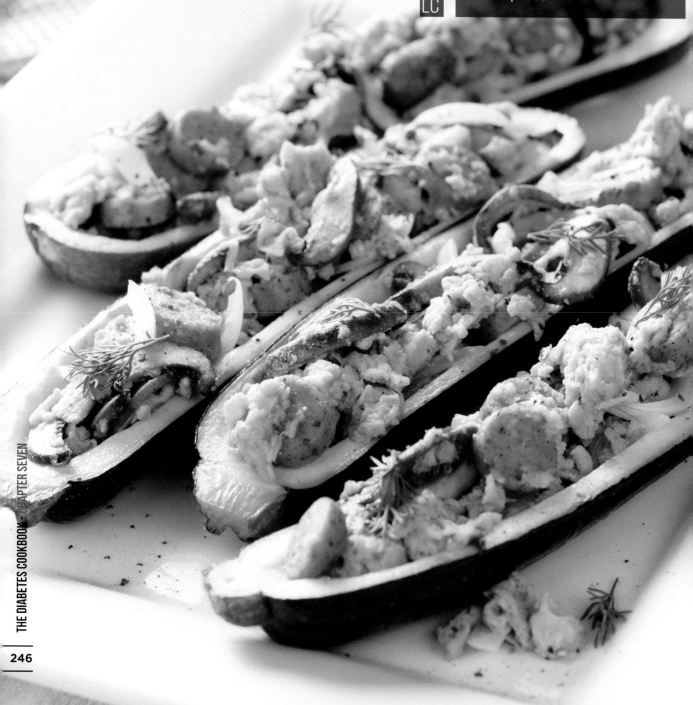

THIS RECIPE IS AN EXAMPLE OF
HOW TO BE CREATIVE WHEN
WORKING MORE LOW-CARB
VEGGIES INTO YOUR DIET.

ZUCCHINI EGG BOATS

LC

- ⏲ 15 minutes
- 🍲 35 minutes
- 🍽 4 servings
- 🥄 1 piece

Nonstick cooking spray
2   medium zucchini
8   ounces sliced mushrooms
1   small onion
4   ounces chicken breakfast sausage
      links (fully cooked as purchased)
4   eggs
2   tablespoons water
1   teaspoon hot sauce
1/4   teaspoon salt
1/4   teaspoon ground black pepper

1. Preheat oven to 400°F. Coat a baking sheet with cooking spray. Slice zucchini in half lengthwise, scoop the seeds out to make a boat, and place on the prepared baking sheet. Roast the zucchini 25 minutes.
2. While the zucchini is roasting, add cooking spray to a medium nonstick sauté pan over medium-high heat. Add mushrooms, onion, and sausage to the pan and sauté 7 minutes, or until mushrooms and onion are tender.
3. In a medium bowl, whisk together eggs, water, hot sauce, salt, and pepper. Pour the egg mixture over the sautéed veggies and sausage, gently stirring over medium-low heat until eggs and vegetable mixture are thoroughly combined, about 4 minutes.
4. Remove the zucchini from the oven and top each zucchini half with a scant cup of the egg mixture.

MAKE IT GLUTEN-FREE: *Confirm all ingredients are gluten-free, including the chicken sausage and hot sauce.*

Nutrition Facts

Serves: 4
Serving Size: 1 piece

Amount per serving

Calories   **160**

Calories from fat 70	
Total fat 8.0 g	
Saturated fat 2.6 g	
Trans fat 0.0 g	
Cholesterol 210 mg	
Sodium 410 mg	
Potassium 570 mg	
Total carbohydrate 8 g	
Dietary fiber 2 g	
Sugars 5 g	
Protein 15 g	
Phosphorus 240 mg	

Choices/Exchanges: 2 Nonstarchy Vegetable, 2 Lean Protein, 1/2 Fat

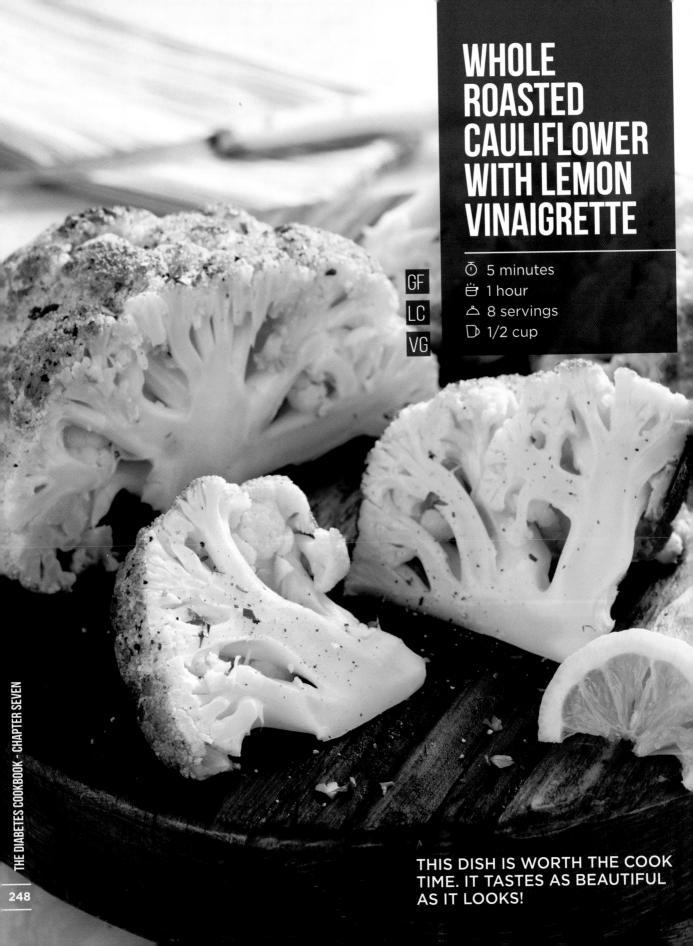

WHOLE ROASTED CAULIFLOWER WITH LEMON VINAIGRETTE

GF
LC
VG

- ⏱ 5 minutes
- 🍲 1 hour
- 🍽 8 servings
- 🥄 1/2 cup

THIS DISH IS WORTH THE COOK TIME. IT TASTES AS BEAUTIFUL AS IT LOOKS!

CAULIFLOWER

2	tablespoons olive oil
1/2	teaspoon salt
1	(2 1/2-pound) whole cauliflower

VINAIGRETTE

Juice of 1/2 lemon
2	tablespoons extra-virgin olive oil
1/2	teaspoon dried parsley
1/8	teaspoon ground black pepper

1. Preheat oven to 425°F.
2. In a small bowl mix together olive oil and salt.
3. Place cauliflower, cut side down, in a large baking dish. Pour olive oil evenly over cauliflower and use your hands to rub the oil and salt mixture into the cauliflower.
4. Place on the middle oven rack, and roast 1 hour (if cauliflower starts getting too dark, then cover with aluminum foil).
5. While cauliflower is roasting, whisk together all the vinaigrette ingredients in a small bowl.
6. When cauliflower is finished roasting, pour vinaigrette evenly over entire head.
7. To serve, cut whole cauliflower in half, then cut each half into 4 pieces.

Nutrition Facts

Serves: 8
Serving Size: 1/2 cup

Amount per serving
Calories 80

Calories from fat 60	
Total fat 7.0 g	
Saturated fat 1.0 g	
Trans fat 0.0 g	
Cholesterol 0 mg	
Sodium 170 mg	
Potassium 260 mg	
Total carbohydrate 4 g	
Dietary fiber 2 g	
Sugars 2 g	
Protein 2 g	
Phosphorus 40 mg	

Choices/Exchanges: 1 Nonstarchy Vegetable, 1 1/2 Fat

SAUTÉED ASPARAGUS, PEPPERS, AND MUSHROOMS

GF
LC
VG

⏱ 10 minutes
☕ 20 minutes
△ 7 servings
▭ 1/2 cup

NONSTARCHY VEGGIES—SUCH AS ASPARAGUS, PEPPERS, AND MUSHROOMS—ARE PACKED WITH VITAMINS AND MINERALS YET LOW IN CALORIES AND CARBOHYDRATES. USE SIMPLE, DELICIOUS IDEAS LIKE THIS RECIPE TO FILL HALF YOUR PLATE WITH NONSTARCHY VEGGIES!

1 1/2	tablespoons olive oil
1	pound asparagus, trimmed and cut into thirds
1/2	cup sliced red onion
8	ounces baby bella mushrooms, sliced
1	medium red bell pepper, chopped
1	clove garlic, minced

1. Heat olive oil in a large sauté pan or wok over medium-high heat. Add asparagus, onion, mushrooms, and pepper, and cook 15–18 minutes, stirring frequently.
2. Add garlic to pan and cook 1 minute, stirring vegetables and garlic to incorporate.

DIETITIAN TIP: *Mix up the variety of nutritious veggies you choose for this easy recipe. Look for packs of chopped, prepared vegetables sold in your grocery store's produce section.*

Nutrition Facts

Serves: 7
Serving Size: 1/2 cup

Amount per serving

Calories 50

Calories from fat 25

Total fat 3.0 g

    Saturated fat 0.4 g

    Trans fat 0.0 g

Cholesterol 0 mg

Sodium 0 mg

Potassium 270 mg

Total carbohydrate 5 g

    Dietary fiber 1 g

    Sugars 2 g

Protein 2 g

Phosphorus 65 mg

Choices/Exchanges: 1 Nonstarchy Vegetable, 1/2 Fat

CILANTRO LIME CAULIFLOWER RICE

GF
LC
VG

- ⏱ 5 minutes
- 🍲 10 minutes
- 🍽 4 servings
- 🍚 1 cup

THIS LOW-CARB "RICE" PAIRS NICELY WITH MEXICAN DISHES SUCH AS CHICKEN OR SHRIMP FAJITAS.

1 (12-ounce) bag frozen cauliflower rice
1 tablespoon olive oil
2 cloves garlic, minced
Juice and zest of 3 limes (juice divided)
1/4 cup chopped fresh cilantro

1. Cook cauliflower rice in microwave according to the directions on the package.
2. Heat the olive oil in a large skillet over medium heat. Add the garlic and cook 30 seconds. Reduce heat to low and add the cauliflower rice.
3. Add the juice of 2 limes and the lime zest, and simmer cauliflower rice 2 minutes. Just before serving, stir in the juice of 1 lime and chopped cilantro.

Nutrition Facts

Serves: 4
Serving Size: 1 cup

Amount per serving
Calories **60**

Calories from fat 30	
Total fat 3.5 g	
Saturated fat 0.6 g	
Trans fat 0.0 g	
Cholesterol 0 mg	
Sodium 30 mg	
Potassium 300 mg	
Total carbohydrate 7 g	
Dietary fiber 2 g	
Sugars 2 g	
Protein 2 g	
Phosphorus 45 mg	

Choices/Exchanges: 1 Nonstarchy Vegetable, 1 Fat

FOR AN EVEN SHORTER PREP TIME,
USE STORE-BOUGHT GUACAMOLE
TO MAKE THIS RECIPE.

GUACAMOLE-STUFFED CHERRY TOMATOES

GF
LC
VG

- ⏱ 15 minutes
- 🍽 12 servings
- 🥄 2 tomatoes

24 cherry tomatoes (round, not grape tomatoes)
1 ripe avocado
Juice of 1 lime
1 clove garlic, minced or grated
2 tablespoons chopped fresh cilantro, divided
1/2 teaspoon salt
1/2 teaspoon ground black pepper

1. Cut out the stem of each cherry tomato, cutting deep enough to make a hole in the middle of the tomato without going through the other end.
2. Scoop out and finely chop the insides of the tomatoes, and reserve for the guacamole. Place each scooped-out tomato upside down on paper towels to drain.
3. In a medium bowl, mash the avocado with a fork and mix in the scooped-out tomato pieces, lime juice, garlic, 1 tablespoon cilantro, salt, and pepper.
4. Scoop or pipe the guacamole into the hollowed-out tomatoes, dividing it equally among all the tomatoes. Sprinkle the remaining cilantro on top of the tomatoes.

Nutrition Facts

Serves: 12
Serving Size: 2 tomatoes

Amount per serving
Calories 25

Calories from fat 20	
Total fat 2.0 g	
Saturated fat 0.3 g	
Trans fat 0.0 g	
Cholesterol 0 mg	
Sodium 100 mg	
Potassium 130 mg	
Total carbohydrate 2 g	
Dietary fiber 1 g	
Sugars 1 g	
Protein 1 g	
Phosphorus 15 mg	

Choices/Exchanges: 1/2 Fat

BACON-WRAPPED SHRIMP

DON'T BE SURPRISED WHEN THESE APPETIZERS ARE DEVOURED AT YOUR NEXT PARTY. THIS CLASSIC TAKE ON SHRIMP PROVES THAT SOMETIMES THE SIMPLEST RECIPES ARE CROWD PLEASERS!

GF
LC

- ⏱ 10 minutes
- 🍲 6 minutes
- 🍽 10 servings
- 🍴 2 shrimp

7   slices bacon
20 raw jumbo shrimp, peeled and deveined
4   small leaves of romaine lettuce

1. Preheat broiler.
2. Cut each bacon slice crosswise into three pieces. Wrap one piece around each shrimp. Repeat for remaining shrimp and bacon. Place on baking sheet and broil 2–3 minutes per side, flipping once.
3. Serve shrimp on lettuce leaves.

DIETITIAN TIP: *This recipe is a portion-controlled way to incorporate the rich flavor of bacon into your next celebration.*

NOTE: *If possible, use fresh (never frozen) shrimp, or shrimp that are free of preservatives (for example, shrimp that have not been treated with salt or STPP [sodium tripolyphosphate]).*

Nutrition Facts

Serves: 10
Serving Size: 2 shrimp

Amount per serving
Calories 90

Calories from fat 50	
Total fat 6.0 g	
Saturated fat 2.2 g	
Trans fat 0.0 g	
Cholesterol 50 mg	
Sodium 130 mg	
Potassium 95 mg	
Total carbohydrate 0 g	
Dietary fiber 0 g	
Sugars 0 g	
Protein 7 g	
Phosphorus 70 mg	

Choices/Exchanges: 1 Lean Protein, 1 Fat

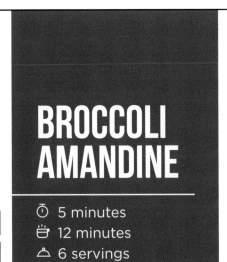

BROCCOLI AMANDINE

⏱ 5 minutes
🍲 12 minutes
△ 6 servings
▷ 1/2 cup

HAVE YOU HAD GREEN BEANS AMANDINE? NOW TRY BROCCOLI AMANDINE. ALMONDS CONTAIN HEART-HEALTHIER MONOUNSATURATED AND POLYUNSATURATED FATS. THE AMERICAN HEART ASSOCIATION RECOMMENDS EATING AT LEAST 4 SERVINGS PER WEEK OF NUTS, LEGUMES, OR SEEDS.

Nonstick cooking spray
1 (12-ounce) bag broccoli florets
1 1/2 tablespoons olive oil
2 cloves garlic, minced
3 tablespoons slivered almonds
1/8 teaspoon ground black pepper
1 tablespoon lemon juice

1. Preheat oven to 425°F. Spray a baking sheet with cooking spray.
2. In a small bowl mix together broccoli, olive oil, garlic, almonds, and pepper. Pour mixture onto baking sheet.
3. Bake 10–12 minutes until broccoli tips are slightly brown.
4. Pour broccoli mixture into a bowl and stir in lemon juice.

Nutrition Facts

Serves: 6
Serving Size: 1/2 cup

Amount per serving
Calories 70

Calories from fat 50

Total fat 6.0 g

Saturated fat 0.7 g

Trans fat 0.0 g

Cholesterol 0 mg

Sodium 15 mg

Potassium 220 mg

Total carbohydrate 4 g

Dietary fiber 2 g

Sugars 1 g

Protein 3 g

Phosphorus 55 mg

Choices/Exchanges: 1 Nonstarchy Vegetable, 1 Fat

FROZEN BANANAS ARE THE SURPRISING BASE FOR THIS SOFT-SERVE "ICE CREAM" THAT'S LOW IN SATURATED FAT. SHOP FOR SMALL RAMEKINS OR CUPS TO MAKE PORTION CONTROL EASY WHEN SERVING DESSERTS LIKE THIS ONE.

STRAWBERRY BANANA "ICE CREAM"

GF
VG

- ⏱ 2 hours, 10 minutes
- 🍽 4 servings
- 🥄 1/2 cup

2 large bananas
1 cup sliced fresh strawberries
2 tablespoons coconut milk

1. Peel bananas and slice into 1/4-inch rounds. Place in a bowl and freeze for at least 2 hours.

2. Once bananas are frozen, add strawberries, bananas, and coconut milk to a blender or food processor. Blend on high speed 30 seconds. Scrape down the sides of the blender and blend on high 30 more seconds. Repeat this process until mixture is smooth and the texture of soft-serve ice cream.

3. You can serve immediately or freeze for 30 minutes.

4. Scoop into 1/2-cup scoops to serve.

Nutrition Facts

Serves: 4
Serving Size: 1/2 cup

Amount per serving
Calories 80

Calories from fat 0

Total fat 0.0 g
    Saturated fat 0.2 g
    Trans fat 0.0 g

Cholesterol 0 mg

Sodium 0 mg

Potassium 310 mg

Total carbohydrate 19 g
    Dietary fiber 3 g
    Sugars 10 g

Protein 1 g

Phosphorus 25 mg

Choices/Exchanges: 1 Fruit

THIS LOW-CARB DISH PAIRS
NICELY WITH JUST ABOUT
EVERYTHING AND TAKES
LITTLE TIME TO MAKE.

CAULIFLOWER RICE SALAD

GF
LC
VG

- ⏱ 15 minutes
- 🍲 30 minutes
- △ 4 servings
- 🥛 1 cup

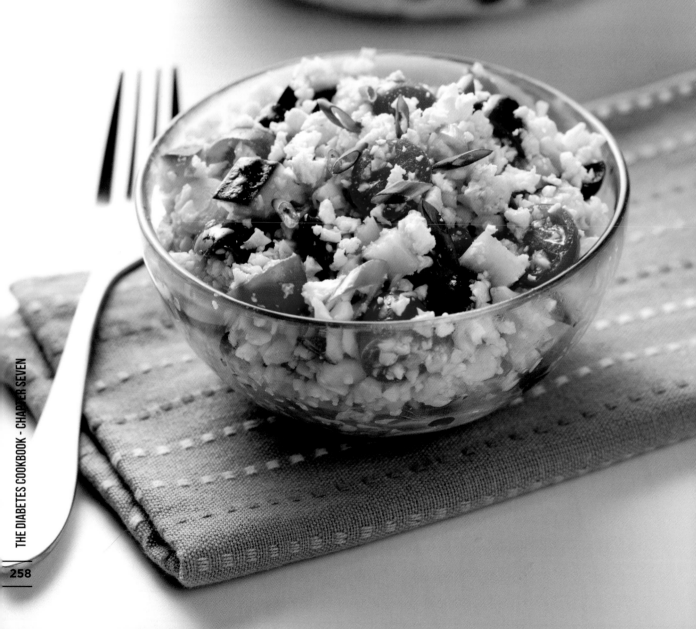

THE DIABETES COOKBOOK - CHAPTER SEVEN

SALAD

12 ounces cauliflower rice (also see Step 1)
1   cup diced cucumber
1   cup grape tomatoes, cut in half
2   green onions, sliced
3   tablespoons sliced kalamata olives

DRESSING

1/4 cup red wine vinegar
2   tablespoons extra-virgin olive oil
1/2 tablespoon Dijon mustard

1. Cauliflower rice can be purchased frozen, or you can make your own by placing cauliflower florets in a food processor and processing until rice-like consistency (be careful not to overprocess).
2. In a salad bowl, combine all salad ingredients.
3. In a small bowl, whisk together dressing ingredients.
4. Pour dressing over salad and serve with reduced-fat feta cheese, if desired.

DIETITIAN TIP: *Cauliflower rice is a new trend, and you will be pleasantly surprised how delicious this low-carb alternative is when used in traditional rice dishes.*

Nutrition Facts

Serves: 4
Serving Size: 1 cup

Amount per serving
Calories 120

Calories from fat 80

Total fat 9.0 g
  Saturated fat 1.3 g
  Trans fat 0.0 g
Cholesterol 0 mg
Sodium 180 mg
Potassium 410 mg
Total carbohydrate 8 g
  Dietary fiber 3 g
  Sugars 3 g
Protein 2 g
Phosphorus 60 mg

Choices/Exchanges: 2 Nonstarchy Vegetable, 1 1/2 Fat

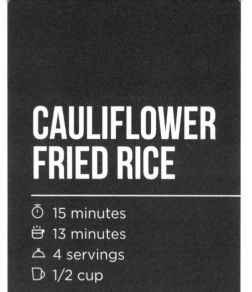

CAULIFLOWER FRIED RICE

⏱ 15 minutes
🍲 13 minutes
🍽 4 servings
🍚 1/2 cup

GF
LC

FINELY CHOPPED CAULIFLOWER CAN BE A REMARKABLE NONSTARCHY SIDE THAT'S LOWER IN CALORIES AND CARBOHYDRATES THAN RICE. OR YOU CAN MAKE IT A MAIN DISH BY ADDING CHICKEN BREAST, SHRIMP, OR TOFU.

3 cups cauliflower florets
1 tablespoon olive oil, divided
2 large carrots, finely diced
3 scallions, chopped
1 teaspoon sesame oil
1 1/2 tablespoons lite, gluten-free soy sauce
1/4 cup fat-free, gluten-free, no-salt-added chicken broth
1/8 teaspoon ground ginger
1/8 teaspoon ground black pepper

1. Place cauliflower in a food processor and process until rice-like consistency; set aside.
2. Heat 1/2 tablespoon olive oil in a nonstick pan over medium-high heat. Add carrots and scallions and sauté 5 minutes.
3. Add remaining 1/2 tablespoon olive oil and sesame oil to pan. Add cauliflower rice and remaining ingredients and reduce heat to medium-low. Cook cauliflower mixture 6–8 minutes, stirring frequently. Cauliflower should be tender but not mushy.

DIETITIAN TIP: *Some grocery stores sell cauliflower rice in the frozen or refrigerated produce section. Look for this convenient option, or use a box grater if you don't have a food processor. If you are avoiding soy due to allergies, coconut aminos can be substituted for soy sauce here.*

Nutrition Facts
Serves: 4
Serving Size: 1/2 cup

Amount per serving
Calories **80**

Calories from fat 45

Total fat 5.0 g
   Saturated fat 0.7 g
   Trans fat 0.0 g
Cholesterol 0 mg
Sodium 260 mg
Potassium 360 mg
Total carbohydrate 8 g
   Dietary fiber 3 g
   Sugars 3 g
Protein 3 g
Phosphorus 55 mg

Choices/Exchanges: 2 Nonstarchy Vegetable, 1 Fat

AVOCADO TUNA SALAD

⏱ 5 minutes
◿ 5 servings
🍽 1/2 cup

GF
LC

THIS MAKES A FAST AND EASY LUNCH OR DINNER. YOU CAN PURCHASE PICO DE GALLO IN THE PRODUCE SECTION OR AT THE DELI COUNTER IN MOST GROCERY STORES. AVOCADOS ARE A GREAT SOURCE OF MONOUNSATURATED FAT, WHICH IS GOOD FOR HEART HEALTH.

1   medium avocado, cut in half
1/2 cup no-salt-added pico de gallo
2   (6.4-ounce) tuna flavorseal pouches, packed in water

1. Remove the pit from the avocado. Use a spoon to scoop out the insides of the avocado and place in a medium bowl. Mash the avocado with a fork or potato masher. Add the pico de gallo and mix well.
2. Add the tuna to the bowl and mix well. Serve the tuna salad with your choice of crackers or lettuce wraps.

Nutrition Facts

Serves: 5
Serving Size: 1/2 cup

Amount per serving
Calories 130

Calories from fat 45

Total fat 5.0 g

   Saturated fat 0.8 g

   Trans fat 0.0 g

Cholesterol 30 mg

Sodium 300 mg

Potassium 340 mg

Total carbohydrate 4 g

   Dietary fiber 3 g

   Sugars 1 g

Protein 18 g

Phosphorus 140 mg

Choices/Exchanges: 3 Lean Protein

BAKED APPLE CHIPS

GF
VG

⏱ 10 minutes
🍲 2 hours
🍽 4 servings
🍴 1/2 apple

EXPERIMENT USING OTHER FRUITS SUCH AS PEARS TO MAKE THESE CHIPS.

2 medium apples (honeycrisp or another sweet apple)
1 teaspoon cinnamon

1. Preheat oven to 200°F. Lay parchment paper on one large or two medium baking sheets.
2. Using a mandoline or knife, thinly slice the apples to make round chips. Discard the seeds.
3. Lay the apple slices on the prepared baking sheet(s) without overlapping. Sprinkle the cinnamon over apples.
4. Bake 1 hour, then flip the apples. Continue baking 1–2 hours, flipping occasionally, until the apple slices are no longer moist. Let cool completely, and then store in airtight container.

Nutrition Facts

Serves: 4
Serving Size: 1/2 apple

Amount per serving
Calories 50

Calories from fat 0

Total fat 0.0 g

   Saturated fat 0.0 g

   Trans fat 0.0 g

Cholesterol 0 mg

Sodium 0 mg

Potassium 100 mg

Total carbohydrate 13 g

   Dietary fiber 2 g

   Sugars 9 g

Protein 0 g

Phosphorus 10 mg

Choices/Exchanges: 1 Fruit

ZUCCHINI NOODLES WITH TURKEY MEATBALLS

THESE ZUCCHINI NOODLES KEEP THE AMOUNT OF CARBOHYDRATES IN THIS DISH LOW. YOU COULD ALSO SAUTÉ THE ZUCCHINI NOODLES IF YOU'D LIKE.

- ⏱ 20 minutes
- 🍳 25 minutes
- 🍽 4 servings
- 🍴 1 zucchini and 3 meatballs

GF

MEATBALLS

	Nonstick cooking spray
1 1/4	pounds lean ground turkey
2	cloves garlic, minced
1	tablespoon dried oregano
1/4	cup finely chopped fresh Italian parsley
1	teaspoon dried minced onion
1	egg, slightly beaten
3	tablespoons almond flour

NOODLES AND SAUCE

4	medium zucchini
2	cups lower-sodium marinara sauce

1. Preheat oven to 375°F. Coat a baking sheet with cooking spray.

2. In a bowl, combine turkey, garlic, oregano, parsley, dried onion, egg, and almond flour and mix well.

3. Form the turkey mixture into 12 meatballs and place them on the baking sheet.

4. Bake the meatballs 25–30 minutes or until cooked through and they reach an internal temperature of 165°F.

5. While the meatballs are cooking, use a julienne peeler, a spiralizer, or mandoline set on the julienne setting to cut the zucchini into noodles. Place the noodles in a large microwave-safe dish, cover with a lid, and microwave on high 2 minutes.

6. Heat the marinara sauce in a large saucepan. Add the cooked meatballs to the sauce and pour sauce with meatballs over zucchini noodles.

Nutrition Facts

Serves: 4

Serving Size: 1 zucchini and 3 meatballs

Amount per serving

Calories 400

Calories from fat 180	
Total fat 20.0 g	
Saturated fat 4.4 g	
Trans fat 0.2 g	
Cholesterol 155 mg	
Sodium 420 mg	
Potassium 1320 mg	
Total carbohydrate 19 g	
Dietary fiber 4 g	
Sugars 11 g	
Protein 35 g	
Phosphorus 445 mg	

Choices/Exchanges: 1/2 Starch, 2 Nonstarchy Vegetable, 4 Lean Protein, 2 1/2 Fat

SUMMER FRUIT SMOOTHIE

GF
VG

WHEN FRESH PRODUCE IS ABUNDANT, TAKE ADVANTAGE OF YOUR LOCAL FARMERS MARKET AND MIX UP THE TYPES OF FRUITS IN THIS SMOOTHIE.

🕐 10 minutes
🍽 4 servings
🥤 1 cup

1   cup fresh blueberries
1   cup fresh strawberries, chopped
2   peaches, peeled, pitted, and chopped
1   (5.3-ounce or 150-gram) container gluten-free dairy-free peach Greek almond-milk yogurt
1   cup unsweetened almond milk
2   tablespoons ground flaxseed
1/2 cup ice

1. Combine all ingredients in a blender and purée until smooth.

Nutrition Facts

Serves: 4
Serving Size: 1 cup

Amount per serving
Calories   **140**

Calories from fat 45

Total fat 5.0 g

   Saturated fat 0.5 g

   Trans fat 0.0 g

Cholesterol 0 mg

Sodium 50 mg

Potassium 330 mg

Total carbohydrate 22 g

   Dietary fiber 4 g

   Sugars 14 g

Protein 5 g

Phosphorus 60 mg

Choices/Exchanges: 1 Fruit, 1/2 Carbohydrate, 1 Fat

BUTTERNUT SQUASH WITH ITALIAN SAUSAGE

- ⏱ 10 minutes
- 🍲 30 minutes
- 🍽 4 servings
- 🥤 1 heaping cup

GF

CUTTING BUTTERNUT SQUASH CAN BE VERY TIME-CONSUMING. SAVE TIME BY USING PREPACKAGED SQUASH IN THIS MOUTHWATERING DISH. SERVE THIS WITH A LARGE GREEN SALAD.

Nonstick cooking spray
2   (12-ounce) packages cubed butternut squash
1/2 small onion, diced
3   gluten-free Italian-style cooked chicken sausage links (3 ounces each), sliced
1   teaspoon olive oil
1/8 teaspoon sage
Pinch cayenne pepper

1. Preheat oven to 425°F. Spray a baking sheet with cooking spray.
2. In a medium bowl, mix together all remaining ingredients.
3. Spread evenly on baking sheet and bake 30–35 minutes or until squash is tender.

Nutrition Facts

Serves: 4
Serving Size: 1 heaping cup

Amount per serving
Calories 180

Calories from fat 60

Total fat 7.0 g
  Saturated fat 1.7 g
  Trans fat 0.0 g
Cholesterol 50 mg
Sodium 360 mg
Potassium 770 mg
Total carbohydrate 19 g
  Dietary fiber 4 g
  Sugars 4 g
Protein 13 g
Phosphorus 150 mg

Choices/Exchanges: 1 Starch, 2 Lean Protein, 1/2 Fat

CHOPPED CHICKEN SALAD

⏱ 15 minutes
🍽 5 servings
🥡 2 cups

GF

THIS SALAD IS DELICIOUS AND TASTES LIKE ONE YOU WOULD ORDER AT A RESTAURANT. IT IS VERSATILE AND CAN BE PACKED FOR LUNCHES OR ROAD TRIPS, OR SERVED FOR LUNCH AT HOME.

SALAD

8	cups chopped romaine lettuce
2	green onions, chopped
2	carrots, shredded
2	cups diced cooked chicken breast
2	hard-boiled eggs, diced
1	large tomato, diced
4	tablespoons cooked bacon pieces
1	avocado, cut in half and the pit removed

DRESSING

1/2	avocado
	Juice of 1 lemon
1/16	teaspoon salt
1	clove garlic

1. In a large salad bowl, add all salad ingredients except avocado and toss.
2. Gently remove the insides of the avocado from shell. Cut avocado into thin slices and lay on top of sald.
3. Place dressing ingredients in a blender and blend until smooth.
4. Divide salad evenly among 5 bowls. Top each with about 2 tablespoons salad dressing.

DIETITIAN TIP: *You can either use leftover chicken breasts for this recipe or purchase a cooked rotisserie chicken from your local grocery store. You can also buy cooked bacon pieces.*

Nutrition Facts

Serves: 5
Serving Size: 2 cups

Amount per serving	
Calories	**250**

Calories from fat 110	
Total fat 12.0 g	
Saturated fat 2.7 g	
Trans fat 0.0 g	
Cholesterol 125 mg	
Sodium 200 mg	
Potassium 790 mg	
Total carbohydrate 12 g	
Dietary fiber 6 g	
Sugars 4 g	
Protein 24 g	
Phosphorus 250 mg	

Choices/Exchanges: 2 Nonstarchy Vegetable, 3 Lean Protein, 1 1/2 Fat

CHICKEN AND VEGETABLE SOUP

- ⏱ 10 minutes
- 🍳 50 minutes
- 🍽 7 servings
- 🍲 About 1 cup

SOUP IS A HEALTHY DISH THAT YOU CAN LOAD WITH LOTS OF VEGGIES. IF DESIRED, YOU CAN ADD SOME BROWN OR WILD RICE TO THIS DISH, BUT IF YOU DO, BE SURE TO ADD SOME EXTRA WATER. THIS SOUP PAIRS NICELY WITH A SALAD.

1	tablespoon olive oil
1	pound boneless skinless chicken breasts
2	carrots, diced
3	stalks celery, diced
1	cup diced mushrooms
32	ounces fat-free, gluten-free, reduced-sodium chicken broth
1/4	teaspoon dried oregano
1/4	teaspoon dried thyme

1. Add the oil to a large soup pot or dutch oven and heat over medium-high heat. Add the chicken and sear 4 minutes on each side. Remove the chicken from the pan and set aside.
2. Add the carrots, celery, and mushrooms to the same pot and sauté over medium-high heat 5 minutes.
3. Add the remaining ingredients, and add the chicken back to the pot. Bring to a boil, reduce heat, and simmer 45 minutes.
4. Remove the chicken from the pot and shred or cut up. Add the chicken back to the pot; stir.

Nutrition Facts

Serves: 7
Serving Size: About 1 cup

Amount per serving
Calories 110

Calories from fat 30

Total fat 3.5 g

    Saturated fat 0.7 g

    Trans fat 0.0 g

Cholesterol 35 mg

Sodium 370 mg

Potassium 370 mg

Total carbohydrate 3 g

    Dietary fiber 1 g

    Sugars 2 g

Protein 16 g

Phosphorus 145 mg

Choices/Exchanges: 1 Nonstarchy Vegetable, 2 Lean Protein

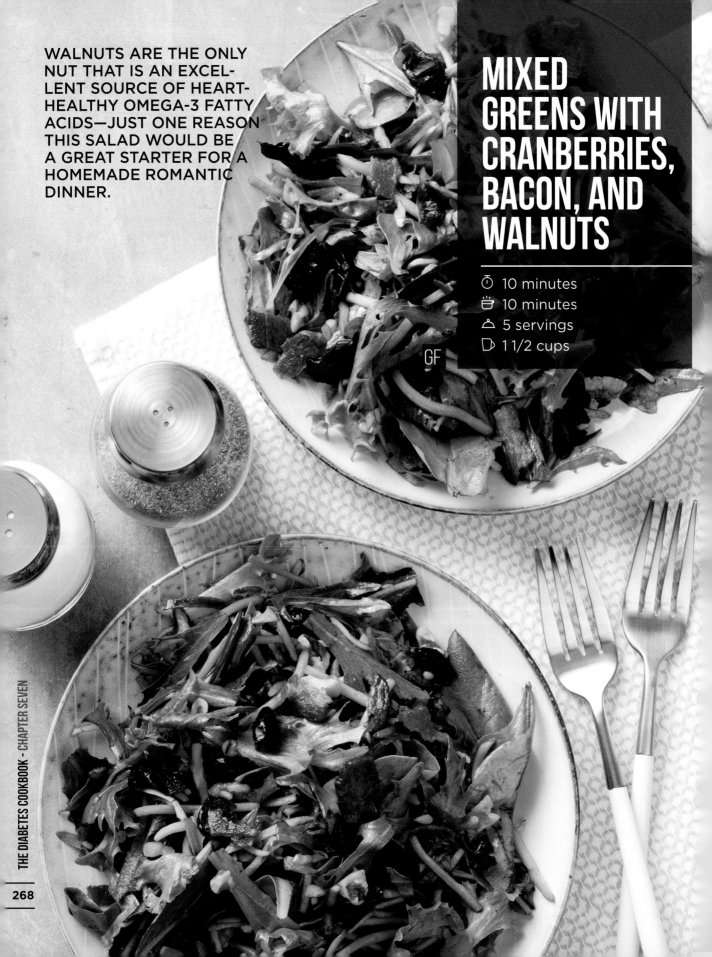

WALNUTS ARE THE ONLY NUT THAT IS AN EXCEL-LENT SOURCE OF HEART-HEALTHY OMEGA-3 FATTY ACIDS—JUST ONE REASON THIS SALAD WOULD BE A GREAT STARTER FOR A HOMEMADE ROMANTIC DINNER.

MIXED GREENS WITH CRANBERRIES, BACON, AND WALNUTS

GF

- ⏱ 10 minutes
- 🍲 10 minutes
- 🍽 5 servings
- 🥄 1 1/2 cups

SALAD

2	slices bacon, cut into 1-inch pieces
1/4	cup chopped walnuts
1	(10-ounce) bag spring lettuce mix
6	ounces broccoli slaw mix
2	tablespoons dried cranberries

DRESSING

2	tablespoons balsamic vinegar
1/2	teaspoon Dijon mustard
1	tablespoon honey or 2 packets artificial sweetener
2 1/2	tablespoons extra-virgin olive oil

1. In a medium skillet, cook the bacon over medium-high heat until done. Place the bacon on a paper towel and set aside.
2. Place the walnuts in a small nonstick skillet on low heat and cook until the walnuts begin to brown, about 4 minutes.
3. In a salad bowl, mix together all the salad ingredients.
4. In a small bowl, whisk together the dressing ingredients. Pour dressing over the salad and toss to coat.

Nutrition Facts

Serves: 5
Serving Size: 1 1/2 cups

Amount per serving

Calories 170

Calories from fat 120

Total fat 13.0 g

 Saturated fat 1.9 g

 Trans fat 0.0 g

Cholesterol 13 mg

Sodium 150 mg

Potassium 280 mg

Total carbohydrate 12 g

 Dietary fiber 3 g

 Sugars 8 g

Protein 5 g

Phosphorus 80 mg

Choices/Exchanges:
1/2 Carbohydrate, 1 Nonstarchy Vegetable, 2 1/2 Fat

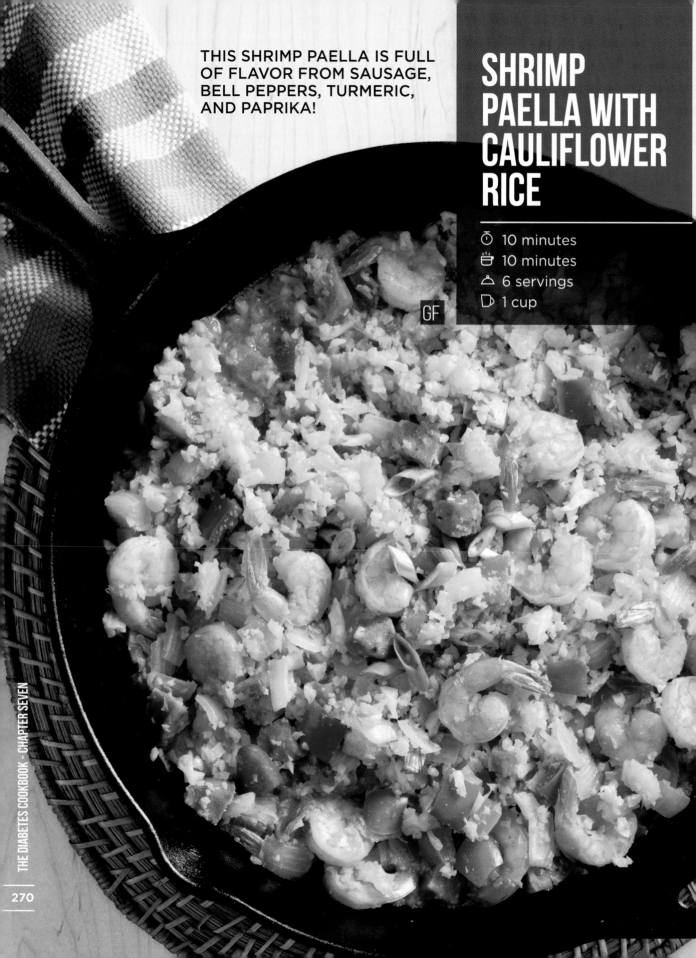

THIS SHRIMP PAELLA IS FULL OF FLAVOR FROM SAUSAGE, BELL PEPPERS, TURMERIC, AND PAPRIKA!

SHRIMP PAELLA WITH CAULIFLOWER RICE

- ⏱ 10 minutes
- 🍲 10 minutes
- 🍽 6 servings
- 🥄 1 cup

GF

Nonstick cooking spray
1   link (3 ounces) fully cooked gluten-free andouille or chorizo chicken sausage, diced
1   large onion, diced
1   red bell pepper, seeded and diced
2   cloves garlic, minced
1/2 teaspoon turmeric
1/2 teaspoon paprika
3   cups fat-free, gluten-free, low-sodium chicken broth
6   cups cauliflower rice (buy frozen and microwave according to the directions on the package)
1/2 teaspoon salt
1/2 teaspoon ground black pepper
12 ounces uncooked peeled and deveined shrimp

1. Spray a large skillet with cooking spray and place over medium-high heat. Add sausage, onion, bell pepper, and garlic. Sauté until onions start to caramelize, about 8 minutes.
2. Stir in turmeric and paprika. Add the broth, cauliflower rice, salt, and pepper. Bring to a boil; then reduce heat to low, cover, and simmer 5 minutes.
3. Add the shrimp to the cauliflower rice, cover, and cook until shrimp are just opaque in center, about 6 minutes.

CHEF TIP: *To save time, buy shrimp that are already peeled and deveined. If frozen, thaw under cold running water.*

NOTE: *If possible, use fresh (never frozen) shrimp, or shrimp that are free of preservatives (for example, shrimp that have not been treated with salt or STPP [sodium tripolyphosphate]).*

Nutrition Facts

Serves: 6
Serving Size: 1 cup

Amount per serving

Calories 130

Calories from fat 20

Total fat 2.0 g	
Saturated fat 0.6 g	
Trans fat 0.0 g	
Cholesterol 80 mg	
Sodium 410 mg	
Potassium 740 mg	
Total carbohydrate 13 g	
Dietary fiber 4 g	
Sugars 6 g	
Protein 16 g	
Phosphorus 225 mg	

Choices/Exchanges: 2 Nonstarchy Vegetable, 2 Lean Protein

SAVOR RICH FALL FLAVORS WITH
THIS DELICIOUS AND FAST SOUP.
USING FROZEN BUTTERNUT SQUASH
IN THIS RECIPE IS A BIG TIME-SAVER—
COOKING THE SQUASH WOULD
NORMALLY TAKE ABOUT AN HOUR.
CHECK THE VEGETABLE SECTION
OF THE FROZEN-FOOD AISLE FOR
FROZEN BUTTERNUT SQUASH.

GF

BUTTERNUT SQUASH SOUP

- ⏱ 10 minutes
- ⏲ 30 minutes
- 🍽 5 servings
- 🥛 1 cup

2	(12-ounce) packages frozen butternut squash
1	tablespoon olive oil
1	onion, diced
1	large carrot, diced
2	cloves garlic, minced
24	ounces fat-free, gluten-free, low-sodium chicken broth
1/2	teaspoon ground black pepper
1/8	teaspoon dried sage

1. Microwave the frozen squash 5 minutes.
2. In a large soup pot, heat the oil over medium-high heat. Add the onion and carrot and sauté 5 minutes, or until onion is clear. Add the garlic and sauté 30 seconds. Add the squash and sauté 3 minutes.
3. Add the remaining ingredients. Bring to a boil, reduce heat, and simmer 15 minutes.
4. After the soup has cooled slightly, transfer it to a blender and blend until smooth or use an immersion blender in the pot to blend until smooth. If desired, return the puréed soup to the pot to reheat before serving.

Nutrition Facts

Serves: 5
Serving Size: 1 cup

Amount per serving
Calories 110

Calories from fat 25

Total fat 3.0 g

    Saturated fat 0.4 g

    Trans fat 0.0 g

Cholesterol 0 mg

Sodium 90 mg

Potassium 690 mg

Total carbohydrate 19 g

    Dietary fiber 4 g

    Sugars 5 g

Protein 4 g

Phosphorus 75 mg

Choices/Exchanges: 1 Starch, 1 Nonstarchy Vegetable, 1/2 Fat

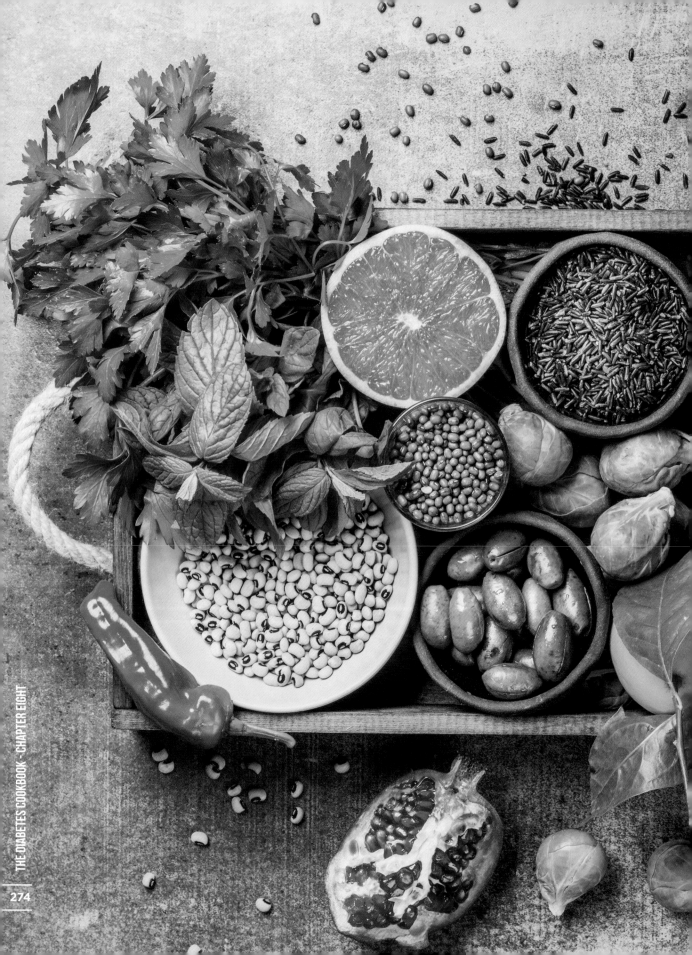

CHAPTER EIGHT

VEGETARIAN AND FLEXITARIAN RECIPES

A VEGETARIAN EATING PATTERN MAY REDUCE THE RISK OF CHRONIC DISEASE; LOWER INTAKE OF SATURATED FAT; AND INCREASE INTAKE OF FRUITS, VEGETABLES, WHOLE GRAINS, FIBER, AND PHYTOCHEMICALS. ALTHOUGH A VEGETARIAN DIET MAY NOT BE FOR EVERYONE, MANY PEOPLE CAN EAT VEGETARIAN MEALS SOME OF THE TIME. BY DEFINITION, A *FLEXITARIAN* IS A PERSON WHOSE DIET IS MOSTLY VEGETARIAN

BUT SOMETIMES INCLUDES MEAT OR POULTRY. IN OTHER WORDS, IT'S POSSIBLE TO REAP THE HEALTH BENEFITS ASSOCIATED WITH VEGETARIANISM BY BEING A FLEXIBLE VEGETARIAN AND NOT ELIMINATING MEAT COMPLETELY. YOU CAN BE A VEGETARIAN MOST OF THE TIME BUT STILL CHOW DOWN ON CHICKEN OR A LEAN BURGER WHEN THE URGE HITS. THIS CHAPTER IS CHOCK-FULL OF VEGETABLE-BASED DISHES AND INCLUDES SOME FISH AND SEAFOOD MEALS, TOO.

VEGGIE GUMBO

⏱ 20 minutes
🍲 50 minutes
△ 6 servings
🥄 1 cup

VG

SERVE THIS GUMBO OVER 1/3 CUP COOKED BROWN RICE OR QUINOA. IF YOU ARE COOKING FOR ONLY ONE OR TWO PEOPLE, YOU CAN EASILY FREEZE LEFTOVERS FROM THIS RECIPE TO SAVE FOR LATER.

2	tablespoons olive oil
2	tablespoons all-purpose flour
1	small onion, diced
1	green bell pepper, seeded and diced
1	red bell pepper, seeded and diced
2	stalks celery, diced
3	cloves garlic, minced
1/2	teaspoon salt
1/2	teaspoon ground black pepper
2	tablespoons salt-free Cajun seasoning
3	cups fat-free reduced-sodium vegetable broth
9	ounces baby spinach
1	(14.5-ounce) can black-eyed peas, drained and rinsed

1. Add the olive oil to a large pot over medium-high heat. Add the flour and cook, stirring, until golden, about 3 minutes.
2. Add the onion, bell peppers, celery, and garlic. Reduce the heat to medium and cook, stirring frequently, until the vegetables soften, 5–7 minutes.
3. Add the salt, black pepper, and Cajun seasoning. Cook 1 minute.
4. Add the vegetable broth, scraping up any browned bits from the bottom of the pot. Bring to a boil, then reduce heat to a simmer and cover.

5. Simmer, covered, 40 minutes, stirring occasionally.
6. Add the spinach and black-eyed peas. Continue to simmer until the spinach is wilted.

Nutrition Facts

Serves: 6
Serving Size: 1 cup

Amount per serving

Calories	**160**

Calories from fat 50	
Total fat 6.0 g	
Saturated fat 0.6 g	
Trans fat 0.0 g	
Cholesterol 0 mg	
Sodium 440 mg	
Potassium 600 mg	
Total carbohydrate 22 g	
Dietary fiber 6 g	
Sugars 5 g	
Protein 6 g	
Phosphorus 130 mg	

Choices/Exchanges: 1 Starch, 2 Nonstarchy Vegetable, 1 Fat

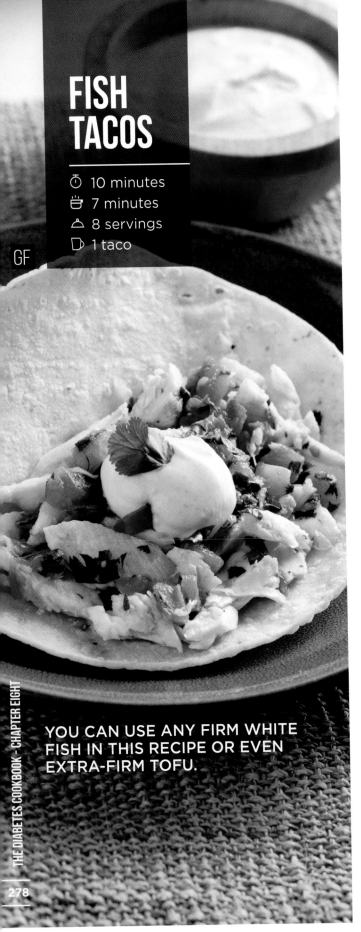

FISH TACOS

- ⏱ 10 minutes
- 🍲 7 minutes
- 🍽 8 servings
- 🍴 1 taco

GF

YOU CAN USE ANY FIRM WHITE FISH IN THIS RECIPE OR EVEN EXTRA-FIRM TOFU.

1/2 cup salsa
Juice of 1 lime
1 tablespoon chopped fresh cilantro
1 teaspoon chili powder
1/4 teaspoon salt
1/4 teaspoon ground black pepper
Nonstick cooking spray
4 halibut fillets (about 1 1/4 pounds)
8 (6-inch) corn tortillas, warmed

SAUCE

1/2 cup fat-free plain Greek yogurt
1 tablespoon hot sauce

1. In a medium bowl combine salsa, lime juice, cilantro, chili powder, salt, and pepper. Set aside
2. Coat a large sauté pan with cooking spray. Sauté fish over medium heat for 2 minutes on each side. Pour salsa mixture over fish and sauté an additional 3 minutes.
3. Remove fish from pan and shred into large pieces, mixing in the salsa mixture.
4. In a small bowl combine the sauce ingredients.
5. Evenly divide fish among 8 tortillas. Top each taco with a dollop of the sauce.

Nutrition Facts

Serves: 8
Serving Size: 1 taco

Amount per serving
Calories 150

Calories from fat 20

Total fat 2.5 g

    Saturated fat 0.4 g

    Trans fat 0.0 g

Cholesterol 25 mg

Sodium 230 mg

Potassium 440 mg

Total carbohydrate 14 g

    Dietary fiber 2 g

    Sugars 1 g

Protein 18 g

Phosphorus 265 mg

Choices/Exchanges: 1 Starch, 2 Lean Protein

CREAM OF CARAMELIZED ONION SOUP

⏱ 20 minutes
🍲 60 minutes
🍽 6 servings
🥣 1 1/4 cups

VG

THIS SOUP IS SO CREAMY IT'S HARD TO BELIEVE IT'S NOT LOADED WITH FAT. THIS RECIPE PROVES THAT HEALTHY EATING CAN BE DELICIOUS AND YOU DON'T HAVE TO FEEL DEPRIVED!

Nonstick cooking spray
2   tablespoons olive oil
3   pounds sweet onions (such as Vidalia), sliced
2   large stalks celery, diced
2   cloves garlic, minced
2   sprigs fresh thyme
1/2 cup dry white wine or 2 tablespoons lemon juice
6   cups fat-free low-sodium vegetable broth
1/2 teaspoon salt-free all-purpose seasoning (such as Spike or Mrs. Dash)
1/2 teaspoon ground black pepper
1/2 cup fat-free half-and-half

1. Add a generous amount of cooking spray and the olive oil to a soup pot over medium-high heat. Add onions and sauté 20 minutes or until onions just begin to caramelize.
2. Add the celery and garlic and continue to cook an additional 25 minutes, stirring regularly until onions are dark golden brown and celery is beginning to caramelize and very soft.
3. Add thyme and white wine. Cook until the wine is almost evaporated, about 5 minutes.
4. Stir in broth, salt-free seasoning, and pepper, and bring to a boil. Then reduce heat to simmer 10 minutes, uncovered. Remove thyme stems.
5. With an immersion or upright blender, blend the soup until very smooth (see Chef Tip).

6. Gently whisk in the half-and-half and serve. Do not boil again after adding the half-and-half or the soup will curdle.

CHEF TIP: *If using an upright blender, be sure to blend the soup in batches so as not to overload the blender and risk getting burned.*

Nutrition Facts

Serves: 6
Serving Size: 1 1/4 cups

Amount per serving	
Calories	**140**
Calories from fat 45	
Total fat 5.0 g	
Saturated fat 0.8 g	
Trans fat 0.0 g	
Cholesterol 0 mg	
Sodium 190 mg	
Potassium 480 mg	
Total carbohydrate 20 g	
Dietary fiber 3 g	
Sugars 13 g	
Protein 2 g	
Phosphorus 170 mg	

Choices/Exchanges: 4 Nonstarchy Vegetable, 1 Fat

CREAM OF ASPARAGUS SOUP

⏱ 15 minutes
🍲 25 minutes
△ 6 servings
🍶 1 1/2 cups

VG

IF USING AN UPRIGHT BLENDER, BE SURE TO BLEND THE SOUP IN BATCHES SO AS NOT TO OVERLOAD THE BLENDER AND RISK GETTING BURNED.

1	tablespoon olive oil
1	large onion, chopped
2	pounds asparagus, ends trimmed and chopped
6	cups fat-free low-sodium vegetable broth
1/4	teaspoon salt
1/2	teaspoon ground black pepper
1/2	cup fat-free plain Greek yogurt

1. Add oil to a soup pot over medium-high heat. Add onion and sauté 5 minutes, or until onion is clear.
2. Add asparagus and sauté another 2–3 minutes. Stir in broth, salt, and pepper, and bring to a boil. Then reduce heat and simmer 20 minutes, uncovered.
3. With an immersion or upright blender, blend the soup until very smooth.
4. Gently whisk in the yogurt (see Chef Tip) and serve.

CHEF TIP: *Do not boil again after adding yogurt or the soup will curdle.*

Nutrition Facts

Serves: 6
Serving Size: 1 1/2 cups

Amount per serving
Calories 80

Calories from fat 20

Total fat 2.5 g

Saturated fat 0.4 g

Trans fat 0.0 g

Cholesterol 0 mg

Sodium 240 mg

Potassium 440 mg

Total carbohydrate 12 g

Dietary fiber 4 g

Sugars 6 g

Protein 5 g

Phosphorus 170 mg

Choices/Exchanges: 2 Nonstarchy Vegetable, 1/2 Fat

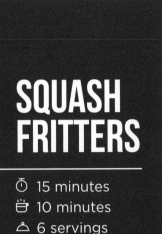

SQUASH FRITTERS

THESE LOW-CARB FRITTERS PROVE THAT COMFORT FOOD CAN BE HEALTHY!

GF
LC
VG

⏱ 15 minutes
🍲 10 minutes
△ 6 servings
🍽 1 fritter

1 cup (1/2 large) grated onion
1 cup grated carrot
2 cups (1 large) grated zucchini
2 cloves garlic, minced
1/2 cup shredded parmesan cheese
1/4 cup almond flour
2 eggs
1 egg white
1/2 teaspoon salt-free all-purpose seasoning (such as Spike or Mrs. Dash)
1/2 teaspoon ground black pepper
1 tablespoon olive oil
Nonstick cooking spray

1. In a medium bowl, mix together onion, carrot, zucchini, garlic, parmesan cheese, almond flour, eggs, egg white, salt-free seasoning, and pepper.
2. Add oil and a generous amount of cooking spray to a nonstick skillet over medium heat.
3. Using a 1/2 cup measure, scoop 1 scoop of the vegetable mixture into the hot pan and use a spatula to spread the fritter about 5 inches in diameter. Cook on each side 4 minutes, lowering the heat if it starts to burn. Respray the pan between each fritter if needed.

4. Repeat this process to make 6 fritters. Drain on a paper towel and serve hot.

Nutrition Facts

Serves: 6
Serving Size: 1 fritter

Amount per serving
Calories 120

Calories from fat 70

Total fat 8.0 g

Saturated fat 1.7 g

Trans fat 0.0 g

Cholesterol 65 mg

Sodium 100 mg

Potassium 310 mg

Total carbohydrate 7 g

Dietary fiber 2 g

Sugars 3 g

Protein 6 g

Phosphorus 115 mg

Choices/Exchanges: 1 Nonstarchy Vegetable, 2 Fat

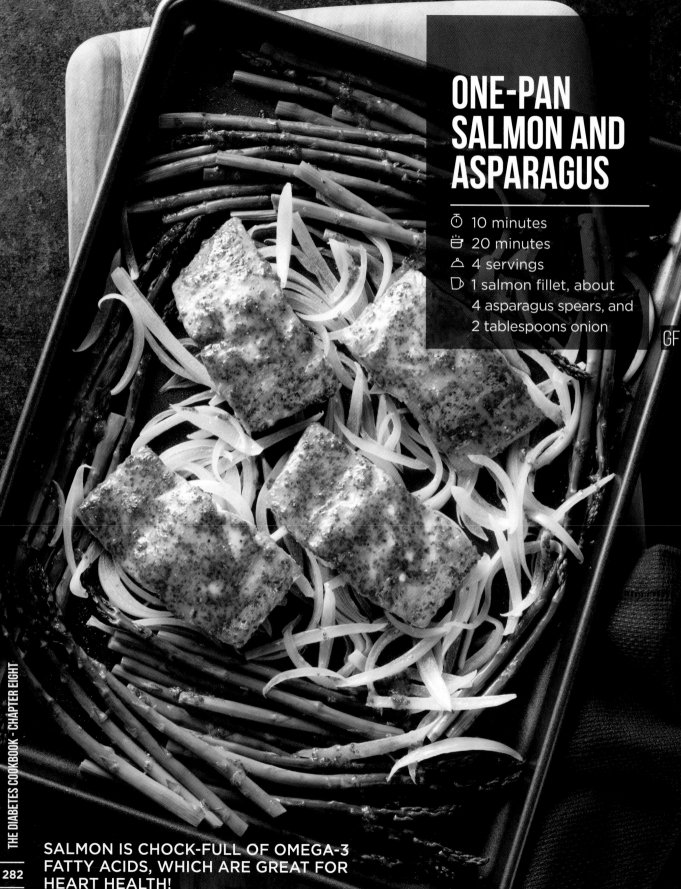

ONE-PAN SALMON AND ASPARAGUS

- 🕐 10 minutes
- 🍲 20 minutes
- 🔔 4 servings
- 🍽 1 salmon fillet, about 4 asparagus spears, and 2 tablespoons onion

GF

SALMON IS CHOCK-FULL OF OMEGA-3 FATTY ACIDS, WHICH ARE GREAT FOR HEART HEALTH!

Nonstick cooking spray
1   medium onion, thinly sliced
4   (4-ounce) skinless salmon fillets
1   pound asparagus, ends trimmed
1/4 cup whole-grain Dijon mustard
1   tablespoon olive oil
1   tablespoon honey
1/2 teaspoon ground black pepper

1. Preheat oven to 400°F.

2. Coat a baking sheet with cooking spray. Place the sliced onion in the middle of the baking sheet. Place the salmon fillets on top of the onion slices, and place the asparagus around the salmon.

3. In a small bowl, whisk together the mustard, olive oil, honey, and pepper.

4. Spread the mustard mixture on top of the salmon fillets and drizzle any extra on the asparagus.

5. Bake 20 minutes. Serve each salmon fillet with the asparagus on the side and the onions on top of the salmon.

Nutrition Facts

Serves: 4

Serving Size: 1 salmon fillet, about 4 asparagus spears, and 2 tablespoons onion

Amount per serving

Calories 260

Calories from fat 120

Total fat 13.0 g

Saturated fat 2.4 g

Trans fat 0.0 g

Cholesterol 60 mg

Sodium 440 mg

Potassium 640 mg

Total carbohydrate 12 g

Dietary fiber 3 g

Sugars 8 g

Protein 25 g

Phosphorus 360 mg

Choices/Exchanges:
1/2 Carbohydrate, 1 Nonstarchy Vegetable, 3 Lean Protein, 1 1/2 Fat

FRESH BLACK BEAN SALSA

⏱ 5 minutes
🍽 8 servings
🍴 10 chips and
   1/4 cup salsa

GF
VG

THIS SALSA IS BETTER THAN ANYTHING YOU WILL BUY AT THE STORE! IT'S DELICIOUS, QUICK, AND USES FRESH INGREDIENTS THAT YOU MIGHT ALREADY HAVE IN YOUR KITCHEN. IF YOU DON'T WANT TO SERVE IT WITH CHIPS, TRY IT WITH CUCUMBERS, CELERY, OR JICAMA. IT ALSO MAKES A GREAT TOPPING FOR TACOS!

1 cup canned black beans, rinsed and drained
2 large tomatoes, diced
1/4 cup finely diced onion
1 clove garlic, minced
Juice of 1 small lime
1/4 cup finely chopped fresh cilantro
80 gluten-free multigrain scoop tortilla chips

1. In a medium bowl, mix together all ingredients except chips.
2. Serve salsa in a bowl with chips on the side.

Nutrition Facts

Serves: 8
**Serving Size: 10 chips and
1/4 cup salsa**

Amount per serving	
Calories	**160**
Calories from fat 50	
Total fat 6.0 g	
Saturated fat 0.9 g	
Trans fat 0.0 g	
Cholesterol 0 mg	
Sodium 125 mg	
Potassium 250 mg	
Total carbohydrate 22 g	
Dietary fiber 4 g	
Sugars 2 g	
Protein 4 g	
Phosphorus 60 mg	

Choices/Exchanges: 1 1/2 Starch, 1 Fat

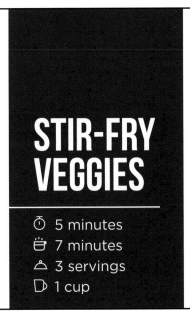

STIR-FRY VEGGIES

- ⏱ 5 minutes
- 🍲 7 minutes
- 🍽 3 servings
- 🥛 1 cup

VG

NEED HELP EATING MORE VEGGIES? GIVE THIS RECIPE A TRY! ADD SOME STIR-FRIED CHICKEN OR TOFU AND SERVE OVER BROWN RICE TO MAKE IT A MEAL.

1/4	cup fat-free low-sodium vegetable broth
1	tablespoon reduced-sodium soy sauce
1/8	teaspoon crushed red pepper flakes
2	teaspoons olive oil
1	(12-ounce) bag carrots and broccoli florets
1	cup stringless sugar snap peas
1	teaspoon sesame seeds

1. In a small bowl, whisk together the vegetable broth, soy sauce, and red pepper flakes.
2. In a large nonstick skillet or wok, heat the oil over medium-high heat. Add the vegetables and cook 5 minutes.
3. Add the vegetable broth mixture to the pan and bring to a simmer. Cook an additional 2 minutes. Sprinkle the stir-fry with sesame seeds and serve.

Nutrition Facts

Serves: 3
Serving Size: 1 cup

Amount per serving
Calories **90**

Calories from fat 35

Total fat 4.0 g

    Saturated fat 0.6 g

    Trans fat 0.0 g

Cholesterol 0 mg

Sodium 250 mg

Potassium 430 mg

Total carbohydrate 13 g

    Dietary fiber 4 g

    Sugars 4 g

Protein 4 g

Phosphorus 110 mg

Choices/Exchanges: 2 Nonstarchy Vegetable, 1 Fat

BUTTERNUT SQUASH ENCHILADAS

THESE ARE A GREAT WAY TO MAKE TRADITIONAL ENCHILADAS INTO A VEGETARIAN TREAT!

GF
VG

- ⏱ 20 minutes
- 🍲 1 hour 15 minutes
- 🍽 8 servings
- 🍴 1 enchilada

Nonstick cooking spray
1/2 butternut squash (about 2 pounds with skin on and seeds in)
1 cup cooked black beans, rinsed and drained if using canned
1 cup shredded reduced-fat mozzarella cheese, divided
2 teaspoons chili powder
1 teaspoon cumin
1/4 teaspoon cayenne pepper
1/2 teaspoon salt
1/4 teaspoon ground black pepper
8 (6-inch) corn tortillas
1 cup diced tomato
1 clove garlic, minced
1 tablespoon gluten-free Mexican-style hot sauce

1. Preheat oven to 375°F. Coat a baking pan with cooking spray.
2. Fill baking pan with 1 inch of water. Lay butternut squash half, cut side down, in the pan and roast 45 minutes.
3. Remove the roasted squash from the skin, discarding skin and seeds, and place squash in a medium bowl.
4. Coat a 9-by-13-inch baking pan with cooking spray. Set aside.
5. Add the black beans, 1/2 cup mozzarella cheese, chili powder, cumin, cayenne pepper, salt, and pepper to the roasted butternut squash. Mix well to incorporate.
6. Wrap the tortillas in a damp paper towel and microwave 30 seconds.
7. Divide the squash mixture evenly among the 8 tortillas and fold to make an enchilada. Place seam side down in the baking pan coated with cooking spray.
8. In a small bowl, mix tomato, garlic, and hot sauce. Pour over the enchiladas and top with remaining 1/2 cup mozzarella cheese.
9. Bake 30 minutes.

CHEF TIP: *You can buy frozen butternut squash in the freezer section of the grocery store and steam until softened. That will save some time in both prep and cooking. Two 10- or 12-ounce packages should work for this recipe.*

Nutrition Facts

Serves: 8
Serving Size: 1 enchilada

Amount per serving
Calories 160

Calories from fat 30

Total fat 3.5 g
  Saturated fat 1.7 g
  Trans fat 0.0 g
Cholesterol 10 mg
Sodium 320 mg
Potassium 400 mg
Total carbohydrate 27 g
  Dietary fiber 6 g
  Sugars 3 g
Protein 8 g
Phosphorus 205 mg

Choices/Exchanges: 2 Starch

ROASTED AND SPICED CHICKPEAS

GF
VG

⏱ 5 minutes
⏲ 60 minutes
△ 6 servings
🥣 1/4 cup

THIS HIGH-FIBER SNACK IS A MUCH HEALTHIER CHOICE THAN CHIPS AND IS A GREAT ALTERNATIVE FOR PEOPLE WITH NUT ALLERGIES. PLACE IN SMALL BOWLS OR RAMEKINS AT YOUR NEXT PARTY.

Nonstick cooking spray
1 (15.5-ounce) can chickpeas (garbanzo beans), rinsed and drained (dry well)
2 tablespoons olive oil, divided
1 teaspoon cinnamon
1 teaspoon cumin
1/4 teaspoon chili powder
1/4 teaspoon salt
1 1/2 tablespoons low-calorie brown sugar blend (such as Splenda)

1. Preheat oven to 400°F. Spray a baking sheet with cooking spray.
2. In a medium bowl mix together chickpeas (garbanzo beans), 1 tablespoon olive oil, cinnamon, cumin, chili powder, and salt.
3. Spread mixture evenly on bakin sheet. Bake 40–45 minutes, stirring every 10 minutes, until chickpeas are crispy and dry.
4. Remove from oven and place in a medium bowl. Add 1 tablespoon olive oil and the brown sugar blend. Mix well.
5. Pour beans on parchment paper and allow to cool 20 minutes.

Nutrition Facts

Serves: 6
Serving Size: 1/4 cup

Amount per serving
Calories 120

Calories from fat 50

Total fat 6.0 g

  Saturated fat 0.7 g

  Trans fat 0.0 g

Cholesterol 0 mg

Sodium 170 mg

Potassium 135 mg

Total carbohydrate 15 g

  Dietary fiber 4 g

  Sugars 4 g

Protein 4 g

Phosphorus 75 mg

Choices/Exchanges: 1 Starch, 1 Fat

THIS RECIPE MAKES A GREAT APPETIZER, BUT ADD SOME LEAN PROTEIN SUCH AS TOFU OR SHRIMP AND YOU HAVE A LIGHT MEAL.

VEGGIE SPRING ROLLS WITH PEANUT SAUCE

GF
LC
VG

- ⏱ 30 minutes
- 🍽 12 servings
- 🍽 1 roll

SPRING ROLLS

1	cup shredded cabbage
1	cup shredded carrots
1	cup peeled, seeded, and diced cucumber
1/4	cup chopped fresh cilantro
1	green onion, chopped
12	spring roll skins

PEANUT SAUCE

1/4	cup peanut butter, heated in microwave 30 seconds
3	tablespoons lite, gluten-free soy sauce
3	tablespoons rice wine vinegar
2	tablespoons hot water
1	tablespoon olive oil
1/4	teaspoon crushed red pepper flakes
1	clove garlic, minced
2	tablespoons chopped fresh cilantro

1. In a medium bowl combine cabbage, carrots, cucumbers, cilantro, and green onion.
2. In a small bowl, whisk together peanut sauce ingredients.
3. Soak a spring roll skin in water 10–15 seconds and remove, shaking off excess water. Place about 1/4 cup of vegetable mixture in the bottom of spring roll skin. Fold the spring roll edge nearest to you to cover the filling. Fold the side edges in tightly. Roll away from you to seal. Repeat procedure for remaining 11 spring rolls.
4. Serve spring rolls with peanut sauce.

CHEF TIP: *To save time, use bagged, shredded cabbage with carrots.*

Nutrition Facts

Serves: 12
Serving Size: 1 roll

Amount per serving
Calories   **80**

Calories from fat 35	
Total fat 4.0 g	
Saturated fat 0.7 g	
Trans fat 0.0 g	
Cholesterol 0 mg	
Sodium 300 mg	
Potassium 110 mg	
Total carbohydrate 9 g	
Dietary fiber 1 g	
Sugars 1 g	
Protein 3 g	
Phosphorus 40 mg	

Choices/Exchanges: 1/2 Starch, 1 Fat

ZUCCHINI AND FRESH CORN SUCCOTASH

GF
VG

⏱ 20 minutes
🍲 13 minutes
🍽 6 servings
🥄 1/2 cup

1	tablespoon olive oil
1	medium onion, diced
2	cloves garlic, minced
1	medium zucchini, diced
4	medium ears fresh sweet corn, cooked and kernels cut off the cob
1	(14.5-ounce) can black beans, drained and rinsed
2	tablespoons chopped fresh parsley
1/2	teaspoon salt
1/4	teaspoon ground black pepper

1. Add the olive oil to a large skillet over medium-high heat. Add the onion and sauté 5–6 minutes or until the onion starts to turn clear.
2. Add the garlic and zucchini and sauté 4–5 more minutes until the zucchini is just starting to soften.
3. Add the corn and sauté 2–3 minutes. Then add remaining ingredients and sauté until heated through.

CHEF TIP: *Cook fresh corn on the cob for this recipe by simmering it in boiling water for 8 minutes. Let the ears of corn cool, and then use a sharp knife to cut the kernels off the cob.*

Nutrition Facts

Serves: 6
Serving Size: 1/2 cup

Amount per serving
Calories 150

Calories from fat 30

Total fat 3.5 g

   Saturated fat 0.5 g

   Trans fat 0.0 g

Cholesterol 0 mg

Sodium 250 mg

Potassium 420 mg

Total carbohydrate 27 g

   Dietary fiber 6 g

   Sugars 6 g

Protein 7 g

Phosphorus 130 mg

Choices/Exchanges: 1 1/2 Starch, 1 Nonstarchy Vegetable, 1/2 Fat

JAPANESE CUCUMBER SALAD

GF
LC
VG

 15 minutes
 2 servings
⬭ 1 cup

SERVE THIS SALAD AS A VEGETABLE SIDE DISH WITH GRILLED FISH OR CHICKEN AND A SIDE OF BROWN RICE.

1 medium cucumber
2 tablespoons rice vinegar
1 tablespoon extra-virgin olive oil
1 teaspoon honey or 1/2 packet artificial sweetener
1/4 teaspoon salt
1 tablespoon sesame seeds, toasted

1. Peel the cucumber to leave alternating green stripes. Slice the cucumber in half lengthwise and scrape the seeds out with a spoon.
2. Using a mandoline, food processor, or knife, slice the cucumber into very thin slices.
3. In a medium bowl, whisk together the vinegar, olive oil, honey or artificial sweetener, and salt.
4. Toss the cucumbers and sesame seeds in the dressing and serve.

CHEF TIP: *You can find a reasonably priced handheld slicer (also called a mandoline) in any kitchen supply store. Using one will make preparing this salad really easy and make the texture consistent.*

Nutrition Facts

Serves: 2
Serving Size: 1 cup

Amount per serving
Calories 120

Calories from fat 80

Total fat 9.0 g

Saturated fat 1.3 g

Trans fat 0.0 g

Cholesterol 0 mg

Sodium 290 mg

Potassium 170 mg

Total carbohydrate 8 g

Dietary fiber 1 g

Sugars 5 g

Protein 1 g

Phosphorus 55 mg

Choices/Exchanges: 1 Nonstarchy Vegetable, 2 Fat

INDIAN VEGETABLE CURRY

⏱ 20 minutes
🍲 20 minutes
🍽 4 servings
🥤 1 1/4 cups

VG

THIS FLAVORFUL CURRY IS PACKED WITH NUTRITIOUS VEGGIES! SERVE THIS DISH OVER BROWN RICE OR IN LETTUCE CUPS.

1	small onion, chopped
4	cloves garlic, roughly chopped
1	jalapeño pepper, seeded and chopped
2	tablespoons water
1	tablespoon olive oil
2	tablespoons sweet curry powder
1	sweet potato, peeled and cut into 1-inch chunks
2	carrots, peeled and cut into 1-inch chunks
1	red bell pepper, seeded and cut into 1-inch chunks
6	ounces (about 2 handfuls) fresh green beans, trimmed and snapped in half
4	scallions (white and green parts), thinly sliced
1/2	cup unsweetened coconut milk beverage
1	cup fat-free low-sodium vegetable broth
1	tablespoon cornstarch
2	tablespoons chopped fresh cilantro
1	teaspoon paprika
1/4	teaspoon salt
1/4	teaspoon ground black pepper

1. Purée the onion, garlic, jalapeño pepper, and water in a blender or food processor to make a paste.
2. Add the oil to a wok or large sauté pan over high heat. Add the onion paste and curry powder to oil and sauté 3–4 minutes, stirring constantly.
3. Add the sweet potatoes and carrots to the paste and sauté 4–5 minutes, stirring constantly.
4. Add the red bell pepper, green beans, and scallions. Sauté 2 minutes.
5. In a separate cup or bowl, whisk together the coconut milk beverage, vegetable broth, and cornstarch. Pour over the vegetables and bring to a boil. Reduce to a simmer. Simmer, covered, 10 minutes.
6. Stir in the cilantro, paprika, salt, and black pepper.

Nutrition Facts

Serves: 4
Serving Size: 1 1/4 cups

Amount per serving
Calories 150

Calories from fat 45

Total fat 5.0 g

    Saturated fat 1.3 g

    Trans fat 0.0 g

Cholesterol 0 mg

Sodium 220 mg

Potassium 630 mg

Total carbohydrate 26 g

    Dietary fiber 7 g

    Sugars 9 g

Protein 4 g

Phosphorus 110 mg

Choices/Exchanges: 1/2 Starch, 3 Nonstarchy Vegetable, 1 Fat

EGG AND AVOCADO TOAST

- ⏱ 5 minutes
- ☕ 5 minutes
- △ 4 servings
- ▭ 1 toast

VG

4 eggs
4 slices (1 1/2 ounces each) hearty whole-grain bread
1 avocado, mashed
1/4 teaspoon salt
1/4 teaspoon ground black pepper
1/4 cup fat-free plain Greek yogurt

1. To poach each egg, fill a 1-cup microwave-safe bowl or teacup with 1/2 cup water. Gently crack an egg into the water, making sure it's completely submerged. Cover with a saucer and microwave on high about 1 minute, or until the white is set and the yolk is starting to set but is still soft (not runny).
2. Toast the bread and spread each piece with 1/4 of the mashed avocado.
3. Sprinkle avocado with salt and pepper. Top each avocado toast with a poached egg. Top each egg with 1 tablespoon Greek yogurt.

DIETITIAN TIP: *Serve these low-cost egg toasts with a green salad tossed in a light balsamic vinaigrette. What a great way to start your day, with protein, veggies, and healthy fat from the avocado.*

Nutrition Facts

Serves: 4
Serving Size: 1 toast

Amount per serving
Calories 250

Calories from fat 110

Total fat 12.0 g
  Saturated fat 2.8 g
  Trans fat 0.0 g
Cholesterol 185 mg
Sodium 380 mg
Potassium 330 mg
Total carbohydrate 26 g
  Dietary fiber 9 g
  Sugars 16 g
Protein 12 g
Phosphorus 240 mg

Choices/Exchanges: 1 1/2 Starch, 1 Medium-Fat Protein, 1 1/2 Fat

HUMMUS DEVILED EGGS

⏱ 15 minutes
🍽 8 servings
🍴 2 egg halves

TRY THIS TWIST ON TRADITIONAL DEVILED EGGS. REPLACE THE YOLK WITH A ZESTY BEAN MIXTURE TO CUT DOWN ON CALORIES, FAT, AND CHOLESTEROL. YOUR GUESTS WILL ENJOY THEM JUST AS MUCH!

8   eggs, hard-boiled and peeled
1   (14.5-ounce) can chickpeas (garbanzo beans), drained and rinsed
2   cloves garlic
Juice and zest of 1 small lemon
1   tablespoon olive oil
1/4   cup fat-free reduced-sodium vegetable broth
1/4   teaspoon salt
1/4   teaspoon ground black pepper
1/4   cup salsa
1   tablespoon chopped fresh parsley

1. Slice hard-boiled eggs in half lengthwise and discard the yolks.
2. Add chickpeas, garlic, lemon juice, lemon zest, olive oil, broth, salt, pepper, salsa, and parsley to a blender or food processor. Process until hummus is smooth.
3. Fill each egg half with a heaping tablespoon of hummus.

CHEF TIP: *To cook perfect hard-boiled eggs, cover fresh eggs with cold water in a soup pot. Put the pot over high heat and immediately start a timer set for 20 minutes. When the water begins to boil, reduce heat to a simmer. While the eggs are simmering, prepare a bowl of ice water and set aside. When the timer goes off, remove eggs from heat, drain, and immediately submerge in the ice water. Let the eggs sit 15–20 minutes in the ice water, then crack and peel.*

MAKE IT GLUTEN-FREE: *Use gluten-free broth and confirm all other ingredients are gluten-free.*

Nutrition Facts

Serves: 8
Serving Size: 2 egg halves

Amount per serving

Calories   **90**

Calories from fat 20	
Total fat 2.5 g	
Saturated fat 0.3 g	
Trans fat 0.0 g	
Cholesterol 0 mg	
Sodium 250 mg	
Potassium 180 mg	
Total carbohydrate 10 g	
Dietary fiber 3 g	
Sugars 2 g	
Protein 7 g	
Phosphorus 60 mg	

Choices/Exchanges: 1/2 Starch, 1 Lean Protein

HEALTHY HOMEMADE GREEN BEAN CASSEROLE

⏲ 5 minutes
🍳 30 minutes
🍽 7 servings
🍴 1/2 cup

VG

THIS IS A DELICIOUS LOWER-CALORIE VERSION OF TRADITIONAL GREEN BEAN CASSEROLE.

CASSEROLE

Nonstick cooking spray
4 spreadable creamy light Swiss cheese wedges (such as Laughing Cow)
1 tablespoon olive oil
1/2 onion, finely diced
1 teaspoon trans fat–free margarine
8 ounces mushrooms, diced
1/8 teaspoon salt
1/4 teaspoon ground black pepper
1/2 cup fat-free reduced-sodium vegetable broth
2 teaspoons cornstarch
2 teaspoons cold water
1/4 cup 1% milk
2 (14.5-ounce) cans no-salt-added cut green beans, drained

CORN FLAKE TOPPING

1 cup corn flakes, crushed
1 2/3 tablespoons trans fat–free margarine, melted

1. Preheat oven to 400°F. Spray a 1 1/2-quart baking dish with cooking spray.
2. Heat spreadable cheese wedges in microwave 30 seconds. Stir, and set aside.
3. In a large sauté pan, heat oil over medium heat. Add onion and sauté 2–3 minutes.
4. Add margarine to sauté pan and melt. Add mushrooms, salt, and pepper and cook 4–5 minutes. Pour vegetable broth into pan and simmer 1 minute.
5. In a small bowl, mix together cornstarch and water; add to vegetable broth mixture and stir 1 minute.
6. Add melted spreadable cheese to sauté pan and mix well. Add milk; stir to incorporate. Cook an additional 2–3 minutes until thick.
7. Remove from heat and stir in green beans. Pour green bean mixture into baking dish.

8. In a small bowl, mix together corn flakes and margarine. Spread corn flake mixture on top of green beans. Bake 15–20 minutes.

MAKE IT GLUTEN-FREE: *Use gluten-free vegetable broth and gluten-free corn flakes.*

Nutrition Facts

Serves: 7
Serving Size: 1/2 cup

Amount per serving	
Calories	**110**
Calories from fat 50	
Total fat 6.0 g	
Saturated fat 1.6 g	
Trans fat 0.0 g	
Cholesterol 6 mg	
Sodium 260 mg	
Potassium 240 mg	
Total carbohydrate 11 g	
Dietary fiber 3 g	
Sugars 4 g	
Protein 4 g	
Phosphorus 130 mg	

Choices/Exchanges: 1/2 Starch, 1 Nonstarchy Vegetable, 1 Fat

VEGETARIAN BAKED BEANS

YOU CAN MAKE THESE BAKED BEANS WITH PINTO BEANS IF YOU PREFER THEM OVER NAVY BEANS.

⏱ 5 minutes
🍲 1 1/4 hours
🍽 9 servings
🥣 1/3 cup

GF
VG

Nonstick cooking spray
1   large onion, diced
2   (14.5-ounce) cans navy beans, rinsed and drained
1   cup fat-free, gluten-free, low-sodium vegetable broth
1/4 cup no-salt-added ketchup
1/4 cup low-calorie brown sugar blend (such as Splenda)
1   tablespoon lite, gluten-free soy sauce
1   tablespoon Dijon mustard
1   teaspoon garlic powder

1. Preheat oven to 350°F. Coat an 8-inch baking pan with cooking spray. Set aside.
2. Mix all ingredients in a large bowl. Pour into prepared baking pan. Cover and bake 45 minutes. Uncover and bake an additional 30–40 minutes or until thickened.

Nutrition Facts

Serves: 9
Serving Size: 1/3 cup

Amount per serving
Calories 120

Calories from fat	0
Total fat 0.0 g	
Saturated fat 0.1 g	
Trans fat 0.0 g	
Cholesterol 0 mg	
Sodium 250 mg	
Potassium 300 mg	
Total carbohydrate 24 g	
Dietary fiber 6 g	
Sugars 6 g	
Protein 5 g	
Phosphorus 95 mg	

Choices/Exchanges: 1 Starch, 1/2 Carbohydrate

CHICKPEA PASTA WITH ROASTED VEGETABLES

⏱ 10 minutes
🍲 25 minutes
🍽 5 servings
🥄 1 1/3 cups

VG

TRY THIS HEALTHY AND DELICIOUS DISH WITH A NEW TYPE OF PASTA MADE FROM CHICKPEAS (GARBANZO BEANS). THE PASTA IS LOADED WITH FIBER, IS LOWER IN CARBS, IS GLUTEN-FREE, AND HAS A LOWER GLYCEMIC INDEX. THE BRAND NAME OF PASTA USED HERE WAS BANZA, AND IT WAS FOUND AT A LOCAL GROCERY STORE.

Nonstick cooking spray
2 medium zucchini, diced
12 ounces broccoli florets
2 tablespoons olive oil
1/2 teaspoon salt
1/4 teaspoon ground black pepper
1 (8-ounce) box chickpea (garbanzo bean) penne pasta
1/2 cup fat-free reduced-sodium vegetable broth
1/4 teaspoon dried oregano
3 tablespoons freshly grated parmesan cheese

1. Preheat oven to 400°F. Spray a baking sheet with cooking spray.
2. Place the zucchini and broccoli in a bowl. Add the olive oil, salt, and pepper; toss to coat and spread on the baking sheet. Bake 20 minutes. Remove the vegetables from the oven.
3. While the vegetables are baking, cook the pasta according to the directions on the package. Do not boil water for pasta; rather, bring the water to near boiling and let the pasta sit in the water 4–6 minutes, stirring occasionally.
4. Drain the pasta after cooking. Add the vegetable broth to pot. Add the pasta, cooked vegetables, and oregano to the pot and mix well.

5. Sprinkle with parmesan cheese and serve immediately.

MAKE IT GLUTEN-FREE: *Use gluten-free vegetable broth and confirm all other ingredients are gluten-free.*

Nutrition Facts

Serves: 5
Serving Size: 1 1/3 cups

Amount per serving
Calories **240**

Calories from fat 80	
Total fat 9.0 g	
Saturated fat 1.5 g	
Trans fat 0.0 g	
Cholesterol 0 mg	
Sodium 400 mg	
Potassium 830 mg	
Total carbohydrate 32 g	
Dietary fiber 9 g	
Sugars 7 g	
Protein 15 g	
Phosphorus 240 mg	

Choices/Exchanges: 1 1/2 Starch, 1 Nonstarchy Vegetable, 1 Lean Protein, 1 1/2 Fat

PEANUT BUTTER PROTEIN BLAST SMOOTHIE

GF
VG

- ⏱ 5 minutes
- 🍽 2 servings
- 🥤 3/4 cup

ENJOY THIS HIGH-PROTEIN SMOOTHIE FOR BREAKFAST, LUNCH, OR A SNACK. ADD A TABLESPOON OF COCOA POWDER TO THIS SMOOTHIE TO MAKE IT EVEN MORE DECADENT!

1	cup skim milk
1	tablespoon natural peanut butter
1	scoop vanilla-flavored low-carb protein powder
1	tablespoon ground flaxseed
1/2	cup ice

1. Combine all ingredients in a blender and purée until smooth and thick.
2. Pour into 2 glasses and serve.

Nutrition Facts

Serves: 2
Serving Size: 3/4 cup

Amount per serving
Calories 180

Calories from fat 70

Total fat 8.0 g

  Saturated fat 1.5 g

  Trans fat 0.0 g

Cholesterol 30 mg

Sodium 85 mg

Potassium 340 mg

Total carbohydrate 12 g

  Dietary fiber 2 g

  Sugars 8 g

Protein 16 g

Phosphorus 260 mg

Choices/Exchanges: 1/2 Fat-Free Milk, 1/2 Carbohydrate, 1 Lean Protein, 1 Fat

PEAR SALAD WITH WALNUTS AND GOAT CHEESE

THIS TASTY FALL SALAD HAS THE PERFECT COMBINATION OF SWEET AND SALTY FROM THE CRISP PEARS AND TANGY GOAT CHEESE.

⏱ 10 minutes
🍽 6 servings
🍲 About 1 cup

GF
VG

1 (10-ounce) bag spring mix lettuce
2 tablespoons crumbled goat cheese
1/2 cup walnuts, toasted
2 medium pears, peeled and diced
8 tablespoons light raspberry walnut vinaigrette salad dressing (such as Ken's Steak House)

1. In a salad bowl mix together all ingredients except for the dressing.
2. Add the dressing and toss to coat.

DIETITIAN TIP: *To toast the walnuts, place in a small nonstick skillet on low heat and cook until the walnuts begin to brown, about 4 minutes. Walnuts are the only nut that provides an excellent source of heart-healthy omega-3 fatty acids.*

Nutrition Facts

Serves: 6
Serving Size: About 1 cup

Amount per serving
Calories 160

Calories from fat 90

Total fat 10.0 g

Saturated fat 1.1 g

Trans fat 0.0 g

Cholesterol 10 mg

Sodium 220 mg

Potassium 270 mg

Total carbohydrate 16 g

Dietary fiber 3 g

Sugars 10 g

Protein 3 g

Phosphorus 65 mg

Choices/Exchanges: 1/2 Fruit, 1/2 Carbohydrate, 2 Fat

QUINOA BLACK BEAN BURGER

DON'T BE AFRAID OF THIS HEALTHY VEGGIE BURGER—IT IS DELICIOUS AND PACKED WITH FIBER AND PROTEIN. BEANS ARE ONE OF THE HEALTHIEST CARBOHYDRATES YOU CAN CHOOSE, AND THIS RECIPE IS A GREAT WAY TO WORK THEM INTO A MEAL.

GF
VG

- ⏱ 10 minutes
- 🍲 25 minutes
- 🍽 9 servings
- 🍔 1 burger

BURGERS

1/2	cup quinoa
1	cup water
2	(15-ounce) cans black beans, rinsed and drained, divided
1/4	cup salsa
1	large egg
1/4	cup certified gluten-free cornmeal
1	teaspoon chili powder
1/2	teaspoon cumin
1/4	teaspoon cayenne pepper
	Nonstick cooking spray

TOPPINGS

9	iceberg lettuce leaves (to use as wraps)
9	tablespoons salsa
1	large avocado, sliced into 9 slices

1. Cook dried quinoa in water according to the directions on the package.

2. Purée 1 can black beans, 1/4 cup salsa, and egg in a blender or food processor until smooth.

3. Pour cooked quinoa in a medium bowl. Add puréed beans, remaining 1 can black beans, cornmeal, chili powder, cumin, and cayenne pepper, and mix together until well blended.

4. Form bean mixture into nine 1/2-inch-thick patties.

5. Coat a large skillet or grill pan with cooking spray and heat over medium heat. Add black bean patties and grill 2–3 minutes per side, until slightly brown.

6. Serve each burger in a lettuce wrap topped with 1 tablespoon salsa and an avocado slice.

Nutrition Facts

Serves: 9
Serving Size: 1 burger

Amount per serving
Calories 170

Calories from fat 40

Total fat 4.5 g

　　Saturated fat 0.8 g

　　Trans fat 0.0 g

Cholesterol 20 mg

Sodium 220 mg

Potassium 450 mg

Total carbohydrate 26 g

　　Dietary fiber 8 g

　　Sugars 3 g

Protein 8 g

Phosphorus 160 mg

Choices/Exchanges: 1 1/2 Starch, 1 Nonstarchy Vegetable, 1 Lean Protein

SPINACH AND PINE NUT QUINOA

GF
VG

⏱ 5 minutes
🍲 20 minutes
🍽 6 servings
🥣 1/2 cup

THIS NUTRITION-PACKED SIDE DISH GOES GREAT WITH FISH, CHICKEN, OR PORK. MAKE THIS RECIPE THE SAME WEEK YOU MAKE THE SPINACH PESTO HALIBUT (PAGE 378) BECAUSE IT USES MANY OF THE SAME INGREDIENTS.

1   cup quinoa
2   cups fat-free low-sodium vegetable broth (or gluten-free broth if cooking gluten-free)
1   tablespoon olive oil
2   cloves garlic, minced
6   ounces baby spinach
1/4   cup pine nuts, toasted
1/8   teaspoon ground black pepper
2   tablespoons freshly grated parmesan cheese

1. Cook quinoa according to the directions on the package, using vegetable broth in place of water.
2. Heat olive oil in a sauté pan over medium-high heat. Add garlic and sauté 30 seconds. Add spinach and sauté about 5 minutes.
3. Pour cooked quinoa in a medium bowl; add spinach and remaining ingredients and mix well.

Nutrition Facts

Serves: 6
Serving Size: 1/2 cup

Amount per serving
Calories **180**

Calories from fat 70

Total fat 8.0 g

   Saturated fat 1.1 g

   Trans fat 0.0 g

Cholesterol 0 mg

Sodium 90 mg

Potassium 430 mg

Total carbohydrate 22 g

   Dietary fiber 3 g

   Sugars 3 g

Protein 7 g

Phosphorus 210 mg

Choices/Exchanges: 1 1/2 Starch, 1 1/2 Fat

SALAD GREENS WITH SPICED PECANS

⏱ 5 minutes
🍳 7 minutes
🍽 4 servings
🥄 About 1 3/4 cups

GF
VG

THE PECANS, WHICH ARE A SOURCE OF HEART-HEALTHY FAT, ARE THE STAR OF THIS SALAD. YOU MIGHT WANT TO MAKE A DOUBLE BATCH OF THE PECANS BECAUSE THEY MAKE A GREAT SNACK, TOO.
IF YOU DON'T LIKE GOAT CHEESE, YOU CAN SUBSTITUTE BLUE CHEESE IN THIS RECIPE.

PECANS

1/2	cup pecan halves
2	teaspoons trans fat–free margarine
1	tablespoon low-calorie brown sugar blend (such as Splenda)
1	tablespoon water
1/4	teaspoon cumin
1/4	teaspoon cinnamon
	Pinch cayenne pepper

SALAD

1	(10-ounce) bag spring mix lettuce
2	ounces goat cheese, crumbled
4	tablespoons light raspberry walnut vinaigrette salad dressing (such as Ken's Steak House)

1. Heat the pecans in a dry skillet over medium heat. Stir frequently until they begin to toast, about 4 minutes. Add the margarine and cook, stirring, until the nuts begin to darken, about 1 minute. Add brown sugar blend, water, cumin, cinnamon, and cayenne pepper. Stir until the sauce thickens and the nuts are glazed, 1–2 minutes.

2. Remove from heat and place pecans on wax paper. Separate pecans with a fork and let cool.

3. In a salad bowl, mix together lettuce, goat cheese, and pecans. Add dressing and toss to coat.

Nutrition Facts

Serves: 4
Serving Size: About 1 3/4 cups

Amount per serving
Calories 170

Calories from fat 120

Total fat 13.0 g
  Saturated fat 2.0 g
  Trans fat 0.0 g
Cholesterol 13 mg
Sodium 160 mg
Potassium 270 mg
Total carbohydrate 11 g
  Dietary fiber 2 g
  Sugars 6 g
Protein 3 g
Phosphorus 70 mg

Choices/Exchanges:
1 Carbohydrate, 2 1/2 Fat

GARLICKY SAUTÉED SPINACH

⏱ 5 minutes
🍲 35 minutes
🍽 4 servings
🍴 1/2 cup

SERVE THIS GARLICKY SAUTÉED SPINACH WITH DIJON SALMON (PAGE 347) FOR A GOURMET MEAL. ROASTED GARLIC MAKES A GREAT APPETIZER, TOO. JUST SERVE ROASTED GARLIC CLOVES WITH WHOLE-WHEAT CROSTINI AND LET YOUR GUESTS SPREAD THE GARLIC ON TOP.

1	head garlic
1	tablespoon olive oil, divided
	Nonstick cooking spray
1/2	cup minced onion
6	cups fresh spinach
1/8	teaspoon salt
1/4	teaspoon ground black pepper

1. Preheat oven to 400°F.

2. Leaving the head of garlic whole, cut off 1/4 to 1/2 inch of the top of head, exposing the individual cloves of garlic. Leave the peel on.

3. Place the garlic head cut side up on a sheet of foil. Drizzle one teaspoon olive oil over the cut side of the garlic head. Fold foil up around the garlic and pinch to seal to make a packet.

4. Bake 30–35 minutes, or until the cloves feel soft.

5. Allow the garlic to cool slightly to the touch. Squeeze the roasted garlic cloves out of their skins into a small bowl and mash with a fork to make a paste.

6. In a large sauté pan, add remaining olive oil and a generous amount of cooking spray over medium-high heat. Add the onion and sauté until just starting to caramelize.

7. Add the roasted garlic paste and stir until the onion is coated. Add the spinach and sauté until the spinach is wilted and coated with the garlic and onion.

8. Season with salt and pepper.

Nutrition Facts

Serves: 4
Serving Size: 1/2 cup

Amount per serving
Calories **60**

Calories from fat 30

Total fat 3.5 g

   Saturated fat 0.5 g

   Trans fat 0.0 g

Cholesterol 0 mg

Sodium 110 mg

Potassium 320 mg

Total carbohydrate 6 g

   Dietary fiber 2 g

   Sugars 1 g

Protein 2 g

Phosphorus 40 mg

Choices/Exchanges: 1 Nonstarchy Vegetable, 1 Fat

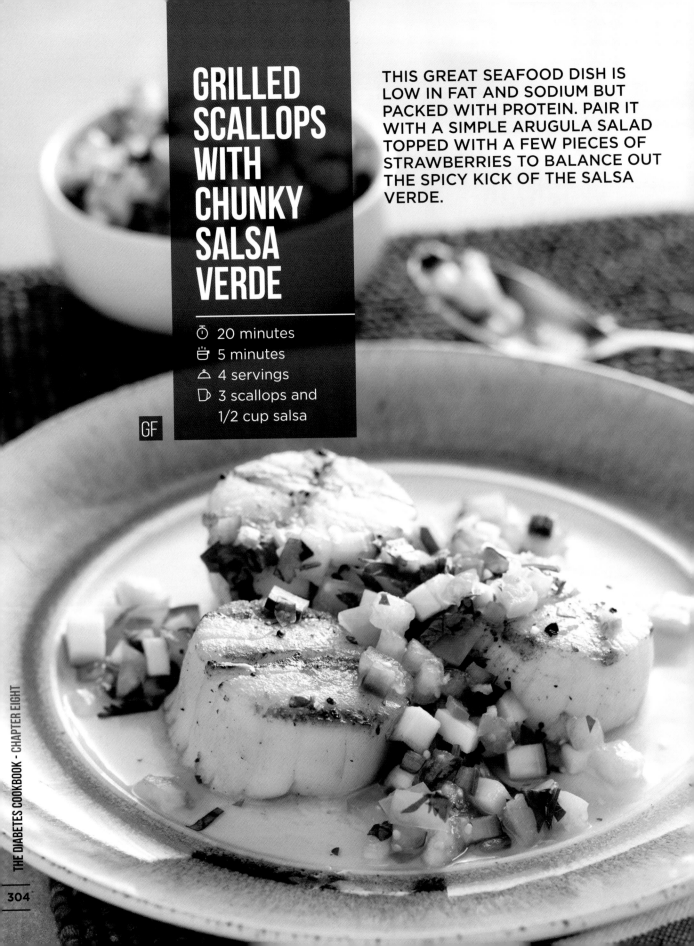

GRILLED SCALLOPS WITH CHUNKY SALSA VERDE

THIS GREAT SEAFOOD DISH IS LOW IN FAT AND SODIUM BUT PACKED WITH PROTEIN. PAIR IT WITH A SIMPLE ARUGULA SALAD TOPPED WITH A FEW PIECES OF STRAWBERRIES TO BALANCE OUT THE SPICY KICK OF THE SALSA VERDE.

- 20 minutes
- 5 minutes
- 4 servings
- 3 scallops and 1/2 cup salsa

GF

SALSA VERDE

1/2	pound tomatillos, husked, rinsed, cut into small dice
1	small jalapeño pepper, seeded, deveined, and minced
1/4	cup chopped fresh cilantro
1	zucchini, seeded, cut into a small dice
2	tablespoons lime juice
1	teaspoon honey or 1/2 packet artificial sweetener
2	cloves garlic, minced

SCALLOPS

12	large sea scallops, tabs removed
1	tablespoon olive oil
1/4	teaspoon salt
1/4	teaspoon ground black pepper

1. Prepare an indoor or outdoor grill.
2. In a medium bowl, mix the tomatillos, jalapeño pepper, cilantro, zucchini, lime juice, honey or artificial sweetener, and garlic. Set aside.
3. Pat the scallops dry with a paper towel. Toss them with the olive oil, salt, and pepper in a medium bowl.
4. Place scallops on grill, flat side down. Turning occasionally, grill until lightly charred and just cooked through, about 2 minutes per side. Serve scallops topped with the chunky salsa verde.

CHEF TIP: *If you can't find tomatillos, you can substitute red or green tomatoes in this recipe.*

NOTE: *Look for sea scallops that are fresh or that have no preservatives, if possible. The nutrition information for the recipe is based on the use of preservative-free scallops.*

Nutrition Facts

Serves: 4
Serving Size: 3 scallops and 1/2 cup salsa

Amount per serving
Calories   **150**

Calories from fat 40	
Total fat 4.5 g	
Saturated fat 0.7 g	
Trans fat 0.0 g	
Cholesterol 30 mg	
Sodium 340 mg	
Potassium 540 mg	
Total carbohydrate 12 g	
Dietary fiber 2 g	
Sugars 5 g	
Protein 16 g	
Phosphorus 350 mg	

Choices/Exchanges:
1/2 Carbohydrate, 1 Nonstarchy Vegetable, 2 Lean Protein

GENERAL TSO'S TOFU WITH BROCCOLI

- ⏱ 35 minutes
- 🍳 30 minutes
- 🍽 4 servings
- 🍱 1 cup

VG

CHINESE FOOD MINUS THE TAKEOUT MENU? IT'S POSSIBLE TO PRODUCE SATISFYING RESULTS THAT KEEP SODIUM AND CALORIES IN CHECK. THIS RECIPE CALLS FOR TOFU THAT'S PATTED DRY AND SPRINKLED WITH CORNSTARCH BEFORE BAKING, SO IT GETS BROWN AND CRISPY WITHOUT DEEP FRYING.

TOFU

Nonstick cooking spray
- 1 (16-ounce) package extra-firm tofu, drained and cut into 1-inch chunks
- 1 teaspoon reduced-sodium soy sauce
- 2 teaspoons rice vinegar
- 1 teaspoon vegetable oil
- 1 clove garlic, minced
- 1/2 teaspoon grated fresh ginger
- 1 tablespoon cornstarch

SAUCE

- 1/2 cup fat-free low-sodium vegetable broth
- 1 tablespoon honey or 2 packets artificial sweetener
- 1 tablespoon reduced-sodium soy sauce
- 1 tablespoon rice vinegar
- 2 teaspoons sesame oil
- 2 teaspoons cornstarch
- 1 1/2 teaspoons tomato paste

- 1/2 teaspoon Asian-style hot sauce, such as sambal oelek
- 2 teaspoons vegetable oil
- 2 scallions, sliced thinly
- 1 clove garlic, minced
- 1/2 teaspoon grated fresh ginger
- 2 cups steamed broccoli

1. Preheat oven to 350°F. Coat baking sheet with cooking spray. Set aside.
2. Pat tofu dry with a paper towel.
3. Combine soy sauce, vinegar, oil, garlic, and ginger in a bowl. Add tofu and toss to coat. Marinate 30 minutes.
4. Sprinkle cornstarch over tofu in the bowl and turn to coat evenly. Spread tofu on the baking sheet in a single layer. Bake 30 minutes, turning frequently, until brown on all sides.
5. While the tofu is baking, whisk together broth, honey or artificial sweetener, soy sauce, vinegar, sesame oil, cornstarch, tomato paste, and hot sauce in small bowl. Set aside.

6. Add vegetable oil to a large sauté pan or wok over medium-high heat. Add scallions, garlic, and ginger, and stir-fry 1 minute. Add sauce mixture and cook 2–3 minutes, or until thickened.

7. Remove tofu from oven and stir into the sauce with the steamed broccoli.

CHEF TIP: *Serve this dish over cooked brown rice.*

Nutrition Facts

Serves: 4
Serving Size: 1 cup

Amount per serving
Calories   210

Calories from fat 100	
Total fat 11.0 g	
Saturated fat 1.3 g	
Trans fat 0.0 g	
Cholesterol 0 mg	
Sodium 280 mg	
Potassium 360 mg	
Total carbohydrate 17 g	
Dietary fiber 3 g	
Sugars 6 g	
Protein 13 g	
Phosphorus 190 mg	

Choices/Exchanges:
1 Carbohydrate, 1 Nonstarchy Vegetable, 1 Medium-Fat Protein, 1 Fat

ROASTED FALL VEGETABLES

GF
LC
VG

⏱ 10 minutes
🍲 25 minutes
🍽 11 servings
🥄 1/2 cup

SO EASY—JUST THREE STEPS FROM START TO FINISH. ROASTING BRINGS OUT THE SWEET FLAVORS IN THESE VEGGIES.

Nonstick cooking spray
1 head cauliflower (about 1 pound), cut into small florets
1 pound Brussels sprouts, trimmed and cut in half
2 cups baby carrots
3 tablespoons olive oil
1/2 teaspoon salt
1/2 teaspoon ground black pepper

1. Preheat oven to 400°F. Spray a baking sheet with cooking spray.
2. In a large bowl, mix together all ingredients. Pour the vegetables onto the prepared baking sheet.
3. Bake on the lower oven rack 25 minutes.

Nutrition Facts

Serves: 11
Serving Size: 1/2 cup

Amount per serving
Calories   **60**

Calories from fat 35

Total fat 4.0 g

    Saturated fat 0.6 g

    Trans fat 0.0 g

Cholesterol 0 mg

Sodium 140 mg

Potassium 290 mg

Total carbohydrate 7 g

    Dietary fiber 3 g

    Sugars 2 g

Protein 2 g

Phosphorus 45 mg

Choices/Exchanges: 1 Nonstarchy Vegetable, 1 Fat

3 cups cubed and chilled seedless watermelon
1/3 cup crumbled reduced-fat feta cheese
7 ounces arugula
1/4 small red onion, thinly sliced
2 tablespoons balsamic vinegar
1 tablespoon extra-virgin olive oil
1/4 teaspoon salt
1/4 teaspoon ground black pepper

1. In a large bowl, toss together watermelon, feta cheese, arugula, and onion.
2. In a medium bowl, whisk together vinegar, olive oil, salt, and pepper.
3. Drizzle the dressing over the salad and toss gently to coat.

WATERMELON, ARUGULA, AND FETA SALAD

GF
LC
VG

⏱ 15 minutes
△ 6 servings
▷ 1 cup

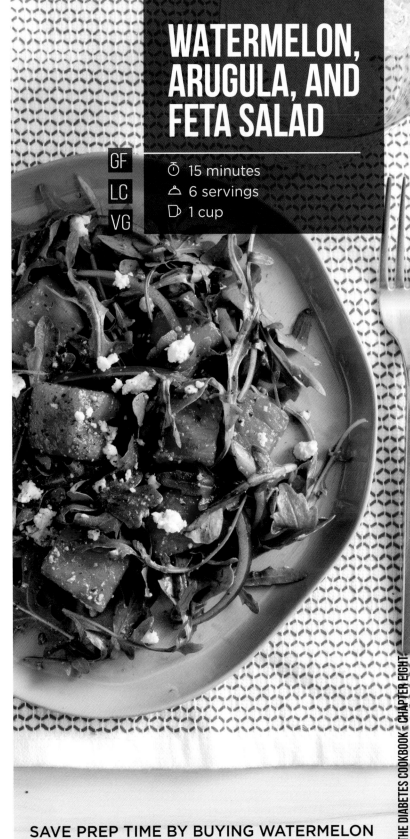

Nutrition Facts

Serves: 6
Serving Size: 1 cup

Amount per serving
Calories **70**

Calories from fat 30

Total fat 3.5 g

  Saturated fat 0.9 g

  Trans fat 0.0 g

Cholesterol 4 mg

Sodium 200 mg

Potassium 230 mg

Total carbohydrate 9 g

  Dietary fiber 1 g

  Sugars 6 g

Protein 3 g

Phosphorus 55 mg

Choices/Exchanges: 1/2 Fruit, 1 Fat

SAVE PREP TIME BY BUYING WATERMELON THAT IS ALREADY CUT AND CUBED.

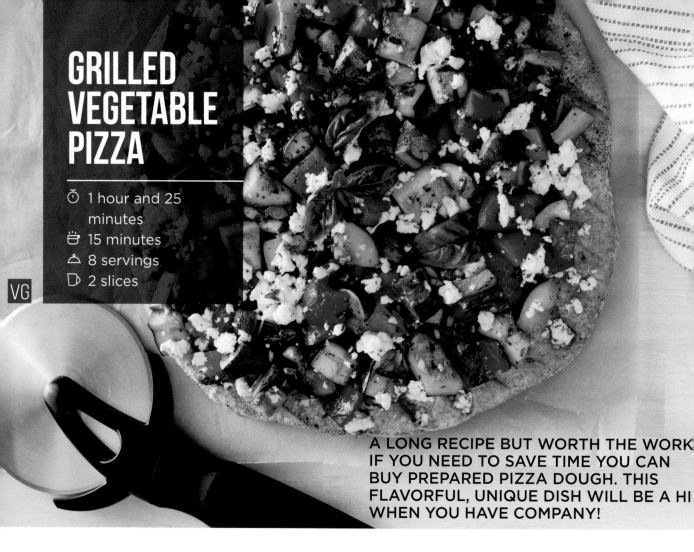

GRILLED VEGETABLE PIZZA

- ⏱ 1 hour and 25 minutes
- 🍲 15 minutes
- 🍽 8 servings
- 🍴 2 slices

VG

A LONG RECIPE BUT WORTH THE WORK. IF YOU NEED TO SAVE TIME YOU CAN BUY PREPARED PIZZA DOUGH. THIS FLAVORFUL, UNIQUE DISH WILL BE A HI WHEN YOU HAVE COMPANY!

PIZZA DOUGH (PREPARE FIRST)

- 1 cup warm water (around 100°F)
- 1 packet active dry yeast
- 1 tablespoon low-calorie brown sugar blend (such as Splenda)
- 2 cups whole-wheat flour
- 1/2 teaspoon salt
- Nonstick cooking spray

PIZZA TOPPINGS (PREPARE SECOND)

- 1 tablespoon olive oil
- 1/4 cup balsamic vinegar
- 2 cloves garlic, grated or minced
- 1 tablespoon minced fresh basil
- 2 medium zucchini, sliced lengthwise into thirds
- 1 yellow bell pepper, seeded and sliced into fourths
- 1 red bell pepper, seeded and sliced into fourths
- 8 baby bella mushrooms (cremini), stemmed
- 3 1/2 ounces reduced-fat feta cheese, divided
- 2 teaspoons dried oregano, divided

1. Set up a mixer fitted with the dough hook attachment. If you do not have a mixer, set up a food processor. You will also need plastic wrap and wax paper eventually for this recipe.

2. Add warm water, yeast, and brown sugar blend to the mixing bowl or food processor bowl and let the yeast bloom 5 minutes. The yeast should begin to get frothy.

3. Add the flour and salt, and mix on low until flour is incorporated. If using a mixer with the dough hook attachment, turn the speed up to medium and knead the dough 5 minutes. If using a food processor, turn the dough onto a clean, floured board or countertop and knead by hand 5–7 minutes. If the dough is too sticky, add a tablespoon of flour at a time until it forms a smooth dough.

4. Coat a large bowl with cooking spray, place the kneaded dough in the bowl, cover, and put in a warm place for 1 hour to rise.

5. While the dough is rising, prepare an indoor or outdoor grill. If using a charcoal grill, preheat oven to 300°F as well.

6. In a medium bowl, whisk together olive oil, vinegar, garlic, and basil. Set aside.

7. Coat the vegetables with cooking spray and grill on both sides 7–9 minutes or until just cooked through.

8. Remove the vegetables from the grill and dice while still warm. Add the warm, diced vegetables to the oil and vinegar dressing and toss to coat. Set aside.

9. Once the dough has risen for 1 hour, punch the dough down and form into a ball. Knead the dough 1 minute and then cover to rest 2 minutes.

10. Once the dough has rested, divide the dough into two balls. Keep the dough you are not working with covered with plastic wrap.

11. Dust your board or countertop with a little bit of flour. Using a rolling pin, roll the dough into an 8- or 9-inch round that is between 1/4 and 1/2 inch thick. Spray a piece of wax paper that is just larger than the crust with cooking spray and lay the pizza crust on the wax paper. Spray another piece of wax paper the same size and lay it, sprayed side down, on top of the crust. Set aside.

12. Repeat this process for the second ball of dough.

13. To cook the pizza, have the crusts, marinated vegetables, and cheese ready at the grill. Turn the grill heat to low and place the two pizza crusts on the grill (or you can do them one at a time for easier management). Let the crust grill 3–4 minutes or until crispy on the bottom. Turn the crust over and divide the vegetable mixture and marinade equally between the two pizzas, spreading to within about 1/2 inch of the edge. Top each pizza with half the feta cheese and close the grill lid. Let the pizza grill another 3–4 minutes. Turn off the grill's flame and leave the lid closed another 2 minutes. If using a charcoal grill, preheat oven to 300°F and move the pizzas to the oven for 5 minutes.

14. Remove the pizzas and top each with 1 teaspoon of dried oregano. Slice each pizza into 8 pieces.

CHEF TIP: *Watch the flame on your grill to make sure it does not burn the pizza. If it starts to burn, turn one side of the burners off and move the pizza to that side, leaving the other burners on to form a convection oven. If using a charcoal grill and it gets too hot, finish the pizza in the oven rather than on the grill.*

Nutrition Facts

Serves: 8
Serving Size: 2 slices

Amount per serving
Calories — **180**

Calories from fat 40	
Total fat 4.5 g	
Saturated fat 1.4 g	
Trans fat 0.0 g	
Cholesterol 5 mg	
Sodium 310 mg	
Potassium 490 mg	
Total carbohydrate 31 g	
Dietary fiber 5 g	
Sugars 5 g	
Protein 9 g	
Phosphorus 220 mg	

Choices/Exchanges: 1 1/2 Starch, 1 Nonstarchy Vegetable, 1 Fat

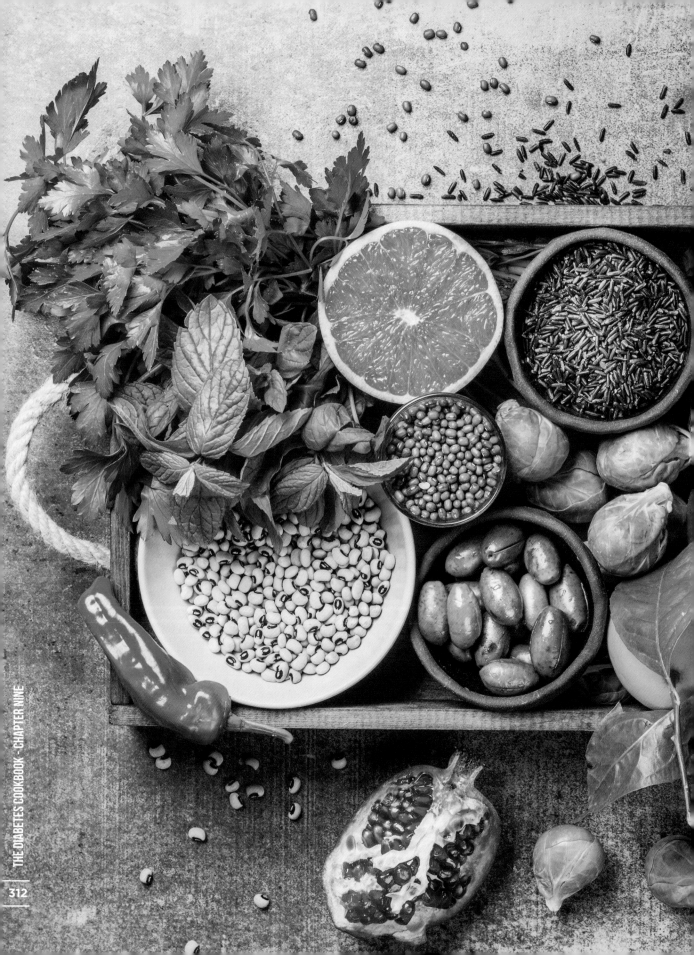

CHAPTER NINE

LOW GLYCEMIC-INDEX RECIPES

THE GLYCEMIC INDEX IS A RANKING OF CARBOHYDRATE FOODS ACCORDING TO THEIR EFFECT ON BLOOD SUGAR LEVELS. THE THEORY IS THAT A FOOD WITH A LOW GLYCEMIC INDEX IS DIGESTED MORE SLOWLY, RESULTING IN A LOWER RISE IN BLOOD SUGAR LEVEL. SUBSTITUTING LOW-GLYCEMIC MEALS FOR HIGH-GLYCEMIC MEALS MAY MODESTLY IMPROVE BLOOD SUGAR CONTROL. THIS CHAPTER IS FULL OF HIGH-FIBER, LOW GLYCEMIC-INDEX MEALS THAT WON'T SPIKE BLOOD SUGARS TOO MUCH. YOU WON'T FIND ANY WHITE FLOUR OR WHITE RICE IN THIS CHAPTER!

GRILLED CHICKEN CAESAR KEBABS

GF

- ⏱ 30 minutes
- 🍳 12 minutes
- 🍽 4 servings
- 🍴 2 cups romaine lettuce and 2 kebabs

8	bamboo skewers
1/2	cup fat-free plain Greek yogurt
1	clove garlic, minced or grated
2	tablespoons lemon juice
2	teaspoons gluten-free Worcestershire sauce
1	tablespoon extra-virgin olive oil
1/4	cup plus 2 tablespoons grated parmesan cheese, divided
1/4	teaspoon salt
1/4	teaspoon ground black pepper
1 1/4	pounds boneless skinless chicken breast, cut into 3/4-inch cubes (aim for 24 pieces of chicken)
2	red bell peppers, seeded and cut into 1-inch pieces (aim for 24 pieces of pepper)
8	cups chopped romaine lettuce
8	kalamata olives, pitted and sliced into fourths

1. Soak the bamboo skewers in warm water for at least 30 minutes.

2. Preheat an indoor or outdoor grill.

3. While the skewers are soaking, whisk together the yogurt, garlic, lemon juice, Worcestershire sauce, olive oil, 2 tablespoons parmesan cheese, salt, and black pepper.

4. Add the chicken pieces to a bowl, pour 3 tablespoons of the dressing over the chicken, and toss to lightly coat. Let the chicken sit 15 minutes. Reserve the extra dressing and be sure it does not come in contact with the raw chicken.

5. Thread alternating pieces of chicken and red bell pepper onto the soaked skewers starting with the chicken and ending with peppers, using 3 pieces of chicken and 3 pieces of red pepper.

6. Grill the kebabs about 10–12 minutes, turning frequently or until the chicken is cooked through and reaches 165°F. Set aside.

7. Toss the romaine lettuce with the remaining salad dressing and serve by placing two cups of salad on a plate, topping with two chicken kebabs, and sprinkling with 8 slices of olive and 1 tablespoon grated parmesan cheese.

CHEF TIP: *This tasty grilling recipe is also packed with vegetables. To make this dish even more colorful, add in some green and yellow bell pepper pieces on your kebabs. To make the dressing more flavorful, consider the option of adding mashed anchovy fillets. If you don't want to purchase anchovy fillets, you can purchase anchovy paste in a tube and use 1 tablespoon of that in the dressing. If you don't want to use anchovy at all, substitute 1 tablespoon Dijon mustard for the anchovy fillets.*

Nutrition Facts

Serves: 4

Serving Size: 2 cups romaine lettuce and 2 kebabs

Amount per serving

Calories	**290**

Calories from fat 100	
Total fat 11.0 g	
Saturated fat 2.7 g	
Trans fat 0.0 g	
Cholesterol 85 mg	
Sodium 420 mg	
Potassium 700 mg	
Total carbohydrate 11 g	
Dietary fiber 4 g	
Sugars 6 g	
Protein 36 g	
Phosphorus 345 mg	

Choices/Exchanges: 2 Nonstarchy Vegetable, 4 Lean Protein, 1 Fat

BAKED PUMPKIN OATMEAL

⏱ 10 minutes
🍲 20 minutes
△ 4 servings
🥣 1 cup

VG

DURING THE FALL MONTHS, YOU'LL SEE PUMPKIN-FLAVORED TREATS RANGING FROM COFFEE TO DOUGHNUTS. TREAT YOURSELF TO A HEALTHY AND DELICIOUS PUMPKIN DISH! THIS OATMEAL IS PERFECT ON A FALL MORNING.

Nonstick cooking spray
2   cups rolled oats
1/4 cup low-calorie brown sugar blend (such as Truvia or Splenda)
1   teaspoon cinnamon
1/8 teaspoon nutmeg
1   teaspoon baking powder
1   cup skim milk
1   teaspoon vanilla extract
1   cup puréed pumpkin
1   tablespoon olive oil
1   egg, beaten

1. Preheat oven to 375°F. Spray a 1 1/2-quart baking dish with cooking spray.
2. In a large bowl, combine oats, brown sugar blend, cinnamon, nutmeg, and baking powder.
3. In a medium bowl, combine milk, vanilla, pumpkin, oil, and egg.
4. Add the pumpkin mixture to the oat mixture; stir well. Pour mixture into baking dish and bake 20 minutes. Serve warm.

MAKE IT GLUTEN-FREE: *Use gluten-free oats and confirm all other ingredients are gluten-free.*

Nutrition Facts

Serves: 4
Serving Size: 1 cup

Amount per serving
Calories   **280**

Calories from fat 70

Total fat 8.0 g

   Saturated fat 1.4 g

   Trans fat 0.0 g

Cholesterol 50 mg

Sodium 140 mg

Potassium 390 mg

Total carbohydrate 43 g

   Dietary fiber 6 g

   Sugars 12 g

Protein 10 g

Phosphorus 390 mg

Choices/Exchanges: 2 Starch, 1 Carbohydrate, 1 Lean Protein, 1/2 Fat

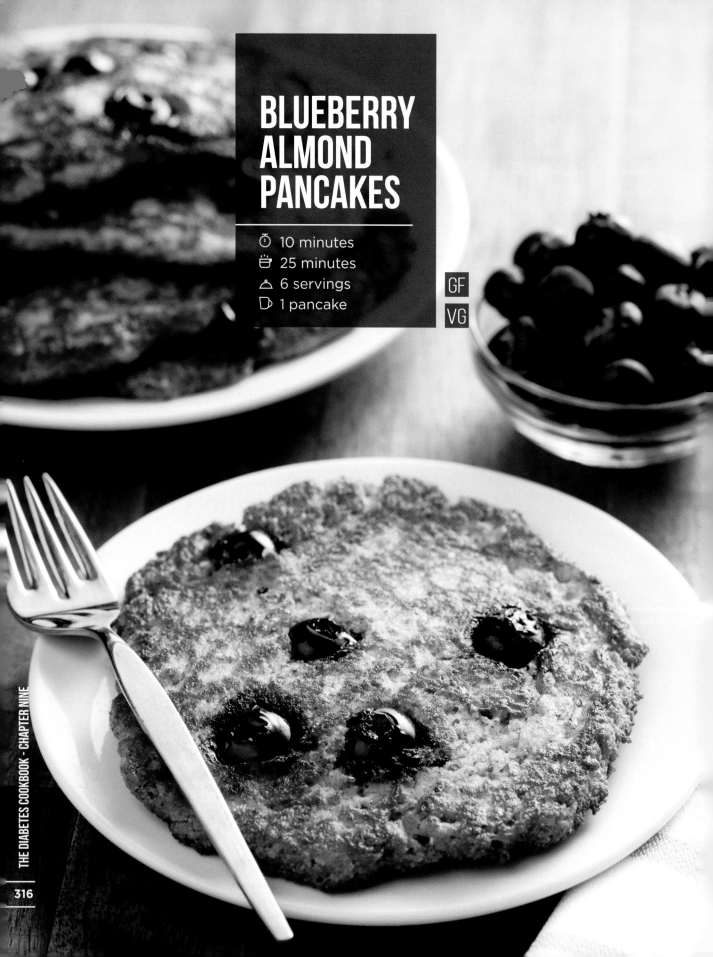

BLUEBERRY ALMOND PANCAKES

- ⏱ 10 minutes
- 🍲 25 minutes
- △ 6 servings
- 🥞 1 pancake

GF
VG

2   eggs
2   egg whites
3/4 cup light ricotta cheese
1/2 teaspoon vanilla extract
1/4 cup unsweetened vanilla almond
     milk
1   large ripe banana
Juice and zest of 1 small lemon
     (2 tablespoons juice, 1 tablespoon
     zest)
1   cup almond flour
1/2 cup ground flaxseed
1   teaspoon baking powder
Nonstick cooking spray
1/2 cup fresh blueberries

1. Add the eggs, egg whites, ricotta cheese, vanilla, almond milk, banana, lemon juice, and lemon zest to a blender. Blend until smooth.
2. In a small bowl, combine the almond flour, ground flaxseed, and baking powder. Add the dry mixture to the liquid mixture in the blender and blend until smooth.
3. Coat a nonstick sauté pan with cooking spray and place over medium heat. Scoop a scant 1/3 cup of the pancake mixture into the pan and top with 4–5 blueberries. Let cook until edges begin to brown (2–3 minutes); then flip the pancake to continue to cook an additional 2–3 minutes. Remove from the pan and repeat the process for the remaining 5 pancakes.

CHEF TIP: *Use a quick-release ice cream scoop to measure and scoop the pancakes for easy release and a uniform size.*

Nutrition Facts

Serves: 6
Serving Size: 1 pancake

Amount per serving
Calories 240

Calories from fat 140

Total fat 16.0 g

Saturated fat 2.6 g

Trans fat 0.0 g

Cholesterol 70 mg

Sodium 200 mg

Potassium 380 mg

Total carbohydrate 16 g

Dietary fiber 6 g

Sugars 6 g

Protein 13 g

Phosphorus 305 mg

Choices/Exchanges: 1/2 Fruit, 1/2 Carbohydrate, 1 Lean Protein, 3 Fat

CAULIFLOWER CHEESE STICKS

⏱ 10 minutes
🍲 40 minutes
🍽 4 servings
🍴 2 cheese sticks

GF
VG

THESE CHEESE STICKS ARE A GREAT LOW-CARB ALTERNATIVE TO BREAD STICKS. YOU WON'T BELIEVE THE TASTE!

Nonstick cooking spray
Parchment paper or silicone baking mat
3 cups cauliflower rice (1 small head of cauliflower)
2 eggs
3/4 cup part-skim mozzarella cheese
1 teaspoon dried oregano
2 cloves garlic, minced
1/8 teaspoon salt
1/4 teaspoon ground black pepper
1/4 cup grated parmesan cheese
1 cup lower-sodium marinara sauce

1. Preheat oven to 425°F. Lay parchment paper or silicone baking mat on a baking sheet. Coat with cooking spray and set aside.
2. If making your own cauliflower rice, blend in the food processor until a rice texture.

3. Place the cauliflower in a microwave-safe container and microwave 10 minutes. Set aside to cool.
4. In a large bowl, combine the cooled cauliflower, eggs, mozzarella cheese, oregano, garlic, salt, and pepper.
5. Spread the mixture into a rectangle 1/2 inch thick on the prepared baking sheet.
6. Bake 25 minutes or until golden brown. Sprinkle the parmesan cheese on top, and put back in the oven for another 5 minutes or until cheese is golden brown.
7. Slice into 8 sticks and serve with 1/4 cup marinara sauce for dipping (see Chef Tip).

CHEF TIP: *When purchasing lower-sodium marinara sauce, look for a sauce that has less than 300 mg sodium per 1/2 cup serving. Also, confirm that the marinara sauce is gluten-free.*

Nutrition Facts

Serves: 4
Serving Size: 2 cheese sticks

Amount per serving

Calories	**170**
Calories from fat 80	
Total fat 9.0 g	
Saturated fat 4.0 g	
Trans fat 0.0 g	
Cholesterol 110 mg	
Sodium 480 mg	
Potassium 540 mg	
Total carbohydrate 11 g	
Dietary fiber 3 g	
Sugars 5 g	
Protein 13 g	
Phosphorus 245 mg	

Choices/Exchanges: 2 Nonstarchy Vegetable, 1 Medium-Fat Protein, 1 Fat

AVOCADO VEGGIE SANDWICH

⏱ 15 minutes
🍽 4 servings
🥪 1 sandwich

THIS IS A VEGGIE SANDWICH, BUT IF YOU WANT MEAT, YOU COULD ADD TURKEY OR CHICKEN.

1	avocado, cut in half and pitted
4	whole-wheat sandwich thins (about 1 1/2 ounces each), top and bottom separated
4	tablespoons sunflower seeds
1/2	large cucumber, sliced
4	radishes, sliced
2	roma tomatoes, sliced

1. Gently remove the insides of the avocado from shell. Cut avocado into thin slices.
2. Spread 1/4 of the avocado slices on the bottom piece of a sandwich thin. Sprinkle with 1 tablespoon sunflower seeds. Top with 4–5 cucumber slices, 4–5 radish slices, and 3 tomato slices. Place top piece of sandwich thin on sandwich.
3. Repeat process for remaining 3 sandwiches.

MAKE IT GLUTEN-FREE: *If you need this recipe to be gluten-free, serve it on whole-grain gluten-free bread.*

Nutrition Facts

Serves: 4
Serving Size: 1 sandwich

Amount per serving
Calories 220

Calories from fat 100

Total fat 11.0 g	
Saturated fat 1.2 g	
Trans fat 0.0 g	
Cholesterol 0 mg	
Sodium 180 mg	
Potassium 500 mg	
Total carbohydrate 28 g	
Dietary fiber 9 g	
Sugars 4 g	
Protein 8 g	
Phosphorus 215 mg	

Choices/Exchanges: 1 1/2 Starch, 1 Nonstarchy Vegetable, 2 Fat

OPEN-FACE SWEET POTATO SANDWICH

⏱ 10 minutes
🍲 25 minutes
🍽 4 servings
🍽 1 sandwich

GF
VG

THIS METHOD CAN BE USED WITH ANY SANDWICH FILLINGS. TRY SLICED TOMATO, BASIL, AND FRESH MOZZARELLA CHEESE, OR TRY HAM WITH SPINACH AND MUENSTER CHEESE.

Nonstick cooking spray
2 medium sweet potatoes
1 small zucchini, thinly sliced lengthwise
1 red bell pepper, seeded and thinly sliced
1 teaspoon salt-free all-purpose seasoning (such as Spike or Mrs. Dash)
2 (1-ounce) slices reduced-fat swiss cheese

1. Preheat oven to 450°F. Coat a baking sheet with cooking spray and set it aside.
2. Thinly slice 1 round edge of a sweet potato lengthwise. Thinly slice the other round edge of the sweet potato lengthwise. Discard those slices.
3. Slice the sweet potato in half lengthwise and peel. Repeat for the other sweet potato. You will have four 1-inch-thick lengthwise slices of sweet potato.
4. Place the sweet potato slices on the prepared baking sheet and spray them with cooking spray. Bake the sweet potatoes 10 minutes; then reduce the heat to 350°F.
5. Flip the sweet potatoes, and then layer equal amounts of thinly sliced zucchini and red bell pepper on each sweet potato. Season with the salt-free seasoning.
6. Cut each slice of swiss cheese in half and top each sweet potato with the swiss cheese. Return the potatoes to the oven for 15 more minutes.
7. Serve immediately.

Nutrition Facts

Serves: 4
Serving Size: 1 sandwich

Amount per serving
Calories 100

Calories from fat 20

Total fat 2.5 g

Saturated fat 1.1 g

Trans fat 0.0 g

Cholesterol 5 mg

Sodium 85 mg

Potassium 420 mg

Total carbohydrate 14 g

Dietary fiber 3 g

Sugars 6 g

Protein 6 g

Phosphorus 130 mg

Choices/Exchanges: 1/2 Starch, 1 Nonstarchy Vegetable, 1/2 Fat

STUFFED ACORN SQUASH

- ⏱ 20 minutes
- 🍲 45 minutes
- 🍽 8 servings
- 🥣 1/4 squash

TRY THIS DISH IN PLACE OF STUFFING OR AS A VEGETABLE SIDE DISH AT THANKSGIVING. YOU CAN ALSO ENJOY IT ANY OTHER NIGHT FOR DINNER. IT'S PACKED WITH FLAVOR AND NUTRITIOUS INGREDIENTS.

Nonstick cooking spray
- 2 medium acorn squash (about 1 1/4 pounds each), halved widthwise and seeded
- 1 tablespoon olive oil
- 8 ounces cremini mushrooms, sliced
- 2 (3-ounce) links fully cooked apple chicken sausage, diced
- 8 ounces kale, stemmed and chopped
- 1/2 teaspoon ground black pepper
- 1/2 cup fat-free low-sodium chicken broth
- 1 cup dry cornbread stuffing

1. Preheat oven to 375°F.
2. Coat a baking pan with nonstick cooking spray and place squash cut side down in the pan. Add about an inch of water and bake 30 minutes.
3. While the squash is baking, add olive oil to a sauté pan over medium-high heat. Sauté mushrooms and chicken sausage until golden brown. Add kale and pepper, and sauté until kale is wilted, about 5–7 minutes.
4. Add the chicken broth and cornbread stuffing to the mushroom mixture and simmer until all the liquid is absorbed.
5. Remove squash from the oven. Turn the squash over in the pan so the cut side is up. Fill each squash with 1/4 of the mushroom and cornbread mixture, and return to the oven. Bake 15 minutes.
6. Cut each squash in half and serve.

CHEF TIP: *Spinach can be substituted for the kale in this recipe.*

Nutrition Facts

Serves: 8
Serving Size: 1/4 squash

Amount per serving
Calories 150

Calories from fat 45

Total fat 5.0 g
   Saturated fat 1.1 g
   Trans fat 0.0 g
Cholesterol 20 mg
Sodium 260 mg
Potassium 570 mg
Total carbohydrate 21 g
   Dietary fiber 5 g
   Sugars 5 g
Protein 6 g
Phosphorus 130 mg

Choices/Exchanges: 1 1/2 Starch, 1 Fat

WILD MUSHROOM SOUP

- ⏱ 15 minutes
- 🍲 30 minutes
- 🍽 6 servings
- 🥤 1 cup

IF YOU CAN'T FIND THE ASSORTED MUSHROOMS THAT THIS RECIPE CALLS FOR, REGULAR WHITE BUTTON MUSHROOMS WORK JUST AS WELL.

1	teaspoon olive oil
1	onion, diced
1	stalk celery, diced
16	ounces assorted mushrooms (such as cremini, shiitake, oyster, and white), sliced
2	cloves garlic, minced
2	tablespoons flour
4	cups fat-free low-sodium chicken broth
1	bay leaf
1/4	teaspoon salt
1/4	teaspoon ground black pepper
1/2	cup evaporated skim milk

1. Add the oil to a soup pot over medium-high heat. Add the onion and celery and sauté until the onion turns clear, about 5 minutes.
2. Add the mushrooms and sauté until soft and all the liquid is evaporated, about 10–12 minutes. Add the garlic and sauté 1 more minute.
3. Add the flour to the mushroom mixture and sauté 2 minutes; then add the broth and stir well, scraping up the bits on the bottom of the pan.
4. Add the bay leaf, salt, and pepper. Bring to a boil; then reduce heat and simmer 10 minutes.
5. Add the evaporated milk and simmer 1 minute. Remove the bay leaf, and purée the soup with an immersion blender or in batches in an upright blender.

CHEF TIP: *Be sure to use evaporated milk and not sweetened condensed milk.*

Nutrition Facts

Serves: 6
Serving Size: 1 cup

Amount per serving
Calories 70

Calories from fat 10

Total fat 1.0 g

    Saturated fat 0.2 g

    Trans fat 0.0 g

Cholesterol 0 mg

Sodium 220 mg

Potassium 560 mg

Total carbohydrate 11 g

    Dietary fiber 1 g

    Sugars 6 g

Protein 7 g

Phosphorus 180 mg

Choices/Exchanges:
1/2 Carbohydrate, 1 Nonstarchy Vegetable

TURKEY BACON-WRAPPED JALAPEÑO POPPERS

THESE SPICY, CREAMY, BACON-WRAPPED TREATS ARE A SURE CROWD PLEASER.

- ⏱ 25 minutes
- 🍲 30 minutes
- 🍽 20 servings
- 🍴 1 popper

GF
LC

Nonstick cooking spray
10   medium-large jalapeño peppers
3/4   cup reduced-fat cream cheese
3   ounces (approximately 1 link) precooked gluten-free andouille-style chicken sausage, diced
10   pieces turkey bacon

1. Preheat oven to 375°F. Coat a baking sheet with cooking spray and set aside.
2. Add the peppers to a large sauté pan filled with one inch of water and cook over high heat. Bring to a boil, turn off the heat, and cover. Let the peppers steam 10 minutes.
3. Remove the peppers from the pan and let them cool to the touch. Cut each pepper in half lengthwise, and remove the ribs and seeds (if you'd like the poppers to be spicier, leave these in or only partially remove them). Wear gloves or use a sandwich bag to protect your hands while handling the peppers. Wash your hands immediately after handling the peppers.
4. Lay the peppers cut side up on a sheet pan.
5. In a small bowl, mix together the cream cheese and diced sausage. Fill each pepper half with 1 tablespoon of the cream cheese mixture.
6. Cut each piece of turkey bacon in half lengthwise. Wrap each pepper with a strip of turkey bacon and place seam side down on the baking sheet or secure the bacon with a toothpick.

7. Bake the poppers 20 minutes. Let them cool to room temperature before serving.

CHEF TIP: *For a sweeter popper, use a colorful array of mini bell peppers instead of jalapeños.*

Nutrition Facts

Serves: 20
Serving Size: 1 popper

Amount per serving
Calories   **50**

Calories from fat 30	
Total fat 3.5 g	
Saturated fat 1.5 g	
Trans fat 0.0 g	
Cholesterol 15 mg	
Sodium 150 mg	
Potassium 130 mg	
Total carbohydrate 3 g	
Dietary fiber 0 g	
Sugars 1 g	
Protein 3 g	
Phosphorus 50 mg	

Choices/Exchanges: 1 Fat

BERRIES AND CREAM

⏱ 5 minutes

🍽 4 servings

🥄 1 cup berries with 2 1/2 tablespoons topping

GF
VG

FRESH BERRIES (A TRUE POWER FOOD!) AND A DOLLOP OF CREAMY TOPPING LET YOU ENJOY SUMMER BY THE SPOONFUL. THIS YUMMY DESSERT TAKES ONLY 5 MINUTES TO PREPARE.

1/2 cup sugar-free vanilla pudding (prepared with skim milk)
4 tablespoons light whipped cream (such as Cabot Sweetened Light Whipped Cream)
2 cups blueberries
2 cups sliced strawberries

1. In a small bowl, mix together the pudding and whipped cream.

2. In a small bowl, mix together the blueberries and strawberries. For each serving, place 1 cup berries in a parfait or juice glass and top with 2 1/2 tablespoons pudding mixture.

DIETITIAN TIP: *A dessert that includes a whole serving of fruit is a great way to get more nutrition while enjoying something sweet. Garnish with mint leaves if desired.*

Nutrition Facts

Serves: 4

Serving Size: 1 cup berries with 2 1/2 tablespoons topping

Amount per serving

Calories **90**

Calories from fat 10

Total fat 1.0 g

Saturated fat 0.5 g

Trans fat 0.0 g

Cholesterol 1 mg

Sodium 95 mg

Potassium 240 mg

Total carbohydrate 19 g

Dietary fiber 3 g

Sugars 13 g

Protein 2 g

Phosphorus 105 mg

Choices/Exchanges: 1 Fruit, 1/2 Fat

ASIAN MEATBALLS

- ⏱ 10 minutes
- 🍲 23 minutes
- 🍽 5 servings
- 🍴 3 meatballs

THERE IS NO NEED FOR STORE-BOUGHT MEATBALLS WITH THIS EASY RECIPE. THESE MEATBALLS MAKE A QUICK AND HEALTHY APPETIZER. YOU CAN SERVE THESE WITH A SIDE OF SOY SAUCE FOR DIPPING.

1	pound lean ground turkey
3	green onions, sliced
2	tablespoons reduced-sodium soy sauce
2	tablespoons oats
1/2	teaspoon garlic powder
1/2	teaspoon ground ginger
1/4	teaspoon ground black pepper
1/4	teaspoon salt

1. Preheat oven to 375°F.
2. In a medium bowl, mix together all ingredients. Shape into 15 balls.
3. Place meatballs on a baking sheet and bake 20 minutes. Turn oven to broil and broil 2–3 minutes to make crisp.

Nutrition Facts

Serves: 5
Serving Size: 3 meatballs

Amount per serving
Calories 160

Calories from fat 60

Total fat 7.0 g

Saturated fat 2.0 g

Trans fat 0.1 g

Cholesterol 70 mg

Sodium 400 mg

Potassium 250 mg

Total carbohydrate 3 g

Dietary fiber 1 g

Sugars 0 g

Protein 18 g

Phosphorus 190 mg

Choices/Exchanges: 3 Lean Protein

CURRIED LENTILS

🕐 15 minutes
🍲 40 minutes
🍽 5 servings
🥄 1 cup

VG

1	tablespoon olive oil
1	medium red onion, cut in half and thinly sliced
2	medium carrots, diced (about 1 1/2 cups diced)
1	medium yellow, red, or orange bell pepper, seeded and diced
1	cup lentils
4	cups fat-free low-sodium vegetable broth
2	tablespoons roasted red curry paste
1	tablespoon peanut butter
1	teaspoon reduced-sodium soy sauce
1/2	teaspoon ground black pepper

1. Add olive oil to a deep sauté pan or medium saucepan over medium heat.
2. Add onion, carrots, and bell pepper to the pan and sauté 7–8 minutes.
3. Add remaining ingredients. Bring to a boil; then reduce heat and simmer 30 minutes, uncovered, stirring frequently.

CHEF TIP: *Roasted red curry paste can be purchased in the aisle of the grocery store that carries Asian foods.*

Nutrition Facts

Serves: 5
Serving Size: 1 cup

Amount per serving
Calories 220

Calories from fat 45

Total fat 5.0 g

Saturated fat 0.7 g

Trans fat 0.0 g

Cholesterol 0 mg

Sodium 410 mg

Potassium 750 mg

Total carbohydrate 34 g

Dietary fiber 11 g

Sugars 8 g

Protein 12 g

Phosphorus 280 mg

Choices/Exchanges: 1 1/2 Starch, 2 Nonstarchy Vegetable, 1 Lean Protein, 1/2 Fat

PORK DUMPLING LETTUCE WRAPS

⏱ 10 minutes
🍲 20–30 minutes
🍽 8 servings
🍴 2 wraps

THE KEY TO LONG-TERM HEALTHY EATING IS VARIETY AND EXPERIMENTING WITH DIFFERENT FLAVORS. THIS RECIPE IS A GREAT EXAMPLE OF A VARIETY OF FLAVORS AND TEXTURES!

Nonstick cooking spray
1 small onion, finely diced
1 cup shredded carrots
4 cups shredded cabbage
3 cloves garlic, minced
1/4 cup water
1 pound lean ground pork (96% lean)
1 tablespoon sesame oil
3 tablespoons red Thai curry paste
2 tablespoons rice vinegar
1/2 teaspoon ground black pepper
2 tablespoons toasted sesame seeds
Water as needed
16 butter lettuce leaves

1. Add cooking spray to a large sauté pan over medium-high heat.
2. Sauté onion, carrots, cabbage, and garlic 4 minutes. Add water, cover, and steam 7 minutes. Remove lid and turn heat up until all the water is evaporated. Set aside to cool slightly.
3. Add vegetables and remaining ingredients except lettuce to a food processor, and blend until smooth.
4. Scoop the pork mixture into 2-inch balls. Add to a large nonstick sauté pan over medium-high heat. Sauté the pork dumplings 3 minutes. Add enough water to just coat the bottom of the pan; then cover and steam the dumplings 4 minutes. Work in batches until all dumplings are done.
5. Serve 2 dumplings in each butter lettuce wrap.

Nutrition Facts

Serves: 8
Serving Size: 2 wraps

Amount per serving
Calories 130

Calories from fat 45	
Total fat 5.0 g	
Saturated fat 1.2 g	
Trans fat 0.0 g	
Cholesterol 35 mg	
Sodium 270 mg	
Potassium 400 mg	
Total carbohydrate 8 g	
Dietary fiber 2 g	
Sugars 3 g	
Protein 14 g	
Phosphorus 150 mg	

Choices/Exchanges: 1 Nonstarchy Vegetable, 2 Lean Protein

SPAGHETTI SQUASH PASTA PRIMAVERA

TO LOWER YOUR CARB INTAKE, SUBSTITUTE SPAGHETTI SQUASH FOR PASTA IN YOUR FAVORITE DISHES!

- ⏱ 5 minutes
- 🍲 About 25 minutes
- 🍽 5 servings
- 🍝 1 1/2 cups

GF

1	(4-pound) spaghetti squash
3	tablespoons olive oil, divided
1	pound boneless skinless chicken breasts, cut into 1-inch cubes
1/4	teaspoon dried oregano
1/4	teaspoon ground black pepper
2	heads broccoli, chopped into florets (about 3 1/2 cups)
1	red bell pepper, diced
2	cloves garlic, minced
3	cups baby spinach
1	cup fat-free, gluten-free, reduced-sodium chicken broth
3	tablespoons freshly grated parmesan cheese

1. Cut spaghetti squash in half lengthwise and remove seeds. Place squash in a microwave-safe baking dish cut side down. Cover loosely with a lid, leaving room to vent. Microwave 10–15 minutes, rotating every 5 minutes. Squash is done when it's soft to the touch. Set aside.

2. While squash is cooking, add 1 1/2 tablespoons olive oil to a large skillet over medium-high heat. Season chicken with oregano and black pepper. Add to pan and cook about 10 minutes, stirring frequently, until chicken is done. Remove from pan and set aside.

3. Heat 1 1/2 tablespoons olive oil over medium-high heat. Add broccoli and red pepper, and sauté 5–7 minutes. Add garlic and sauté 30 seconds. Add spinach and chicken broth, and cook an additional 4 minutes.

4. Use a fork to scoop out the spaghetti squash. Add the squash noodles and the chicken back to pan. Heat 2 minutes, mixing well. Top with parmesan cheese.

Nutrition Facts

Serves: 5
Serving Size: 1 1/2 cups

Amount per serving
Calories 270

Calories from fat 110

Total fat 12.0 g
  Saturated fat 2.3 g
  Trans fat 0.0 g
Cholesterol 55 mg
Sodium 260 mg
Potassium 750 mg
Total carbohydrate 18 g
  Dietary fiber 5 g
  Sugars 7 g
Protein 24 g
Phosphorus 245 mg

Choices/Exchanges: 4 Nonstarchy Vegetable, 2 Lean Protein, 1 1/2 Fat

SAVORY STUFFED PUMPKINS

○ 15 minutes
○ 70 minutes
○ 4 servings
○ 1 pumpkin

WOW YOUR DINNER COMPANIONS AND PAIR THIS CHARMING MAIN DISH WITH A NONSTARCHY VEGETABLE OR SALAD FOR A COMPLETE MEAL. TO MAKE THIS VEGETARIAN, SIMPLY OMIT THE SAUSAGE AND USE VEGETABLE BROTH INSTEAD OF CHICKEN BROTH.

4   small (1-pound) sugar pie pumpkins
1   cup water
Nonstick cooking spray
1   small onion (1/2 cup), minced
2   stalks celery, diced small
2   large eggs
1   cup fat-free low-sodium chicken broth
2   cups cubed whole-wheat bread
2   (3-ounce) links fully cooked apple
     chicken sausage, diced
1/4 cup shredded parmesan cheese
1/2 teaspoon ground black pepper
1   tablespoon chopped fresh thyme

1. Preheat oven to 375°F. Cut the tops off the pumpkins (save the tops), and place the pumpkins facedown in a 9-by-13-inch baking dish. Pour the water over the pumpkins and bake 30 minutes. Remove the pumpkins from the pan and set them aside to cool slightly. Discard the water.
2. While the pumpkins are baking, coat a small sauté pan with cooking spray and place over medium heat. Add the onion and celery and sauté about 7 minutes, until softened; set aside to cool.
3. In a medium bowl, combine the remaining ingredients and mix until the bread is coated and starting to soften. Stir in the onion and celery mixture.

4. Place the pumpkins cut side up in the baking dish and gently scoop out the seeds, taking care not to remove too much of the pumpkin flesh. Divide the filling mixture evenly among the pumpkins and cap with the pumpkin tops. Bake 30 minutes. Remove the tops and bake 10 more minutes. If desired, serve with the tops.

Nutrition Facts

Serves: 4
Serving Size: 1 pumpkin

Amount per serving

Calories	**250**

Calories from fat 60

Total fat 7.0 g

   Saturated fat 2.5 g

   Trans fat 0.0 g

Cholesterol 125 mg

Sodium 450 mg

Potassium 1000 mg

Total carbohydrate 30 g

   Dietary fiber 5 g

   Sugars 10 g

Protein 17 g

Phosphorus 305 mg

Choices/Exchanges: 1 1/2 Starch, 1/2 Carbohydrate, 2 Lean Protein

CRUSTLESS ASPARAGUS AND PEPPER MINI QUICHES

YOU CAN FREEZE THESE MINI QUICHES ONCE THEY HAVE BAKED AND COOLED. REHEAT IN A TOASTER OVEN OR MICROWAVE FOR A GREAT BREAKFAST OR LUNCH ON THE GO!

GF
LC
VG

- ⏲ 15 minutes
- 🍲 30 minutes
- 🍽 12 servings
- 🍽 1 quiche

Nonstick cooking spray
1   tablespoon olive oil
1   bunch asparagus, trimmed and diced
1   small onion, diced
1   yellow bell pepper, seeded and diced
1/2 teaspoon salt
1/4 teaspoon ground black pepper
2   eggs
6   egg whites
1/3 cup skim milk
6   spreadable creamy light Swiss cheese wedges (such as Laughing Cow), halved

1. Preheat oven to 375°F.
2. Spray a muffin pan with cooking spray.
3. Add olive oil and a generous amount of cooking spray to a medium sauté pan. Sauté asparagus, onion, and bell pepper 7–9 minutes or until cooked through. Season with salt and black pepper, and set aside to cool slightly.
4. In a medium bowl, whisk together eggs, egg whites, and milk.
5. Evenly distribute the sautéed vegetables among 12 muffin cups. Cups should be 1/2 to 3/4 full. Gently pour egg mixture over the vegetables in each muffin cup, distributing evenly. Cups should be full but not overflowing.
6. Gently press 1/2 cheese wedge into the middle of each quiche. Repeat for the remaining 11 quiches.
7. Bake 20 minutes. Serve immediately.

Nutrition Facts

Serves: 12
Serving Size: 1 quiche

Amount per serving
Calories **60**

Calories from fat 25	
Total fat 3.0 g	
Saturated fat 0.9 g	
Trans fat 0.0 g	
Cholesterol 35 mg	
Sodium 230 mg	
Potassium 160 mg	
Total carbohydrate 4 g	
Dietary fiber 1 g	
Sugars 2 g	
Protein 5 g	
Phosphorus 110 mg	

Choices/Exchanges: 1 Lean Protein, 1/2 Fat

BLACK BEAN AND MANGO SALSA LETTUCE WRAPS

THIS RECIPE USES LOWER-CARB BUTTER LETTUCE LEAVES AS A SUBSTITUTE FOR A TORTILLA WRAP. IF YOU DON'T LIKE YOUR FOOD SPICY, USE A CHOPPED GREEN BELL PEPPER INSTEAD OF THE JALAPEÑO PEPPER.

⏱ 10 minutes
△ 5 servings
▭ 1/2 cup or 2 lettuce cups

GF
VG

1	(15-ounce) can black beans, rinsed and drained
1	mango, peeled, diced, and hard center squeezed to release 1 tablespoon juice
1/2	small red onion, diced
1	medium jalapeño pepper, seeded and minced (see Chef Tip)
1	large red bell pepper, seeded and diced
2	tablespoons red wine vinegar
1	tablespoon olive oil
1	tablespoon honey or 2 packets artificial sweetener
10	leaves butter lettuce or 20 leaves Belgian endive

1. Combine all ingredients except lettuce in a medium bowl. Refrigerate for at least 1 hour, or up to 2 days to marinate (the longer, the better).

2. If using butter lettuce leaves, arrange them on a large plate and fill each leaf with 1/4 cup salad mixture. If using the Belgian endive leaves, arrange them on a large plate and fill each one with 1/8 cup (2 tablespoons) salad mixture.

ALTERNATIVE SERVING SUGGESTION: *Use jicama instead of lettuce for serving. Peel a jicama and slice into 1/4-inch-thick rounds; then slice the rounds into triangles (eighths) to resemble tortilla chips. Serve like chips and salsa using the raw jicama chips instead of tortilla chips.*

CHEF TIP: *Be careful when cutting jalapeño peppers. The seeds and veins inside the peppers are where the heat resides. Consider wearing gloves during this step and be careful not to touch your face or eyes when handling hot peppers. If jalapeños are too hot for you, substitute with a green bell pepper.*

Nutrition Facts

Serves: 5
Serving Size: 1/2 cup or 2 lettuce cups

Amount per serving
Calories **150**

Calories from fat 30	
Total fat 3.5 g	
Saturated fat 0.5 g	
Trans fat 0.0 g	
Cholesterol 0 mg	
Sodium 65 mg	
Potassium 420 mg	
Total carbohydrate 27 g	
Dietary fiber 6 g	
Sugars 14 g	
Protein 6 g	
Phosphorus 95 mg	

Choices/Exchanges: 1 Starch, 1/2 Fruit, 1 Nonstarchy Vegetable, 1/2 Fat

THAI LEMONGRASS BEEF SKEWERS

○ 1 hour
⏱ 10 minutes
△ 12 servings
▢ 1 skewer

LC

FOR ANOTHER FUN APPETIZER USING THIS RECIPE, REMOVE THE COOKED BEEF FROM THE SKEWERS AND SERVE IN LETTUCE CUPS WITH A DASH OF THAI-STYLE HOT SAUCE.

12	bamboo skewers
2	teaspoons artificial sweetener
2	tablespoons reduced-sodium soy sauce
1	teaspoon ground black pepper
2	cloves garlic, minced
2	stalks lemongrass, minced
2	pounds lean beef tenderloin, cut into 1-inch chunks
1	cup chopped fresh basil (Thai basil if you can find it)
1	cup chopped fresh cilantro
2	limes, cut into 6 wedges each

1. Soak bamboo skewers in warm water for at least 30 minutes.
2. In a medium bowl, whisk the artificial sweetener, soy sauce, pepper, garlic, and lemongrass. Add the beef and marinate in the refrigerator for at least 1 hour (up to 4 hours).
3. Prepare an indoor or outdoor grill.
4. Remove beef from marinade and divide pieces evenly among 12 skewers. Discard marinade.
5. Grill the skewers about 5 minutes per side.
6. Garnish the skewers with basil, cilantro, and a lime wedge.

Nutrition Facts

Serves: 12
Serving Size: 1 skewer

Amount per serving
Calories 100

Calories from fat 35

Total fat 4.0 g

    Saturated fat 1.5 g

    Trans fat 0.0 g

Cholesterol 40 mg

Sodium 75 mg

Potassium 220 mg

Total carbohydrate 1 g

    Dietary fiber 0 g

    Sugars 0 g

Protein 14 g

Phosphorus 115 mg

Choices/Exchanges: 2 Lean Protein

BROCCOLI CHEESE BITES

- ⏱ 20 minutes
- 🍲 25 minutes
- 🍽 6 servings
- 🍴 5 pieces

VG

THESE BITES ARE A GREAT SNACK OR APPETIZER AND AN EXCELLENT WAY TO ADD MORE VEGETABLES TO YOUR HEALTHY EATING PLAN.

Nonstick cooking spray
2   heads broccoli (about 1 1/2 pounds), trimmed
1   egg
1   egg white
1/3 cup reduced-fat shredded cheddar or Mexican-style cheese
1/3 cup bread crumbs
1/2 cup chopped onion
1/4 teaspoon ground black pepper

1. Preheat oven to 400°F. Coat 1 large (or 2 small) baking sheets with cooking spray. Set aside.

2. Steam the broccoli for approximately 10–12 minutes, until soft. Set aside to cool about 10 minutes.

3. When cooled, add the broccoli and remaining ingredients to a blender or food processor and pulse to combine. Do not overmix; the mixture should be slightly chunky, not a paste. Let the mixture rest 10 minutes.

4. After the mixture has rested, stir it, and drop by tablespoonfuls onto the prepared baking sheet.

5. Lightly spray the top of each ball with cooking spray. Bake 15 minutes. Turn the pieces over and bake an additional 10 minutes, or until golden brown.

CHEF TIP: *Serve these broccoli bites with your favorite Greek yogurt dip.*

Nutrition Facts

Serves: 6
Serving Size: 5 pieces

Amount per serving
Calories   **100**

Calories from fat 25

Total fat 3.0 g
    Saturated fat 1.2 g
    Trans fat 0.0 g

Cholesterol 35 mg

Sodium 150 mg

Potassium 420 mg

Total carbohydrate 13 g
    Dietary fiber 3 g
    Sugars 3 g

Protein 7 g

Phosphorus 140 mg

Choices/Exchanges: 1/2 Starch, 2 Nonstarchy Vegetable, 1/2 Fat

BRUSSELS SPROUTS SLAW

LC
VG

- ⏱ 20 minutes
- 🍲 5 minutes
- 🍽 9 servings
- 🍴 1/2 cup

THIS RECIPE IS BEST MADE SEVERAL HOURS (OR A DAY) AHEAD OF TIME TO ALLOW THE BRUSSELS SPROUTS TO ABSORB THE DRESSING THOROUGHLY, BUT IT CAN BE SERVED IMMEDIATELY IF NEEDED.

6	cups water
1	pound fresh Brussels sprouts
2	scallions, minced
1/4	cup rice wine vinegar
1	tablespoon Dijon mustard
1	tablespoon reduced-sodium soy sauce
2	tablespoons artificial sweetener
1/4	cup light mayonnaise
1/4	teaspoon ground black pepper
1/2	cup slivered almonds, toasted

1. In a large pot, bring 6 cups of water to a boil. Add Brussels sprouts and blanch in the boiling water 1 minute. Remove the sprouts from the boiling water and run under cold water to stop the cooking. Dry the sprouts with a clean towel.

2. Trim the stems on the Brussels sprouts and slice in half lengthwise. Using the slicing blade on a food processor, process the Brussels sprouts to shred them. You can also do this with the slicing side of a box grater or with a very sharp knife.

3. In a medium bowl, whisk together scallions, vinegar, mustard, soy sauce, artificial sweetener, mayonnaise, and pepper.

4. Add the shredded Brussels sprouts and toasted almonds to the dressing and mix well.

MAKE IT GLUTEN-FREE: *Use gluten-free soy sauce and confirm all other ingredients are gluten-free.*

Nutrition Facts

Serves: 9
Serving Size: 1/2 cup

Amount per serving

Calories 80

Calories from fat 45

Total fat 5.0 g

    Saturated fat 0.5 g

    Trans fat 0.0 g

Cholesterol 0 mg

Sodium 160 mg

Potassium 230 mg

Total carbohydrate 7 g

    Dietary fiber 2 g

    Sugars 2 g

Protein 3 g

Phosphorus 65 mg

Choices/Exchanges: 1 Nonstarchy Vegetable, 1 Fat

ROASTED CHICKEN AND ARUGULA SALAD

TRY THIS BUDGET-FRIENDLY DISH FOR LUNCH OR DINNER THIS WEEK. TO MINIMIZE PREP TIME, COOK THE CHICKEN AND MAKE THE DRESSING AHEAD OF TIME.

⏱ 15 minutes
🍲 30 minutes
🍽 4 servings
🥣 2 1/2 cups

GF

2	pounds bone-in, skin-on chicken breasts
1	tablespoon salt-free all-purpose seasoning (such as Spike or Mrs. Dash)
1/4	cup balsamic vinegar
1	clove garlic, minced or grated
1	tablespoon Dijon mustard
1	tablespoon honey or 2 packets artificial sweetener
2	tablespoons extra-virgin olive oil
1/2	teaspoon salt
1/4	teaspoon ground black pepper
6	cups arugula
1/2	small onion, thinly sliced (equivalent to 1/2 cup)
1/4	cup golden raisins

1. Preheat oven to 375°F. Lay the chicken breasts skin side up on a sheet pan and season with the salt-free seasoning.
2. Roast the chicken 30 minutes or until the internal temperature is 165°F. Set the chicken aside to cool.
3. In a large salad bowl, whisk together the vinegar, garlic, mustard, honey or artificial sweetener, olive oil, salt, and pepper.
4. Peel the skin off the chicken and remove the bones, and discard the skin and bones. Cut the chicken into 1-inch chunks.
5. Toss the chicken, arugula, onion, and golden raisins in the dressing and serve.

Nutrition Facts

Serves: 4
Serving Size: 2 1/2 cups

Amount per serving
Calories   **320**

Calories from fat 100

Total fat 11.0 g

   Saturated fat 2.1 g

   Trans fat 0.0 g

Cholesterol 95 mg

Sodium 480 mg

Potassium 530 mg

Total carbohydrate 18 g

   Dietary fiber 1 g

   Sugars 13 g

Protein 36 g

Phosphorus 290 mg

Choices/Exchanges: 1/2 Fruit, 1/2 Carbohydrate, 5 Lean Protein

SWEET POTATO AND SPINACH CHICKEN TACOS

○ 5 minutes
🍲 20 minutes
△ 4 servings
◠ 1 taco

GF

UNEXPECTED TACO FILLINGS ARE ALL THE RAGE ON THE FOOD TRUCK SCENE. MAKE THESE RICH AND SAVORY VERSIONS AT HOME! FOR THE CHICKEN, USE LEFTOVER COOKED CHICKEN OR PURCHASE A COOKED ROTISSERIE CHICKEN. PICO DE GALLO—A FRESH SALSA—IS FOUND IN MOST GROCERY STORES IN THE REFRIGERATED AREA OF THE DELI OR PRODUCE SECTIONS AND ADDS A LOT OF FLAVOR AND TEXTURE TO THIS RECIPE.

1 1/2	tablespoons olive oil
1	clove garlic, minced
24	ounces baby spinach
1	large (8-ounce) sweet potato, peeled and diced
1/4	teaspoon cumin
1/4	teaspoon ground black pepper
4	tablespoons water
1	cup shredded cooked chicken
4	(6-inch) corn tortillas, heated
4	teaspoons reduced-fat sour cream
1/2	cup fresh no-salt-added pico de gallo (purchased)

1. In a large nonstick pan, heat the oil over medium heat. Add the garlic and sauté 30 seconds. Add the spinach and sauté 3-4 minutes.
2. Add the sweet potato, cumin, pepper, and water to the pan. Sauté 2 minutes. Cover, reduce heat to low, and cook 8 minutes.
3. Add the chicken to the pan and mix to incorporate. Heat 2 minutes.
4. Fill each tortilla with 1/4 of the chicken and sweet potato mixture. Top with 1 teaspoon sour cream and 2 tablespoons pico de gallo.

DIETITIAN TIP: *To reduce carbs further, use lettuce wraps in place of corn tortillas.*

Nutrition Facts

Serves: 4
Serving Size: 1 taco

Amount per serving
Calories   **250**

Calories from fat 90

Total fat 10.0 g

    Saturated fat 2.0 g

    Trans fat 0.0 g

Cholesterol 35 mg

Sodium 190 mg

Potassium 1300 mg

Total carbohydrate 28 g

    Dietary fiber 7 g

    Sugars 4 g

Protein 18 g

Phosphorus 265 mg

Choices/Exchanges: 1 1/2 Starch, 1 Nonstarchy Vegetable, 2 Lean Protein, 1/2 Fat

MINI BAKED CRAB CAKES

THESE CRAB CAKES MAKE A GREAT PARTY APPETIZER OR ARE DELICIOUS ON TOP OF A SALAD OF FIELD GREENS WITH LIGHT BALSAMIC VINAIGRETTE.

- ⏱ 5 minutes
- 🍳 10 minutes
- 🍽 5 servings
- 🍴 2 crab cakes

CRAB CAKE

Nonstick cooking spray
1	slice whole-wheat bread (about 1 ounce)
2	egg whites
1	tablespoon hot pepper sauce
2	scallions, minced
1/4	teaspoon salt
1/4	teaspoon ground black pepper
2	(6-ounce) cans fancy white (or lump) crabmeat, drained

DIPPING SAUCE

1/2	cup reduced-sugar apricot preserves
1	teaspoon Thai-style chili garlic sauce (or other hot sauce)
1	teaspoon reduced-sodium soy sauce

1. Preheat oven to 425°F. Coat a baking sheet with cooking spray.
2. In a medium bowl, tear the whole-wheat bread into small (pea-size) pieces. Add the egg whites, hot pepper sauce, scallions, salt, and pepper, and mix well until bread is softened; then fold in the crabmeat.
3. Portion 10 patties onto the baking sheet. Spray the patties liberally with cooking spray and bake on the top rack of the oven 5 minutes. Flip the patties with the spatula and spray again with cooking spray. Bake an additional 5 minutes.
4. Remove from the oven and let the crab cakes rest 5 minutes before serving.
5. To make a dipping sauce for mini baked crab cakes, in a bowl combine reduced-sugar apricot preserves with Thai-style chili garlic sauce (or other hot sauce), and reduced-sodium soy sauce.
6. Heat in the microwave for 30 seconds.
7. Serve crab cakes with dipping sauce.

Nutrition Facts

Serves: 5
Serving Size: 2 crab cakes

Amount per serving
Calories 100

Calories from fat 15	
Total fat 1.5 g	
Saturated fat 0.3 g	
Trans fat 0.0 g	
Cholesterol 40 mg	
Sodium 450 mg	
Potassium 310 mg	
Total carbohydrate 14 g	
Dietary fiber 1 g	
Sugars 9 g	
Protein 8 g	
Phosphorus 150 mg	

Choices/Exchanges:
1 Carbohydrate, 1 Lean Protein

CRAB CAKE BURGERS

THESE BURGERS ARE GREAT WITH A GREEN SALAD WITH CILANTRO LIME VINAIGRETTE.

- ⏱ 10 minutes
- 🍲 15 minutes
- 🍽 6 servings
- 🍴 1 burger

CRAB CAKES

Nonstick cooking spray
1/4 cup minced onion
2 (6-ounce) cans lump crabmeat, drained
1/2 cup bread crumbs
1 egg
1 egg white
1/2 teaspoon hot sauce
1/4 teaspoon ground black pepper
1 tablespoon olive oil

SAUCE

1/4 cup light mayonnaise
1/4 cup fat-free plain Greek yogurt
1 tablespoon adobo sauce from canned chipotle peppers
1/2 cup frozen corn kernels, thawed
6 large lettuce leaves
1 1/2 cups shredded lettuce
1 ripe tomato, cut into 6 slices
1 ripe avocado, seeded, peeled, and cut into 12 slices

1. Coat a small nonstick skillet with cooking spray and place over medium-high heat. Add onion and sauté 2–3 minutes or until onion is clear. Set aside to cool.
2. In a medium bowl combine crabmeat, bread crumbs, egg, egg white, hot sauce, and pepper. Mix well until all ingredients are incorporated. Stir in cooled onion.
3. Add oil and a generous amount of cooking spray to a large nonstick skillet over medium-high heat. Form crab mixture into 1/2-inch-thick patties using a heaping 1/4 cup. Fry about 4–5 minutes on each side or until golden brown.

4. In a small bowl, whisk together mayonnaise, yogurt, adobo sauce, and corn.
5. Place each crab cake on a lettuce leaf. Place 1/4 cup lettuce, 1 tomato slice, and 2 avocado slices on top of each crab cake, and then top with 2 tablespoons of sauce.

Nutrition Facts

Serves: 6
Serving Size: 1 burger

Amount per serving	
Calories	**190**
Calories from fat 90	
Total fat 10.0 g	
Saturated fat 1.6 g	
Trans fat 0.0 g	
Cholesterol 70 mg	
Sodium 370 mg	
Potassium 490 mg	
Total carbohydrate 17 g	
Dietary fiber 3 g	
Sugars 3 g	
Protein 10 g	
Phosphorus 190 mg	

Choices/Exchanges: 1/2 Starch, 1 Nonstarchy Vegetable, 1 Lean Protein, 1 1/2 Fat

EGGS FLORENTINE

- ⏱ 15 minutes
- 🍲 5 minutes
- 🍽 4 servings
- ☕ 1/2 English muffin, 1 poached egg, and 2 tablespoons sauce

VG

HERE'S A HEALTHY VERSION OF EGGS BENEDICT WHERE THE HAM IS REPLACED BY PERFECTLY SAUTÉED SPINACH AND THE HOLLANDAISE SAUCE IS ON THE LIGHTER SIDE.

Nonstick cooking spray
1 teaspoon olive oil
4 cups baby spinach
1 clove garlic, minced
1 egg yolk
1/2 teaspoon lemon juice
2 tablespoons fat-free low-sodium vegetable broth
1/4 cup fat-free plain yogurt
1/4 teaspoon salt
Dash ground black pepper
2 light whole-wheat English muffins, split and lightly toasted
4 eggs, poached (see Chef Tip)

1. Add cooking spray and olive oil to a sauté pan over medium heat. Add spinach and sauté until wilted. Stir in the garlic and sauté 1 additional minute.
2. Prepare a double boiler with a heatproof bowl. Add the egg yolk, lemon juice, and vegetable broth, whisking constantly until hot but not curdled. Remove from heat and whisk in yogurt, salt, and pepper.
3. Top each English muffin half with 1/4 of spinach mixture, 1 poached egg, and 2 tablespoons sauce.

CHEF TIP: *Try poaching eggs in the microwave. Fill a 1-cup microwave-safe bowl or teacup with 1/2 cup water. Gently crack an egg into the water, making sure it's completely submerged. Cover with a saucer and microwave on high about 1 minute, or until the white is set but the yolk is still soft. Use a slotted spoon to transfer the egg to a plate.*

Nutrition Facts

Serves: 4

Serving Size: 1/2 English muffin, 1 poached egg, and 2 tablespoons sauce

Amount per serving

Calories 160

Calories from fat 70

Total fat 8.0 g

Saturated fat 2.2 g

Trans fat 0.0 g

Cholesterol 230 mg

Sodium 330 mg

Potassium 330 mg

Total carbohydrate 16 g

Dietary fiber 5 g

Sugars 2 g

Protein 11 g

Phosphorus 235 mg

Choices/Exchanges: 1 Starch, 1 Medium-Fat Protein, 1/2 Fat

KALE AND QUINOA SALAD

⏱ 15 minutes
🍽 10 servings
🥄 1/2 cup

IT'S IDEAL TO DRESS THIS SALAD AND LET IT SIT AT ROOM TEMPERATURE ABOUT 30 MINUTES TO LET THE KALE WILT A BIT AND ABSORB THE DRESSING. TOSS AGAIN JUST BEFORE SERVING.

1	cup tricolored quinoa (or any one color of quinoa)
1 1/2	cups water
1/4	cup white balsamic or white raspberry balsamic vinegar
1	clove garlic, grated or minced
1	tablespoon Dijon mustard
1	tablespoon honey or 2 packets artificial sweetener
1	tablespoon chopped fresh parsley
1/2	teaspoon salt
1/4	teaspoon ground black pepper
1/4	cup extra-virgin olive oil
4	cups chopped fresh kale leaves
1/4	cup dried cranberries
2	tablespoons sunflower seeds
1	(3-ounce) package crumbled reduced-fat feta cheese

1. Rinse the dry quinoa in a strainer under cold running water. Combine the rinsed quinoa and water in a medium saucepan and bring to a boil. Reduce to a simmer and cover. Cook the quinoa 12–15 minutes until all the liquid is absorbed. Turn off the heat and leave the lid on 10 minutes to steam. Spread the quinoa on a sheet pan to cool.
2. In a large salad bowl, whisk together the vinegar, garlic, mustard, honey or artificial sweetener, parsley, salt, and pepper. Add the olive oil and whisk until emulsified.
3. In the same bowl, toss together the kale, cranberries, sunflower seeds, feta cheese, and cooled quinoa until coated with dressing.

Nutrition Facts

Serves: 10
Serving Size: 1/2 cup

Amount per serving
Calories   **160**

Calories from fat 70

Total fat 8.0 g
   Saturated fat 1.6 g
   Trans fat 0.0 g
Cholesterol 8 mg
Sodium 260 mg
Potassium 160 mg
Total carbohydrate 19 g
   Dietary fiber 2 g
   Sugars 6 g
Protein 5 g
Phosphorus 135 mg

Choices/Exchanges: 1/2 Starch, 1/2 Carbohydrate, 2 Fat

CRISPY ASIAN KALE

THIS IS AN INCREDIBLE SNACK AND A GREAT ALTERNATIVE TO CHIPS. USE IT AS A SIDE DISH OR AS A PARTY APPETIZER!

LC
VG

- ⏱ 5 minutes
- 🍲 15 minutes
- △ 6 servings
- ▷ 1 1/2 cups

Nonstick cooking spray
1 tablespoon olive oil
1 tablespoon reduced-sodium soy sauce
1 tablespoon low-calorie brown sugar blend (such as Splenda)
1 teaspoon garlic powder
1 (16-ounce) bag ready-to-cook kale

1. Preheat oven to 350°F. Coat two large baking sheets with cooking spray.
2. In a large bowl, whisk together the olive oil, soy sauce, brown sugar blend, and garlic powder.
3. Toss the kale in the dressing to coat, and spread kale in one layer on the baking sheets. Do not overload the baking sheets with kale. Use a third baking sheet if needed.
4. Bake 10–15 minutes or until the kale is crispy.

MAKE IT GLUTEN-FREE: *Use gluten-free soy sauce and confirm all other ingredients are gluten-free.*

Nutrition Facts

Serves: 6
Serving Size: 1 1/2 cups

Amount per serving
Calories 70

Calories from fat 25	
Total fat 3.0 g	
Saturated fat 0.4 g	
Trans fat 0.0 g	
Cholesterol 0 mg	
Sodium 120 mg	
Potassium 380 mg	
Total carbohydrate 9 g	
Dietary fiber 3 g	
Sugars 3 g	
Protein 4 g	
Phosphorus 75 mg	

Choices/Exchanges: 2 Nonstarchy Vegetable, 1/2 Fat

MOLE PORK TENDERLOIN WITH ZUCCHINI AND REFRIED BLACK BEANS

⏱ 20 minutes
🍳 25 minutes
🍽 6 servings
🍴 3 ounces pork,
1/4 cup black beans,
and 1/2 cup zucchini

THIS DISH IS A GREAT EXAMPLE OF THE DIABETES PLATE METHOD AT WORK—LEAN PROTEIN (PORK TENDERLOIN), STARCHY BEANS, AND LOW-CARB ZUCCHINI. TO ADD SOME DAIRY, GARNISH THE PORK TENDERLOIN WITH FAT-FREE PLAIN GREEK YOGURT.

PORK

1   tablespoon prepared mole sauce
Juice and zest of 1 small orange (1/4 cup juice, 1 tablespoon zest)
2   cloves garlic, minced or grated
1/4   cup water
Nonstick cooking spray
1 1/4 pounds pork tenderloin, trimmed of all visible fat

BEANS

1   teaspoon olive oil
1   small onion, diced
1   clove garlic, chopped
1   (15.5-ounce) can black beans, drained and rinsed
1/4   cup water

ZUCCHINI

3   medium zucchini, diced (about 4 cups)
1/2   teaspoon chili powder
1/2   teaspoon garlic powder
1/4   teaspoon cayenne pepper
1/4   teaspoon ground black pepper
1/4   teaspoon salt
Juice of 1 lime (1/4 cup juice)

1. Preheat oven to 375°F.
2. In a small bowl, whisk together the mole sauce, orange juice, orange zest, garlic, and water.
3. Coat an oven-safe sauté pan with cooking spray over medium-high heat.
4. Sear the pork tenderloin in the sauté pan until brown on all sides. Pour the mole sauce over the pork and cover completely with sauce. Put the pan in the oven and roast 20 minutes, turning the pork every 5 minutes.
5. While the pork is roasting, add olive oil to a medium nonstick sauté pan over medium heat. Add onion, garlic, and black beans and sauté 5 minutes or until the onion is softened.
6. Add the bean mixture and water to a blender and blend until smooth. Return the beans to the pan and sauté until slightly thickened, about 2 minutes. Set aside.
7. Add cooking spray to another medium nonstick sauté pan over medium heat. Add the zucchini and sauté 3–4 minutes or until the zucchini begins to soften. Add the chili powder, garlic powder, cayenne pepper, black pepper, salt, and lime juice. Sauté 2 more minutes.
8. Let the pork tenderloin rest 5 minutes before slicing. Slice the pork into 18 slices and toss the pieces in any remaining mole sauce.
9. Build your plate with three slices pork tenderloin (about 3 ounces), 1/4 cup black beans, and 1/2 cup zucchini.

Nutrition Facts

Serves: 6

Serving Size: 3 ounces pork, 1/4 cup black beans, and 1/2 cup zucchini

Amount per serving

Calories 230

Calories from fat 45

Total fat 5.0 g

    Saturated fat 1.4 g

    Trans fat 0.0 g

Cholesterol 65 mg

Sodium 210 mg

Potassium 860 mg

Total carbohydrate 18 g

    Dietary fiber 5 g

    Sugars 5 g

Protein 29 g

Phosphorus 320 mg

Choices/Exchanges: 1 Starch, 1 Nonstarchy Vegetable, 3 Lean Protein

CHICKEN AND BEAN CASSOULET

WANT WINTER COMFORT FOOD? TRY CASSOULET! THIS RECIPE FOR SLOW-COOKED FRENCH CASSEROLE REPLACES THE TRADITIONAL PORK AND DUCK INGREDIENTS WITH TURKEY KIELBASA AND CHICKEN THIGHS.

- ⏱ 15 minutes
- 🍲 30 minutes
- 🍽 8 servings
- 🍴 1 chicken thigh and 1/2 cup stew

Nonstick cooking spray
1 1/2 pounds boneless skinless chicken thighs, cut into 8 large pieces
1/4 teaspoon salt
1/2 teaspoon ground black pepper
6 ounces reduced-fat turkey kielbasa, diced
1 onion, diced
2 cloves garlic, minced
2 carrots, diced
1 tablespoon tomato paste
2 sprigs fresh thyme
1 1/2 cups fat-free low-sodium chicken broth
1 (15-ounce) can cannellini (white kidney) beans, drained and rinsed

1. Coat a large sauté pan with cooking spray and place over high heat. Season the chicken on both sides with salt and pepper. Sear the chicken on both sides until golden brown, about 5 minutes; then remove from pan and set aside.
2. Turn heat down to medium. Add kielbasa and sauté 3 minutes. Remove from pan and set aside.
3. Add onion, garlic, and carrots. Sauté 3–4 minutes; then add tomato paste, thyme, and chicken broth. Scrape the brown bits from the bottom of the pan and bring to a boil. Reduce to a simmer, and then add the chicken and sausage back to the pan with any accumulated juices. Cover and simmer 8 minutes. Remove the lid and simmer 5 minutes. Remove the chicken and set aside.
4. Add the beans. Turn heat to high. Simmer 5 more minutes until liquid is slightly reduced. Remove thyme stems.
5. To serve, place a chicken thigh in the bottom of a bowl and pour 1/2 cup stew over it.

CHEF TIP: *This recipe freezes well. Portion servings into freezer-safe containers and freeze up to 6 months.*

Nutrition Facts

Serves: 8
Serving Size: 1 chicken thigh and 1/2 cup stew

Amount per serving	
Calories	**190**
Calories from fat 60	
Total fat 7.0 g	
Saturated fat 1.9 g	
Trans fat 0.0 g	
Cholesterol 90 mg	
Sodium 410 mg	
Potassium 460 mg	
Total carbohydrate 11 g	
Dietary fiber 3 g	
Sugars 2 g	
Protein 21 g	
Phosphorus 230 mg	

Choices/Exchanges: 1/2 Starch, 1 Nonstarchy Vegetable, 3 Lean Protein

QUINOA WITH CRANBERRIES AND PINE NUTS

QUINOA IS A WHOLE GRAIN THAT CAN BE USED IN PLACE OF RICE IN MANY RECIPES. IT IS HIGHER IN PROTEIN THAN OTHER GRAINS AND IS A GOOD SOURCE OF FIBER.

⏱ 5 minutes
🍲 20 minutes
🍽 6 servings
🥄 1/2 cup

1 cup quinoa
2 cups fat-free reduced-sodium chicken broth
1/2 cup dried cranberries
3 tablespoons pine nuts, toasted
1 teaspoon dried parsley

DRESSING

2 tablespoons balsamic vinegar
1/2 teaspoon Dijon mustard
1 clove garlic, minced
3 tablespoons extra-virgin olive oil
1/4 teaspoon ground black pepper

1. Thoroughly rinse the quinoa in a fine mesh sieve under cold running water.
2. Heat the chicken broth in a pot over medium-high heat and bring it to a boil. Stir in the quinoa; then cover the pot, reduce the heat, and simmer 15 minutes. Add the cranberries, cover, and cook 5 more minutes.
3. Turn off the heat and let the quinoa stand 5 minutes. Fluff with a fork.
4. While the quinoa is cooking, whisk together all the dressing ingredients.
5. Pour the dressing over the cooked quinoa. Add the toasted pine nuts and mix well. Pour the quinoa into a serving bowl and sprinkle with parsley. Serve warm or cold.

MAKE IT GLUTEN-FREE: *Confirm all ingredients are gluten-free, including the chicken broth.*

Nutrition Facts

Serves: 6
Serving Size: 1/2 cup

Amount per serving
Calories **240**

Calories from fat 110	
Total fat 12.0 g	
Saturated fat 1.4 g	
Trans fat 0.0 g	
Cholesterol 0 mg	
Sodium 210 mg	
Potassium 270 mg	
Total carbohydrate 31 g	
Dietary fiber 3 g	
Sugars 10 g	
Protein 6 g	
Phosphorus 185 mg	

Choices/Exchanges: 1 1/2 Starch, 1/2 Fruit, 2 Fat

TOASTED QUINOA AND CABBAGE SALAD

YOU CAN USE ANY COLOR QUINOA FOR THIS SALAD, BUT RED QUINOA WILL GIVE IT A NICE POP OF COLOR. QUINOA NOT ONLY IS A WHOLE GRAIN BUT IT ALSO PROVIDES SOME PROTEIN.

○ 10 minutes
🍲 15 minutes
🍽 6 servings
🍴 1 1/2 cups

VG

1/2	cup red quinoa
1	cup fat-free low-sodium vegetable broth
3/4	cup fat-free plain Greek yogurt
1	tablespoon extra-virgin olive oil
2	tablespoons rice wine vinegar
1	tablespoon dry dill
1	teaspoon garlic powder
1/4	teaspoon salt
1/2	teaspoon ground black pepper
1	(14-ounce) package coleslaw mix (shredded cabbage and carrots)
1	(15-ounce) can chickpeas (garbanzo beans), drained and rinsed

1. Thoroughly rinse the quinoa in a fine mesh sieve under cold running water.
2. Add the quinoa to a medium saucepan over medium-high heat. Sauté until all water evaporates (about 5 minutes) and the quinoa begins to pop. Add the vegetable broth and bring to a boil. Reduce to a simmer and cover. Cook 15 minutes or until all water is absorbed. Set the quinoa aside to cool.
3. In a large bowl, whisk together yogurt, olive oil, vinegar, dill, garlic powder, salt, and pepper.
4. Add quinoa and remaining ingredients to bowl. Toss to coat.

MAKE IT GLUTEN-FREE: *Confirm all ingredients are gluten-free, including the broth.*

Nutrition Facts

Serves: 6
Serving Size: 1 1/2 cups

Amount per serving

Calories — **180**

Calories from fat 40

Total fat 4.5 g

    Saturated fat 0.6 g

    Trans fat 0.0 g

Cholesterol 0 mg

Sodium 220 mg

Potassium 460 mg

Total carbohydrate 27 g

    Dietary fiber 6 g

    Sugars 5 g

Protein 9 g

Phosphorus 205 mg

Choices/Exchanges: 1 1/2 Starch, 1 Nonstarchy Vegetable, 1 Fat

DIJON SALMON

⏱ 10 minutes
🍲 15 minutes
🍽 4 servings
🥡 1 salmon fillet

YOU CAN USE FROZEN SALMON FILLETS FOR THIS RECIPE, BUT BE SURE THEY ARE COMPLETELY THAWED BEFORE USING. THE BEST WAY TO THAW THE FISH IS IN THE REFRIGERATOR OVERNIGHT, SO PLAN AHEAD.

2	slices whole-wheat bread
1/4	cup chopped fresh parsley
2	tablespoons olive oil
1/4	cup Dijon mustard
2	cloves garlic, minced or grated
1/4	cup minced onion
1	tablespoon low-calorie brown sugar blend (such as Splenda)
4	(4-ounce) skinless salmon fillets
1/4	teaspoon ground black pepper

Nonstick cooking spray

1. Preheat oven to 375°F.
2. Toast the bread, and then place the toast and chopped parsley in a food processor and pulse to make bread crumbs. Do not overmix.
3. In a medium bowl, whisk together olive oil, mustard, garlic, onion, and brown sugar blend.
4. Season each side of the 4 salmon fillets with pepper.
5. Coat a baking sheet with cooking spray. Place salmon fillets on baking sheet and divide the sauce mixture evenly among each fillet. Sprinkle bread crumbs evenly on top of each fillet.
6. Bake the fillets 15 minutes or until salmon is tender and flakes with a fork.

MAKE IT GLUTEN-FREE: *To make this recipe gluten-free, omit bread crumbs (just use minced parsley) and verify that the other ingredients you are using are gluten-free.*

Nutrition Facts

Serves: 4
Serving Size: 1 salmon fillet

Amount per serving
Calories **300**

Calories from fat 140

Total fat 16.0 g

    Saturated fat 2.9 g

    Trans fat 0.0 g

Cholesterol 60 mg

Sodium 490 mg

Potassium 500 mg

Total carbohydrate 14 g

    Dietary fiber 2 g

    Sugars 4 g

Protein 25 g

Phosphorus 345 mg

Choices/Exchanges: 1/2 Starch, 1/2 Carbohydrate, 3 Lean Protein, 2 Fat

SWEET POTATO BASKETS WITH EGGS

🕐 10 minutes
⏱ 40 minutes
🍽 12 servings
🥣 1 basket

LC

THESE ELEGANT AND DELICIOUS BASKETS ARE PERFECT FOR A SUNDAY BRUNCH OR HOLIDAY. THIS RECIPE PROVIDES LEAN PROTEIN FROM THE EGG SUBSTITUTE (SUCH AS EGG BEATERS) AND HEALTHY CARBOHYDRATES FROM THE SWEET POTATOES.

Nonstick cooking spray
1 large sweet potato (16 ounces), peeled
5 slices (1/2 ounce each) deli-style ham, diced small
1 1/4 cups southwest-style egg substitute (such as Egg Beaters)
1/4 teaspoon ground black pepper

1. Preheat oven to 425°F. Spray muffin tins with cooking spray.
2. Grate the sweet potato using the largest grating size on grater. Place grated potato in a towel or cheesecloth to absorb excess liquid.
3. Use your hands to press a thin layer of grated sweet potato evenly into the bottoms and sides of 12 muffin cups. Spray the grated sweet potato in the muffin cups with cooking spray and bake on lower oven rack for 25 minutes.
4. While the sweet potato cups are baking, sauté the ham in a pan over medium heat 3 minutes.
5. In a medium bowl, mix the egg substitute, ham, and pepper.
6. Remove the sweet potato cups from the oven. Pour the egg mixture into the cups, dividing it evenly to fill each cup about 2/3 full. Bake 12–15 minutes, until the eggs are cooked through.

MAKE IT GLUTEN-FREE: *Confirm all ingredients are gluten-free, including the egg substitute and ham.*

Nutrition Facts

Serves: 12
Serving Size: 1 basket

Amount per serving
Calories 40

Calories from fat 0

Total fat 0.0 g
   Saturated fat 0.1 g
   Trans fat 0.0 g
Cholesterol 0 mg
Sodium 130 mg
Potassium 160 mg
Total carbohydrate 6 g
   Dietary fiber 1 g
   Sugars 2 g
Protein 4 g
Phosphorus 40 mg

Choices/Exchanges: 1/2 Starch

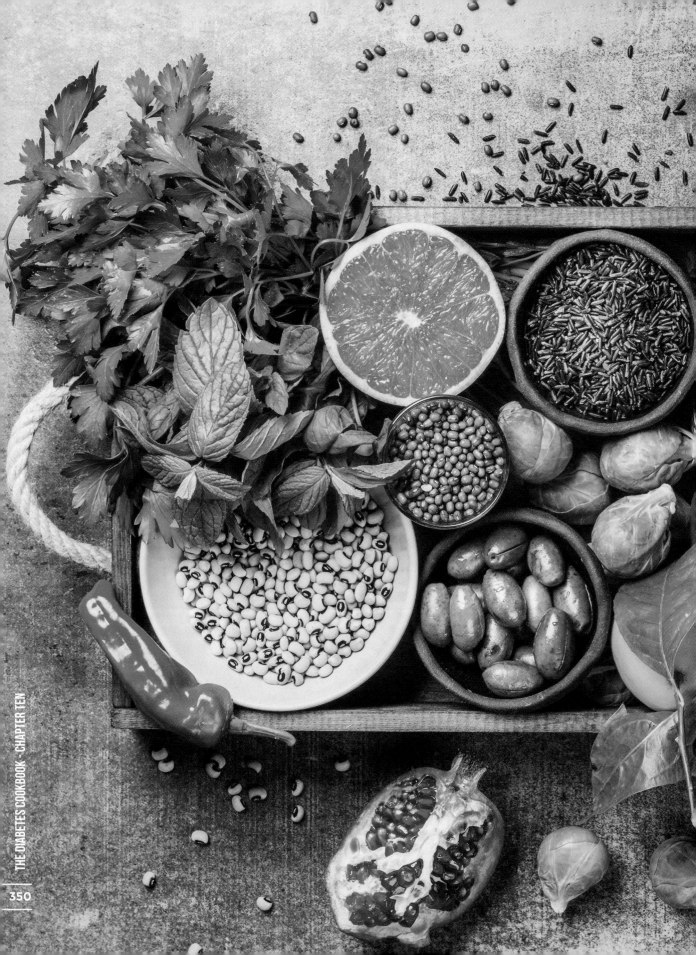

CHAPTER TEN

MEDITERRANEAN RECIPES

A MEDITERRANEAN-STYLE, MONOUNSATURATED FATTY ACID (MUFA)–RICH EATING PATTERN MAY BENEFIT BLOOD SUGAR CONTROL AND CARDIOVASCULAR RISK FACTORS AND IS AN EFFECTIVE ALTERNATIVE TO A LOWER-FAT, HIGHER-CARBOHYDRATE EATING PATTERN IN PEOPLE WITH TYPE 2 DIABETES. A MEDITERRANEAN DIET INCLUDES ABUNDANT PLANT FOODS SUCH AS FRUITS, VEGETABLES, BEANS, NUTS, SEEDS, AND WHOLE GRAINS ALONG WITH MINIMALLY

PROCESSED, FRESH, AND LOCALLY GROWN FOODS SUCH AS FRESH FRUIT FOR DESSERT. OLIVE OIL AND OLIVES ARE THE PRIMARY FAT IN THE MEDITERRANEAN DIET, AND IT IS LOWER IN DAIRY PRODUCTS, SUCH AS CHEESE AND YOGURT. RED MEAT IS CONSUMED INFRE-QUENTLY. WINE CONSUMP-TION IS LOW TO MODERATE, AND WINE IS GENERALLY CONSUMED WITH MEALS. YOU'LL FEEL LIKE YOU'VE ESCAPED TO ITALY AND GREECE IN THIS CHAPTER, WITH DISHES LOADED WITH FISH, NUTS, OLIVES, AND WHOLE GRAINS (AND MAYBE A GLASS OF RED WINE, TOO)!

TURKEY BOLOGNESE

⏱ 10 minutes
🍲 35 minutes
🍽 6 servings
🍴 3/4 cup sauce and 1/2 cup cooked pasta

YOU CAN REDUCE THE AMOUNT OF CARBOHYDRATES IN THIS RECIPE BY SUBSTITUTING ZUCCHINI NOODLES FOR THE PENNE.

1	onion, chopped
1	carrot, chopped
1	stalk celery, chopped
3	cloves garlic
1	tablespoon olive oil
20	ounces lean ground turkey
1	cup dry red wine (such as Pinot Noir)
1	(25-ounce) jar reduced-sodium tomato basil pasta sauce
1	tablespoon dried parsley
1/2	teaspoon ground black pepper
8	ounces whole-wheat penne pasta
6	tablespoons grated parmesan cheese

1. Add onion, carrot, celery, and garlic to a food processor and grind until very fine.
2. Heat oil in a large sauté pan over high heat. Add vegetables and sauté 5 minutes or until vegetables begin to caramelize.
3. Add the ground turkey and sauté until turkey is just cooked through, about 4 minutes.
4. Add the wine and boil until almost all the wine has evaporated, about 5 minutes. Scrape the bottom of the pan to incorporate any brown bits on the bottom of the pan.
5. Add the pasta sauce, parsley, and pepper. Reduce heat and simmer 10 minutes, stirring occasionally.
6. While the sauce is simmering, cook pasta according to the directions on the package, omitting salt.

7. Serve 3/4 cup sauce over 1/2 cup cooked pasta. Top each serving with 1 tablespoon parmesan cheese.

Nutrition Facts

Serves: 6
Serving Size: 3/4 cup sauce and 1/2 cup cooked pasta

Amount per serving
Calories **400**

Calories from fat 120

Total fat 13.0 g

Saturated fat 4.3 g

Trans fat 0.1 g

Cholesterol 75 mg

Sodium 410 mg

Potassium 750 mg

Total carbohydrate 40 g

Dietary fiber 7 g

Sugars 4 g

Protein 26 g

Phosphorus 340 mg

Choices/Exchanges: 2 1/2 Starch, 1 Nonstarchy Vegetable, 3 Lean Protein, 1 Fat

WALNUT LENTIL SALAD

⏱ 20 minutes
🍲 10 minutes
🍽 8 servings
🍴 1 cup

GF
VG

THIS IS A GREAT SALAD TO USE UP THE VEGGIES IN YOUR FRIDGE. TRY ADDING CHOPPED CUCUMBER, BROCCOLI, PEA PODS, OR CARROTS TO THIS SALAD. YOU COULD ALSO MIX IN LEFTOVER PROTEINS SUCH AS GRILLED CHICKEN, SHRIMP, OR TOFU.

2 cups lentils (any color)
6 cups water
Juice and zest of 1 large lemon
1 clove garlic, minced or grated
1 tablespoon minced fresh parsley
1 teaspoon sweet curry powder
1 tablespoon honey or 2 packets artificial sweetener
1/4 cup extra-virgin olive oil
1 medium yellow or orange bell pepper, seeded and diced
1 cup grape tomatoes, halved
1/2 cup toasted chopped walnuts
2 cups mesclun or mixed baby field greens

1. Rinse the lentils in a fine mesh sieve under cold running water until the water runs clear.
2. Add the lentils and 6 cups of water to a large stockpot and bring the water to a boil. Once boiling, reduce the heat and simmer 10 minutes. Drain the lentils, run under cold water to cool, and drain well.
3. In a large salad bowl, whisk together the lemon zest, lemon juice, garlic, parsley, curry powder, honey or artificial sweetener, and olive oil.
4. Add the remaining ingredients and lentils and toss to coat.

Nutrition Facts

Serves: 8
Serving Size: 1 cup

Amount per serving
Calories 290

Calories from fat 110

Total fat 12.0 g
  Saturated fat 1.5 g
  Trans fat 0.0 g
Cholesterol 0 mg
Sodium 15 mg
Potassium 690 mg
Total carbohydrate 34 g
  Dietary fiber 12 g
  Sugars 6 g
Protein 14 g
Phosphorus 290 mg

Choices/Exchanges: 2 Starch, 1 Nonstarchy Vegetable, 1 Lean Protein, 1 1/2 Fat

FRUIT SALAD WITH HONEY YOGURT

GF
VG

- ⏱ 10 minutes
- △ 8 servings
- ▷ 1 cup

FRUIT IS FULL OF ANTIOXIDANTS, VITAMINS, AND FIBER. IF YOU WANT TO TAKE THIS DISH ON A ROAD TRIP, PACK THE FRUIT IN SMALL, INDIVIDUAL PLASTIC CONTAINERS AND KEEP THEM IN A COOLER.

2   cups strawberries, hulled and sliced
2   cups watermelon, cut into small chunks
2   cups cantaloupe, cut into small chunks
1   cup green grapes
1   cup blueberries
2   (6-ounce) containers fat-free honey-flavored Greek yogurt

1. In a large bowl, mix all the fruit.
2. Place 1 cup fruit salad in a small bowl or parfait dish. Top each fruit salad with 1 1/2 ounces Greek yogurt.

DIETITIAN TIP: *There is nothing like fresh fruit in the summertime. Just make sure to count the carbohydrates as part of your meal plan. Fresh fruit is hard to find when you are on the road, so be prepared and pack your own.*

Nutrition Facts

Serves: 8
Serving Size: 1 cup

Amount per serving
Calories 100

Calories from fat 0

Total fat 0.0 g

    Saturated fat 0.0 g

    Trans fat 0.0 g

Cholesterol 0 mg

Sodium 25 mg

Potassium 320 mg

Total carbohydrate 20 g

    Dietary fiber 2 g

    Sugars 17 g

Protein 5 g

Phosphorus 85 mg

Choices/Exchanges: 1 Fruit, 1/2 Fat-Free Milk

MINI ARTICHOKE CAKES

⏱ 10 minutes
🍲 20 minutes
🍽 10 servings
🍴 1 muffin cup

THESE ARTICHOKE CAKES ARE A UNIQUE AND TASTY APPETIZER OR SNACK. BEST OF ALL, YOU CONTROL THE PORTION SIZE BY MAKING THEM IN MUFFIN TINS.

Nonstick cooking spray
1   (14-ounce) can artichokes, packed in water, drained, and chopped
1   tablespoon olive oil
2   egg whites, slightly beaten
1/2 cup shredded part-skim mozzarella
2   tablespoons freshly grated parmesan cheese
2   tablespoons certified gluten-free cornmeal

1. Preheat oven to 350°F. Line muffin tins with muffin papers and spray with cooking spray.
2. In a medium bowl mix together all ingredients.
3. Spoon artichoke mixture evenly into 10 muffin cups. Bake 20–23 minutes until lightly golden on top.

Nutrition Facts

Serves: 10
Serving Size: 1 muffin cup

Amount per serving
Calories 50

Calories from fat 20

Total fat 2.5 g

Saturated fat 0.9 g

Trans fat 0.0 g

Cholesterol 3 mg

Sodium 125 mg

Potassium 80 mg

Total carbohydrate 4 g

Dietary fiber 1 g

Sugars 0 g

Protein 3 g

Phosphorus 50 mg

Choices/Exchanges: 1 Nonstarchy Vegetable, 1/2 Fat

REDUCED-CARB NONALCOHOLIC SANGRIA

GF
LC
VG

⏱ 10 minutes
🍽 7 servings
🥤 1/2 cup

HERE IS A NONALCOHOLIC VERSION OF OUR REDUCED-CARB SANGRIA (PAGE 358). SUBSTITUTE THE DIET LEMONADE DRINK WITH A DIET FRUIT PUNCH DRINK IF YOU'D LIKE.

2 cups club soda
1/4 cup fresh lime juice
1/4 cup fresh lemon juice
1/2 cup artificial sweetener
1 lemon, sliced
1 lime, sliced
1 cup prepared diet lemonade drink (such as Crystal Light Lemonade)

1. Mix all ingredients together in a punch bowl or large pitcher. Refrigerate until ready to serve.
2. To serve, pour into glasses over ice.

Nutrition Facts

Serves: 7
Serving Size: 1/2 cup

Amount per serving
Calories 15

Calories from fat 0

Total fat 0.0 g

Saturated fat 0.0 g

Trans fat 0.0 g

Cholesterol 0 mg

Sodium 25 mg

Potassium 30 mg

Total carbohydrate 4 g

Dietary fiber 0 g

Sugars 2 g

Protein 0 g

Phosphorus 5 mg

Choices/Exchanges: Free food

REDUCED-CARB SANGRIA

GF
LC
VG

⏱ 10 minutes
🍽 12 servings
🥤 1/2 cup

THIS DRINK CAN BE MADE WITH RED OR WHITE WINE. SUBSTITUTE A DRY RED WINE (SUCH AS MERLOT OR PINOT NOIR) FOR THE WHITE WINE AND SUBSTITUTE A DIET FRUIT PUNCH DRINK FOR THE DIET LEMONADE DRINK. A NONALCOHOLIC VERSION OF THIS SANGRIA IS ON PAGE 357.

2   cups dry white wine (such as sauvignon blanc or pinot grigio)
2   cups club soda
1/4   cup fresh lime juice
1/4   cup fresh lemon juice
1/2   cup artificial sweetener
1   lemon, sliced
1   lime, sliced
1   cup prepared diet lemonade drink (such as Crystal Light Lemonade)

1. Mix all ingredients together in a punch bowl or large pitcher. Refrigerate until ready to serve.
2. To serve, pour into glasses over ice.

Nutrition Facts

Serves: 12
Serving Size: 1/2 cup

Amount per serving
Calories   **40**

Calories from fat 0

Total fat 0.0 g

   Saturated fat 0.0 g

   Trans fat 0.0 g

Cholesterol 0 mg

Sodium 15 mg

Potassium 45 mg

Total carbohydrate 3 g

   Dietary fiber 0 g

   Sugars 2 g

Protein 0 g

Phosphorus 10 mg

Choices/Exchanges: 1/2 Alcohol

GARLIC GREEN BEANS

GF
LC
VG

 5 minutes
 10 minutes
△ 4 servings
▷ 3/4 cup

IF YOU MAKE VEGETABLES TASTE GREAT, PEOPLE WILL EAT THEM AND IT WILL BE A CINCH TO MAKE HALF YOUR PLATE VEGGIES! THIS RECIPE PROVES SIMPLE CAN BE DELICIOUS!

1	pound frozen green beans
2	tablespoons olive oil
2	cloves garlic, minced
1/4	teaspoon ground black pepper

1. Microwave green beans according to package directions.
2. Heat oil in a large skillet over medium-high heat. Add garlic and sauté 30 seconds. Add green beans, sprinkle with pepper, and cook 5 minutes, stirring frequently.

Nutrition Facts

Serves: 4
Serving Size: 3/4 cup

Amount per serving
Calories 100

Calories from fat 60

Total fat 7.0 g

    Saturated fat 1.0 g

    Trans fat 0.0 g

Cholesterol 0 mg

Sodium 0 mg

Potassium 150 mg

Total carbohydrate 8 g

    Dietary fiber 3 g

    Sugars 2 g

Protein 2 g

Phosphorus 30 mg

Choices/Exchanges: 2 Nonstarchy Vegetable, 1 Fat

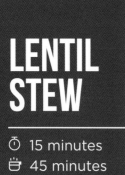

LENTIL STEW

⏱ 15 minutes
🍲 45 minutes
🍽 6 servings
🥣 1 cup

GF
VG

YOU CAN PLAY AROUND WITH DIFFERENT TYPES OF LENTILS IN THIS STEW—TRY RED, YELLOW, OR BROWN LENTILS.

1	tablespoon olive oil
1	onion, diced
2	stalks celery, diced
3	small or 2 medium carrots, peeled and diced
1	jalapeño pepper, seeded and minced
2	cloves garlic, minced
1	cup dried lentils
4	cups fat-free, gluten-free, low-sodium vegetable broth
1	cup water
1	bay leaf
1/2	teaspoon salt
1/4	teaspoon ground black pepper
4	cups baby spinach

1. Add oil to a soup pot over medium-high heat. Add the onion, celery, carrots, and jalapeño pepper, and sauté until the onion turns clear, about 5 minutes.
2. Add the garlic and sauté 1 additional minute.
3. Stir in the lentils and add the vegetable broth and water.
4. Add the bay leaf, salt, and black pepper. Bring to a boil. Then reduce to a simmer. Simmer covered 40 minutes.
5. Remove the bay leaf and stir in the spinach until the spinach is wilted.

Nutrition Facts

Serves: 6
Serving Size: 1 cup

Amount per serving
Calories 160

Calories from fat 25

Total fat 3.0 g

    Saturated fat 0.4 g

    Trans fat 0.0 g

Cholesterol 0 mg

Sodium 330 mg

Potassium 680 mg

Total carbohydrate 26 g

    Dietary fiber 9 g

    Sugars 6 g

Protein 9 g

Phosphorus 230 mg

Choices/Exchanges: 1 Starch, 2 Nonstarchy Vegetable, 1/2 Fat

SAUTÉED CINNAMON APPLES

GF
VG

- 7 minutes
- 15 minutes
- 4 servings
- 1/2 cup

FAST, NUTRITIOUS, AND IT SMELLS LIKE APPLE PIE—WHAT'S NOT TO LIKE? MAKE THIS SLICED FRUIT WITH CINNAMON, VANILLA, AND HONEY FOR YOUR NEXT QUICK DESSERT. FOR EVEN MORE FLAVOR, TOP WITH TOASTED CHOPPED WALNUTS.

1	tablespoon trans fat–free margarine
2	large Granny Smith apples, peeled, cored, and sliced
1/2	teaspoon cinnamon
1	teaspoon vanilla extract
3	tablespoons water
1	tablespoon honey or 2 packets artificial sweetener

1. Heat margarine in a sauté pan over medium-high heat. Add apples and sauté 3 minutes, stirring frequently.
2. Add remaining ingredients. Reduce heat to low and simmer 12 minutes, stirring occasionally.

DIETITIAN TIP: *Fruit is a great choice for dessert. Just make sure to work the carbohydrate into your meal plan. Also, you can cook these longer for a softer apple, if desired.*

Nutrition Facts

Serves: 4
Serving Size: 1/2 cup

Amount per serving
Calories 90

Calories from fat 20

Total fat 2.5 g

Saturated fat 0.6 g

Trans fat 0.0 g

Cholesterol 0 mg

Sodium 25 mg

Potassium 105 mg

Total carbohydrate 18 g

Dietary fiber 2 g

Sugars 15 g

Protein 0 g

Phosphorus 10 mg

Choices/Exchanges: 1 Fruit, 1/2 Fat

GREEK CHICKEN PITAS

⏱ 15 minutes
🍽 5 servings
🍴 1 pita with 1 cup chicken mixture

SALAD

1 1/2	cups diced cooked chicken breast
1 1/2	cups seeded and diced cucumbers
1/2	cup grape tomatoes, cut in half
15	kalamata olives, chopped
2	tablespoons crumbled reduced-fat feta cheese
1/3	cup finely diced red onion
1/2	teaspoon dried oregano
3	tablespoons olive oil
2	tablespoons red wine vinegar
5	whole-wheat pita halves, slit open

1. In a medium bowl mix together all ingredients except pita halves.
2. Scoop about 1 cup chicken mixture into each pita half.

DIETITIAN TIP: *You can use a rotisserie chicken purchased from your local grocery store deli in this recipe. If desired, make a dipping sauce with plain yogurt and fresh dill.*

Nutrition Facts

Serves: 5
Serving Size: 1 pita with 1 cup chicken mixture

Amount per serving
Calories **330**

Calories from fat 120	
Total fat 13.0 g	
Saturated fat 2.2 g	
Trans fat 0.0 g	
Cholesterol 35 mg	
Sodium 470 mg	
Potassium 310 mg	
Total carbohydrate 34 g	
Dietary fiber 5 g	
Sugars 2 g	
Protein 20 g	
Phosphorus 225 mg	

Choices/Exchanges: 2 Starch, 1 Nonstarchy Vegetable, 2 Lean Protein, 1 1/2 Fat

SHEET-PAN OLIVE CHICKEN

GF
LC

- ⏱ 70 minutes
- 🍲 30 minutes
- 🍽 4 servings
- 🥘 1 chicken breast with 8 olives

WHO SAYS CHICKEN HAS TO BE BORING AND BLAND? THIS RECIPE WILL BECOME ONE OF YOUR FAVORITE CHICKEN RECIPES.

MARINADE

1/4	cup red wine vinegar
3	tablespoons olive oil
3	teaspoons dried oregano
1/4	teaspoon ground black pepper
24	reduced-sodium pimiento-stuffed olives
8	garlic-stuffed olives
1	pound boneless skinless chicken breast, pounded thin
	Nonstick cooking spray

1. In a medium bowl whisk together vinegar, olive oil, oregano, and pepper. Add olives and mix well.
2. Place chicken in a large plastic freezer bag. Pour marinade over chicken and marinate 1 hour or overnight in refrigerator.
3. Preheat oven to 350°F. Spray a baking sheet with cooking spray. Place chicken on baking sheet and pour marinade evenly over chicken. Bake chicken 30 minutes or until done.

Nutrition Facts

Serves: 4

Serving Size: 1 chicken breast with 8 olives

Amount per serving

Calories 270

Calories from fat 160

Total fat 18.0 g

    Saturated fat 3.2 g

    Trans fat 0.0 g

Cholesterol 65 mg

Sodium 430 mg

Potassium 230 mg

Total carbohydrate 3 g

    Dietary fiber 1 g

    Sugars 0 g

Protein 24 g

Phosphorus 180 mg

Choices/Exchanges: 3 Lean Protein, 3 Fat

ROASTED CARROTS WITH TAHINI YOGURT SAUCE

DESPITE WHAT MANY PEOPLE BELIEVE, CARROTS ARE A RELATIVELY LOW-CARB VEGETABLE.

- ⏱ 10 minutes
- 🍲 45 minutes
- 🍽 8 servings
- 🥄 1/2 cup

GF
VG

Nonstick cooking spray
1 tablespoon gluten-free tahini paste
1 cup fat-free plain Greek yogurt
1 tablespoon chopped fresh parsley
2 tablespoons olive oil
1 tablespoon mild chili powder
2 teaspoons cumin
1/2 teaspoon ground black pepper
2 pounds baby carrots

1. Preheat oven to 400°F. Coat a baking sheet with cooking spray.
2. In a small bowl, whisk together tahini paste, yogurt, and parsley. Keep refrigerated until ready to use.
3. In large bowl, mix together the olive oil, chili powder, cumin, and pepper. Toss with the baby carrots until coated and spread in an even layer on the prepared baking sheet.
4. Bake 45 minutes, stirring occasionally.
5. Pour tahini yogurt mixture over warm carrots and toss again to coat.

Nutrition Facts

Serves: 8
Serving Size: 1/2 cup

Amount per serving
Calories 110

Calories from fat 45

Total fat 5.0 g
  Saturated fat 0.7 g
  Trans fat 0.0 g
Cholesterol 0 mg
Sodium 100 mg
Potassium 440 mg
Total carbohydrate 13 g
  Dietary fiber 4 g
  Sugars 6 g
Protein 4 g
Phosphorus 95 mg

Choices/Exchanges: 2 Nonstarchy Vegetable, 1 Fat

ROASTED VEGGIE BRUSCHETTA BITES

⏱ 15 minutes
🍲 18 minutes
🍽 11 servings
🥄 2 crackers

LC
VG

THIS FLAVORFUL APPETIZER IS A GREAT WAY TO WORK MORE VEGETABLES INTO YOUR DIET. YOU CAN MIX UP THE VEGGIES IN THE RECIPE IF YOU HAVE OTHERS ON HAND. TRY ZUCCHINI, TOMATOES, OR EVEN EGGPLANT.

Nonstick cooking spray
15 asparagus spears
1 cup mushrooms, sliced
1 red bell pepper, diced
2 cloves garlic
1 1/2 tablespoons olive oil
22 multigrain crackers
2 tablespoons freshly grated parmesan cheese

1. Preheat oven to 400°F. Spray a baking sheet with cooking spray.
2. Place asparagus, mushrooms, and red pepper on baking sheet. Add garlic and olive oil and toss to coat. Bake 15–18 minutes.
3. Remove from oven. Cool vegetables slightly and chop finely. Scoop a spoonful of veggies onto a cracker. Repeat for remaining crackers.
4. Place bruschetta bites on a serving platter and sprinkle with parmesan cheese.

MAKE IT GLUTEN-FREE: *Use gluten-free crackers and confirm all other ingredients are gluten-free.*

Nutrition Facts

Serves: 11
Serving Size: 2 crackers

Amount per serving
Calories 45

Calories from fat 20

Total fat 2.5 g

    Saturated fat 0.4 g

    Trans fat 0.0 g

Cholesterol 0 mg

Sodium 30 mg

Potassium 110 mg

Total carbohydrate 5 g

    Dietary fiber 1 g

    Sugars 1 g

Protein 1 g

Phosphorus 40 mg

Choices/Exchanges:
1/2 Carbohydrate, 1/2 Fat

CRUSTLESS MEDITERRANEAN QUICHE

- ⏱ 15 minutes
- 🍲 45 minutes
- 🍽 8 servings
- 🍴 1 slice

GF
LC
VG

SERVE THIS QUICHE WITH A
MESCLUN SALAD TOSSED WITH
A BALSAMIC VINAIGRETTE.

Nonstick cooking spray
1 tablespoon olive oil
1 medium onion, peeled and diced
1 medium red bell pepper, seeded and diced
1 medium zucchini, shredded
1/2 teaspoon salt
1/2 teaspoon ground black pepper
6 large eggs
1 1/2 cups 1% milk
2 ounces herb and garlic goat cheese
1/2 teaspoon minced fresh thyme
1 teaspoon Dijon mustard
8 pitted kalamata olives, minced

1. Preheat oven to 400°F. Coat a 9- or 10-inch pie pan with cooking spray. Place on a baking sheet and set aside.
2. Add olive oil to a small nonstick sauté pan. Add onion, bell pepper, zucchini, salt, and pepper, and sauté 10–12 minutes or until there is no more liquid in the pan. Set aside to cool.
3. In a mixing bowl, whisk together eggs, milk, cheese, thyme, mustard, and olives.
4. Pour cooled vegetable mixture into the prepared pie pan and spread to cover the bottom of the pan. Pour the egg mixture over the vegetables.
5. Bake 30–35 minutes or until center is set. Let cool 10 minutes before slicing. Slice into 8 pie wedges.

Nutrition Facts

Serves: 8
Serving Size: 1 slice

Amount per serving
Calories 140

Calories from fat 70

Total fat 8.0 g
 Saturated fat 2.9 g
 Trans fat 0.0 g
Cholesterol 150 mg
Sodium 310 mg
Potassium 260 mg
Total carbohydrate 7 g
 Dietary fiber 1 g
 Sugars 5 g
Protein 8 g
Phosphorus 155 mg

Choices/Exchanges: 1 Nonstarchy Vegetable, 1 Medium-Fat Protein, 1 Fat

GREEK BEAN SALAD

GF LC VG

- ⏱ 15 minutes
- 🍽 7 servings
- 🥄 1/2 cup

BEANS ARE ONE OF THE HEALTHIEST CARBOHYDRATE SOURCES OUT THERE. THEY ARE FULL OF FIBER AND OTHER NUTRIENTS. IF YOU NEED TO EAT A GLUTEN-FREE DIET, BEANS CAN BE A STAPLE IN YOUR MEAL PLAN.

SALAD

1	(15.5-ounce) can cannellini (white kidney) beans, rinsed and drained
1	cup grape tomatoes, cut in half
1/4	cup diced red onion
1/4	cup diced green bell pepper
1/4	cup crumbled reduced-fat feta cheese
6	kalamata olives, pitted and chopped

DRESSING

1/4	cup red wine vinegar
1/4	cup extra-virgin olive oil
1/2	teaspoon dried oregano
1/4	teaspoon ground black pepper

1. In a medium salad bowl, combine the salad ingredients.
2. In a small bowl, whisk together the dressing ingredients. Pour the dressing over the salad and toss to coat. Serve cold.

Nutrition Facts

Serves: 7
Serving Size: 1/2 cup

Amount per serving
Calories 140

Calories from fat 80

Total fat 9.0 g

    Saturated fat 1.5 g

    Trans fat 0.0 g

Cholesterol 9 mg

Sodium 130 mg

Potassium 220 mg

Total carbohydrate 10 g

    Dietary fiber 3 g

    Sugars 1 g

Protein 4 g

Phosphorus 75 mg

Choices/Exchanges: 1/2 Starch, 2 Fat

ROASTED CAULIFLOWER

⏱ 10 minutes
🍲 15–20 minutes
🍽 6 servings
🍴 1/2 cup

NOT A BIG VEGGIE FAN? TRY ROASTING YOUR VEGETABLES. ROASTING VEGETABLES IS ONE OF THE EASIEST AND TASTIEST WAYS TO PREPARE THEM.

Nonstick cooking spray
1   large head cauliflower, cut into small florets
2   tablespoons olive oil
1/4   teaspoon ground black pepper
1/4   teaspoon salt

1. Preheat oven to 425°F. Spray a baking sheet with cooking spray.
2. In a small bowl, mix together the cauliflower, olive oil, pepper, and salt. Spread the mixture on the baking sheet.
3. Bake 15–20 minutes, until the cauliflower tips are slightly brown and tender.

Nutrition Facts
Serves: 6
Serving Size: 1/2 cup

Amount per serving
Calories **80**

Calories from fat 45

Total fat 5.0 g

   Saturated fat 0.8 g

   Trans fat 0.0 g

Cholesterol 0 mg

Sodium 140 mg

Potassium 420 mg

Total carbohydrate 7 g

   Dietary fiber 3 g

   Sugars 3 g

Protein 3 g

Phosphorus 60 mg

Choices/Exchanges: 1 Nonstarchy Vegetable, 1 Fat

GREEK CHICKEN SALAD

⏱ 15 minutes

🍽 4 servings

🍴 About 2 heaping cups

WANT TO EAT A RESTAURANT-STYLE SALAD AT HOME? THIS SALAD IS FULL OF FLAVOR AND EASILY MEETS THE GOAL OF MAKING HALF YOUR PLATE VEGGIES WITH ITS LETTUCE, TOMATOES, AND CUCUMBERS.

SALAD

1 (9-ounce) bag romaine lettuce
1 medium cucumber, peeled and diced
2 roma tomatoes, diced
16 kalamata olives, pitted and cut in half
1/2 small red onion, thinly sliced
1/4 cup crumbled reduced-fat feta cheese
2 cups diced cooked chicken
16 baked whole-wheat pita chips (about 1 1/2 ounces)

DRESSING

1/4 cup red wine vinegar
3 tablespoons extra-virgin olive oil
1/4 teaspoon Dijon mustard
1/2 teaspoon oregano
1/8 teaspoon ground black pepper

1. In a medium bowl, mix together all salad ingredients except the pita chips.
2. In a small bowl, whisk together the dressing ingredients.
3. Pour the dressing over the salad and toss to coat.
4. Enjoy the pita chips on the side or break into bits and sprinkle over the salad for added crunch.

DIETITIAN TIP: *The chicken in this recipe provides a lean meat/protein source. Pick up a rotisserie chicken from your local grocery store deli for a real time-saver.*

CHEF TIP: *Make your own pita chips! Use 1 whole-wheat pita (6 1/2-inch diameter or about 2 ounces). Cut the pita in half, and then cut each half into quarters. Separate each piece, for a total of 16 pieces. Place on a rimmed baking sheet and spray lightly with olive oil non-stick cooking spray. Turn over each piece and spray the other side. Bake at 375°F about 10 minutes or until crisp.*

Nutrition Facts

Serves: 4

Serving Size: About 2 heaping cups

Amount per serving

Calories	**340**
Calories from fat 170	
Total fat 19.0 g	
Saturated fat 3.9 g	
Trans fat 0.0 g	
Cholesterol 65 mg	
Sodium 410 mg	
Potassium 530 mg	
Total carbohydrate 16 g	
Dietary fiber 4 g	
Sugars 3 g	
Protein 25 g	
Phosphorus 235 mg	

Choices/Exchanges: 1/2 Starch, 1 Nonstarchy Vegetable, 3 Lean Protein, 3 Fat

SPINACH PESTO CHICKEN SALAD WRAP

- ⏱ 15 minutes
- ☕ 35 minutes
- 🍽 5 servings
- 🍱 1 wrap

TRYING TO LOWER YOUR BLOOD PRESSURE BY WATCHING SODIUM INTAKE? USE HERBS SUCH AS BASIL AND OTHER INGREDIENTS SUCH AS LEMON, GARLIC, AND PEPPER FOR A LOT OF FLAVOR. WITH THE SPINACH, THIS WRAP IS ALSO A GREAT WAY TO WORK IN MORE VEGETABLES.

Nonstick cooking spray
1 pound boneless skinless chicken breasts
1/2 teaspoon ground black pepper, divided
1 teaspoon dried basil
3 cups baby spinach (large stems removed)
2 tablespoons pine nuts, toasted
2 tablespoons fresh lemon juice
1/4 cup light mayonnaise
1 tablespoon olive oil
2 tablespoons freshly grated parmesan cheese
1/4 teaspoon garlic powder
5 (6-inch) corn tortillas

1. Preheat oven to 350°F. Spray a baking sheet with cooking spray.
2. Season the chicken breasts with 1/4 teaspoon pepper and the basil. Bake 35 minutes or until done. Put the chicken breasts in the refrigerator to cool.
3. In a food processor, combine the spinach, pine nuts, lemon juice, and mayonnaise. Lightly pulse. With the machine running, add the olive oil, blending until the mixture is creamy. Stir in the parmesan cheese, garlic powder, and 1/4 teaspoon pepper.
4. Cut the cooked chicken into 1/2-inch pieces and shred. In a medium bowl, combine the chicken and pesto sauce; mix well.
5. Serve 1/2 cup chicken salad in each tortilla. Fold in the two sides of the tortilla and roll like a burrito. You can serve these immediately or wrap tightly in plastic wrap and refrigerate.

Nutrition Facts

Serves: 5
Serving Size: 1 wrap

Amount per serving
Calories 250

Calories from fat 100

Total fat 11.0 g
   Saturated fat 2.0 g
   Trans fat 0.0 g
Cholesterol 55 mg
Sodium 200 mg
Potassium 340 mg
Total carbohydrate 15 g
   Dietary fiber 2 g
   Sugars 1 g
Protein 23 g
Phosphorus 270 mg

Choices/Exchanges: 1 Starch, 3 Lean Protein, 1 Fat

STUFFED CHICKEN AND VEGETABLE RAGOUT

⏱ 20 minutes
🍲 60 minutes
🍽 4 servings
🍴 1 chicken breast and 1 cup vegetables and sauce

GF

FILLING

Nonstick cooking spray
Zest of 1 lemon
    (1 teaspoon zest)
1/3 cup crumbled reduced-fat feta cheese
1   tablespoon drained capers
1/2 teaspoon dried oregano
1   clove garlic, minced
4   (4-ounce) boneless skinless chicken breasts

SPICE RUB

1   tablespoon paprika
2   teaspoons dried oregano
1   teaspoon garlic powder
1/4 teaspoon salt
1/2 teaspoon ground black pepper

VEGETABLE RAGOUT

2   medium zucchini, cut into 1-inch chunks
8   ounces cremini (baby portobello) mushrooms, sliced
1   pint (10 ounces) cherry tomatoes, halved
1   (15-ounce) can cannellini (white kidney) beans, rinsed and drained
2   cloves garlic, minced
1   tablespoon olive oil
Juice of 1 lemon
    (1/4 cup juice)

1. Preheat oven to 375°F. Coat a 9-by-13-inch baking or casserole dish with cooking spray.
2. In a small bowl, combine lemon zest, feta cheese, capers, oregano, and garlic.
3. Slice a pocket in the side of each chicken breast with a sharp knife. Be sure not to slice all the way through the chicken breast, just far enough to make a pocket 3–4 inches long. Divide the filling mixture evenly among the four breasts and fill each pocket. Do not overfill. Press down on each breast to slightly seal the pocket opening.

4. In a small bowl, combine paprika, oregano, garlic powder, salt, and pepper. Rub each chicken breast on both sides with the spice rub so that the entire breast is coated. Set aside.

5. Add zucchini, mushrooms, tomatoes, cannellini beans, garlic, olive oil, and 1/4 cup lemon juice to the baking dish. Toss the vegetables and beans to coat.

6. Place the chicken breasts on top of the vegetables and put in the oven to bake.

7. Bake 30–40 minutes (depending on the size of the chicken breasts) or until the internal temperature of the chicken and filling is 165°F. Check the temperature after 30 minutes and every 5 minutes after until it reaches 165°F.

8. Remove the chicken from the pan and place on a cutting board. Cover with foil and let it rest 15 minutes.

9. Turn the oven up to 400°F. Return the vegetables to the oven and continue to bake 15 minutes (while chicken is resting).

10. Slice chicken and serve over the vegetables.

Nutrition Facts

Serves: 4

Serving Size: 1 chicken breast and 1 cup vegetables and sauce

Amount per serving

Calories 310

Calories from fat 80	
Total fat 9.0 g	
Saturated fat 2.3 g	
Trans fat 0.0 g	
Cholesterol 70 mg	
Sodium 480 mg	
Potassium 1210 mg	
Total carbohydrate 26 g	
Dietary fiber 8 g	
Sugars 6 g	
Protein 35 g	
Phosphorus 430 mg	

Choices/Exchanges: 1 Starch, 2 Nonstarchy Vegetable, 4 Lean Protein

BAKED CHICKEN WITH ARTICHOKE TOPPING

GF
LC

⏱ 5 minutes
🍲 35 minutes
🍽 4 servings
🥡 1 chicken breast

CHICKEN IS A LEAN PROTEIN SOURCE AND SHOULD MAKE UP A QUARTER OF YOUR PLATE. PEOPLE COMPLAIN OF GETTING BORED WITH CHICKEN, BUT THIS RECIPE IS BURSTING WITH FLAVOR.

Nonstick cooking spray
4   (4-ounce) boneless skinless chicken breasts
2   tablespoons fresh lemon juice
1/2 teaspoon garlic powder
1/4 teaspoon ground black pepper
1   tablespoon olive oil
1   clove garlic, minced
1   (15-ounce) can artichoke hearts, drained and chopped
1/3 cup fat-free, gluten-free, reduced-sodium chicken broth
3   tablespoons grated parmesan cheese

1. Preheat oven to 350°F. Spray a baking sheet with cooking spray.
2. Place the chicken breasts in a plastic freezer bag or between plastic wrap. Use a mallet or rolling pin and pound the chicken breasts until they are 1/2 inch thick.
3. Squeeze the lemon juice over the chicken breasts and season with garlic powder and pepper. Bake the chicken 25 minutes.
4. While the chicken is baking, warm the olive oil in a skillet over medium-high heat. Add the garlic and cook 1 minute. Add the artichoke hearts and cook about 3 minutes. Add the chicken broth and simmer 5 minutes. Stir in the parmesan cheese.

5. Remove the chicken from the oven. Spread the artichoke mixture evenly over the chicken breasts. Bake 10 more minutes or until the chicken is done.

Nutrition Facts

Serves: 4
Serving Size: 1 chicken breast

Amount per serving	
Calories	**220**
Calories from fat 60	
Total fat 7.0 g	
Saturated fat 1.9 g	
Trans fat 0.0 g	
Cholesterol 70 mg	
Sodium 340 mg	
Potassium 400 mg	
Total carbohydrate 9 g	
Dietary fiber 3 g	
Sugars 1 g	
Protein 28 g	
Phosphorus 250 mg	

Choices/Exchanges: 2 Nonstarchy Vegetable, 4 Lean Protein

PESTO CHICKEN KEBABS

⏱ 20 minutes
🍲 7 minutes
🍽 4 servings
🍴 2 kebabs

A QUICK AND EASY RECIPE, THESE KEBABS OFFER A GREAT SOURCE OF PROTEIN. THESE KEBABS WOULD BE GREAT SERVED OVER QUINOA OR CAULIFLOWER RICE.

8	bamboo skewers
1	tablespoon olive oil
2	cloves garlic, minced
1	cup packed fresh basil leaves (1 bunch basil)
1/4	cup pine nuts, toasted
1/8	teaspoon ground black pepper
2	tablespoons freshly grated parmesan cheese
1 1/4	pounds boneless skinless chicken breast, cut into 3/4-inch cubes (aim for 24 pieces of chicken)
2	zucchini, cut into 1-inch pieces (aim for 24 pieces of zucchini)
24	cherry tomatoes

1. Soak the bamboo skewers in warm water for at least 30 minutes.
2. Preheat an indoor or outdoor grill.
3. While the skewers are soaking, blend the olive oil, garlic, basil, pine nuts, pepper, and parmesan cheese in a blender or food processor.
4. Thread alternating pieces of chicken, zucchini, and tomato onto the soaked skewers, starting with the chicken, using 3 pieces of chicken, 3 pieces of zucchini, and 3 tomatoes.
5. Brush the kebabs with the basil mixture, coating well.
6. Grill the kebabs about 7 minutes, brushing with the basil mixture until it is all used. Turn the kebabs frequently until the chicken is cooked through and reaches an internal temperature of 165°F.

Nutrition Facts

Serves: 4
Serving Size: 2 kebabs

Amount per serving
Calories 290

Calories from fat 130	
Total fat 14.0 g	
Saturated fat 2.3 g	
Trans fat 0.0 g	
Cholesterol 80 mg	
Sodium 115 mg	
Potassium 830 mg	
Total carbohydrate 9 g	
Dietary fiber 3 g	
Sugars 5 g	
Protein 34 g	
Phosphorus 350 mg	

Choices/Exchanges: 2 Nonstarchy Vegetable, 4 Lean Protein, 1 Fat

QUICK CHICKPEA DIP

GF
LC
VG

- ⏱ 10 minutes
- 🍽 16 servings
- 🍴 2 tablespoons dip plus 2 cucumber rounds

BEANS ARE ONE OF THE HEALTHIEST CARBOHYDRATES YOU CAN EAT. THEY ARE FULL OF FIBER AND ARE A GOOD SOURCE OF PROTEIN. START ADDING MORE BEANS TO YOUR DIET WITH THIS QUICK AND DELICIOUS RECIPE.

1 can (16-ounce) chickpeas (garbanzo beans), rinsed and drained
2 tablespoons light mayonnaise
Juice of 1/2 lemon
1/4 cup diced red pepper
1/4 cup diced celery
Pinch ground black pepper
Pinch cayenne pepper (use paprika if you prefer less spicy)
2 cucumbers, peeled and sliced into rounds

1. In a small bowl, coarsely mash chickpeas with a potato masher, leaving some beans whole.
2. Add remaining ingredients except cucumbers and mix well.
3. Spoon about 1 tablespoon dip onto each cucumber round.

Nutrition Facts

Serves: 16
Serving Size: 2 tablespoons dip plus 2 cucumber rounds

Amount per serving
Calories **35**

Calories from fat 10

Total fat 1.0 g

Saturated fat 0.1 g

Trans fat 0.0 g

Cholesterol 0 mg

Sodium 45 mg

Potassium 95 mg

Total carbohydrate 6 g

Dietary fiber 2 g

Sugars 1 g

Protein 2 g

Phosphorus 35 mg

Choices/Exchanges:
1/2 Carbohydrate

EGGPLANT PARMESAN

VG

- ⏱ 20 minutes
- 🍲 40 minutes
- 🍽 10 servings
- 🍴 1 slice eggplant

YES, YOU CAN MAKE CRISPY, CHEESY EGGPLANT PARMESAN THE WHOLE FAMILY WILL LOVE—WITH WHOLE GRAINS AND WITHOUT DEEP FRYING!

1/2	cup flour
1/2	teaspoon dried basil
1/4	teaspoon ground black pepper
3	egg whites, beaten
1	cup whole-wheat panko bread crumbs
1/4	cup freshly grated parmesan cheese
1	medium (1 pound) eggplant, sliced into 10 1/2-inch-thick rounds
1	tablespoon olive oil
	Nonstick cooking spray
1	(24.5-ounce) jar reduced-sodium marinara sauce
1/4	cup shredded part-skim mozzarella cheese

1. Preheat oven to 350°F.
2. In a medium bowl, combine flour, basil, and pepper. In another medium bowl, add egg whites. In a third medium bowl, combine bread crumbs and parmesan cheese.
3. Dredge both sides of eggplant slices in flour mixture, then egg whites, then bread crumb mixture, coating well. Set aside.
4. Add oil and cooking spray to a large nonstick skillet over medium-high heat. Cook eggplant in batches, about 2 minutes per side. Use additional cooking spray with each batch.
5. Place the eggplant slices in the bottom of a 9-by-13-inch baking dish. Pour pasta sauce over the eggplant to cover all slices. Sprinkle mozzarella cheese over the top and bake 30 minutes, until cheese is melted and slightly golden.

DIETITIAN TIP: *Serve with a green salad and whole-wheat pasta for a complete meal. For a lower-carb option, use zucchini noodles or spaghetti squash instead of pasta.*

Nutrition Facts

Serves: 10

Serving Size: 1 slice eggplant

Amount per serving

Calories	**150**

Calories from fat 50	
Total fat 6.0 g	
Saturated fat 1.2 g	
Trans fat 0.0 g	
Cholesterol 6 mg	
Sodium 240 mg	
Potassium 320 mg	
Total carbohydrate 20 g	
Dietary fiber 3 g	
Sugars 5 g	
Protein 6 g	
Phosphorus 75 mg	

Choices/Exchanges: 1 Starch, 1 Nonstarchy Vegetable, 1 Fat

SPINACH PESTO HALIBUT

⏱ 15 minutes
🍲 10 minutes
🍽 4 servings
🍴 1 halibut fillet

GF
LC

THE DELICIOUS SPINACH PESTO IN THIS RECIPE COULD ALSO BE USED AS A SPREAD ON TURKEY OR CHICKEN SANDWICHES OR WRAPS. IF YOU DON'T LIKE HALIBUT, YOU CAN SUBSTITUTE COD OR TILAPIA.

Nonstick cooking spray
4   (4-ounce) halibut fillets
5   cups baby spinach, divided
2   tablespoons pine nuts, toasted
1   tablespoon lemon juice
1   teaspoon light mayonnaise
3   tablespoons olive oil
2   tablespoons freshly grated parmesan
1/8 teaspoon ground black pepper

1. Spray grill with cooking spray. Preheat grill.
2. Cook halibut over medium-high heat 4–5 minutes on each side.
3. Place 1 cup spinach, pine nuts, lemon juice, and mayonnaise in a food processor and lightly pulse. While processing, slowly add olive oil until the mixture is creamy.
4. Pour the pesto mixture in a bowl and add parmesan cheese and pepper.
5. Put 1 cup spinach on each of 4 plates; top with a grilled halibut fillet.
6. Spread pesto mixture evenly over grilled halibut fillets.

Nutrition Facts

Serves: 4
Serving Size: 1 halibut fillet

Amount per serving
Calories   **260**

Calories from fat 150	
Total fat 17.0 g	
Saturated fat 2.4 g	
Trans fat 0.0 g	
Cholesterol 40 mg	
Sodium 130 mg	
Potassium 740 mg	
Total carbohydrate 2 g	
Dietary fiber 1 g	
Sugars 0 g	
Protein 26 g	
Phosphorus 310 mg	

Choices/Exchanges: 4 Lean Protein, 2 Fat

CAPRESE TURKEY BURGER

CAPRESE SALAD IS TASTY AND REFRESHING, WITH ITS MIXTURE OF TOMATOES, FRESH MOZZARELLA, AND FRESH BASIL. NOW COMBINE THESE FLAVORS IN A BURGER FOR A MOUTHWATERING MEAL—THIS ISN'T YOUR EVERYDAY BURGER. HEALTHY EATING CAN BE DELICIOUS!

- ⏱ 15 minutes
- 🍳 8 minutes
- 🍽 6 servings
- 🍔 1 burger

1	pound lean ground turkey
1/2	teaspoon garlic powder
1/4	teaspoon ground black pepper
6	tablespoons ketchup
3	tablespoons balsamic vinegar
6	whole-grain sandwich thins
6	thick tomato slices
2	ounces fresh mozzarella, cut into 6 thin slices
18	fresh basil leaves

1. Prepare an indoor or outdoor grill.
2. In a medium bowl, mix turkey, garlic powder, and pepper. Divide turkey into 6 equal portions and shape into patties.
3. Place patties on grill rack, and grill 3–4 minutes per side or until juices run clear.
4. In a small bowl, whisk together ketchup and balsamic vinegar.
5. Place burger on sandwich thin and top with 1 tablespoon ketchup mixture, 1 tomato slice, 1 slice cheese, and 3 basil leaves. Repeat process for remaining 5 burgers.

MAKE IT GLUTEN-FREE: *Use gluten-free bread or lettuce wraps in this recipe and confirm all other ingredients are gluten-free.*

Nutrition Facts

Serves: 6
Serving Size: 1 burger

Amount per serving
Calories 270

Calories from fat 80	
Total fat 9.0 g	
Saturated fat 3.0 g	
Trans fat 0.1 g	
Cholesterol 65 mg	
Sodium 420 mg	
Potassium 430 mg	
Total carbohydrate 27 g	
Dietary fiber 6 g	
Sugars 8 g	
Protein 22 g	
Phosphorus 280 mg	

Choices/Exchanges: 1 1/2 Starch, 3 Lean Protein, 1/2 Fat

GREEK SALAD PIZZA

⏱ 15 minutes
🍲 15 minutes
🍴 4 servings
🍽 1/2 pizza

Nonstick cooking spray
2   (6-inch) whole-wheat pitas (not pocket type)
1   tablespoon olive oil
4   teaspoons balsamic vinegar
1/2 cup thinly sliced red onion
1   tablespoon chopped pitted kalamata olives
1   cup chopped fresh spinach
1/2 cup chopped artichoke hearts, drained and rinsed
1   cup diced cooked chicken breast
1/3 cup reduced-fat feta cheese
1   teaspoon dried oregano

1. Preheat oven to 375°F. Coat a baking sheet with cooking spray. Set aside.
2. Drizzle each pita with a little olive oil, using up the full tablespoon.
3. Drizzle each pita with 2 teaspoons balsamic vinegar.
4. Layer each pita with 1/4 cup red onion, 1/2 tablespoon olives, 1/2 cup spinach, 1/4 cup artichokes, 1/2 cup chicken, and half the feta cheese.
5. Sprinkle the top of each pita with dried oregano. Place on the prepared baking sheet.
6. Bake 15 minutes. Cut each pita in half and serve.

CHEF TIP: *You can serve this pizza with homemade tzatziki sauce. Just grate 1 small cucumber and 1 clove garlic into 1/2 cup fat-free plain Greek yogurt and mix to make the tzatziki.*

Nutrition Facts

Serves: 4
Serving Size: 1/2 pizza

Amount per serving
Calories **220**

Calories from fat 70

Total fat 8.0 g
  Saturated fat 1.8 g
  Trans fat 0.0 g
Cholesterol 35 mg
Sodium 450 mg
Potassium 300 mg
Total carbohydrate 22 g
  Dietary fiber 5 g
  Sugars 2 g
Protein 17 g
Phosphorus 210 mg

Choices/Exchanges: 1 Starch, 1 Nonstarchy Vegetable, 2 Lean Protein, 1/2 Fat

PORK SOUVLAKI

- ⏱ 10 minutes
- 🍲 15 minutes
- 🍽 4 servings
- 🥄 3 ounces pork, 1/2 whole-grain pita, and 1/4 cup tzatziki

SOUVLAKI

8	bamboo skewers
1	pound pork tenderloin
1/4	cup lemon juice
1	tablespoon olive oil
4	cloves garlic, minced or grated
1	tablespoon dried oregano
1/4	teaspoon ground black pepper

Nonstick cooking spray

TZATZIKI

1/2	cup fat-free plain Greek yogurt
1	large cucumber, peeled, seeded, and grated
1	clove garlic, minced or grated
1	tablespoon fresh lemon juice
1/4	teaspoon salt
1/4	teaspoon ground black pepper
2	whole-grain pocket-style pitas, cut in half

1. Soak bamboo skewers in warm water for at least 30 minutes. While the skewers are soaking, cut pork tenderloin into 1-inch cubes.

2. In large bowl, whisk together lemon juice, olive oil, garlic, oregano, and pepper. Add pork and stir to coat.

3. Marinate 10 minutes (can be made ahead of time and marinated up to 24 hours in the refrigerator). While the pork is marinating, preheat the broiler. Coat a baking sheet with cooking spray or line with foil. Set aside.

4. Thread pork onto 8 skewers and lay skewers on the baking sheet so they are not touching. Brush the skewers with remaining marinade, using all the marinade.

5. Place the skewers in the broiler 6 inches away from heat. Broil 6 minutes; turn the skewers; and cook an additional 6 minutes.

6. In a small bowl, whisk together yogurt, cucumber, garlic, lemon juice, salt, and pepper to make the tzatziki sauce. Spread 1/4 cup tzatziki sauce inside each pita half.

7. Remove pork from 2 skewers and stuff inside a pita pocket half. Repeat for remaining 3 pita pocket halves.

CHEF TIP: *Souvlaki can be made with any meat of your choice. Try it with chicken, shrimp, or lamb.*

Nutrition Facts

Serves: 4

Serving Size: 3 ounces pork, 1/2 whole-grain pita, and 1/4 cup tzatziki

Amount per serving

Calories 260

Calories from fat 60	
Total fat 7.0 g	
Saturated fat 1.6 g	
Trans fat 0.0 g	
Cholesterol 60 mg	
Sodium 350 mg	
Potassium 560 mg	
Total carbohydrate 21 g	
Dietary fiber 3 g	
Sugars 2 g	
Protein 28 g	
Phosphorus 305 mg	

Choices/Exchanges: 1 Starch, 1 Nonstarchy Vegetable, 3 Lean Protein, 1/2 Fat

ANTIPASTO SALAD

⏱ 10 minutes
🛎 4 servings
🍽 2 cups

GF
LC

DO YOU NEED A QUICK, TASTY, DIFFERENT SALAD FOR A SUMMER PICNIC? HERE IS THE ANSWER. ADD CANNED ARTICHOKE HEARTS IF YOU'D LIKE.

SALAD

1	(10-ounce) bag romaine lettuce
8	ounces gluten-free low-sodium deli-style turkey, cut into strips
2	slices (2/3 ounce each) reduced-fat provolone cheese, cut into 1/2-inch strips
1	tablespoon freshly grated parmesan cheese
1/4	cup green olives, pitted and chopped
1/4	cup sun-dried tomatoes
2	roasted red peppers, cut into 1/2-inch strips

DRESSING

1/4	cup red wine vinegar
2	tablespoons extra-virgin olive oil
1/2	teaspoon Dijon mustard
1/4	teaspoon freshly ground black pepper
1	shallot, minced

1. In a salad bowl, mix together all salad ingredients.
2. In a small bowl, whisk together dressing ingredients. Pour dressing over salad and toss to coat.

Nutrition Facts

Serves: 4
Serving Size: 2 cups

Amount per serving
Calories   **210**

Calories from fat 100

Total fat 11.0 g

  Saturated fat 2.5 g

  Trans fat 0.0 g

Cholesterol 40 mg

Sodium 390 mg

Potassium 550 mg

Total carbohydrate 9 g

  Dietary fiber 3 g

  Sugars 5 g

Protein 19 g

Phosphorus 225 mg

Choices/Exchanges: 2 Nonstarchy Vegetable, 2 Lean Protein, 1 1/2 Fat

MEDITERRANEAN TURKEY WRAP

- ⏱ 15 minutes
- ⌓ 4 servings
- ▭ 1 wrap

DON'T WASTE YOUR MONEY ON FAST FOOD AT LUNCH. MAKE THIS QUICK WRAP INSTEAD, AND YOU WILL DISCOVER THAT HEALTHY EATING DOES NOT HAVE TO BE BLAND OR BORING!

8	tablespoons prepared hummus
4	whole-wheat wraps, heated
8	ounces no-salt-added deli-style turkey
1/2	large cucumber, peeled and diced (about 1 cup)
2	roma tomatoes, diced (about 1 cup)
1/4	cup crumbled reduced-fat feta cheese

1. Spread 2 tablespoons hummus on a wrap.
2. Top with 2 ounces turkey, 1/4 cup cucumber, 1/4 cup tomatoes, and 1 tablespoon feta cheese. Fold wrap to close. Repeat for remaining 3 wraps.

MAKE IT GLUTEN-FREE: *Use gluten-free wraps and confirm all other ingredients are gluten-free.*

Nutrition Facts

Serves: 4
Serving Size: 1 wrap

Amount per serving
Calories **250**

Calories from fat 50	
Total fat 6.0 g	
Saturated fat 1.4 g	
Trans fat 0.0 g	
Cholesterol 40 mg	
Sodium 490 mg	
Potassium 470 mg	
Total carbohydrate 30 g	
Dietary fiber 10 g	
Sugars 3 g	
Protein 28 g	
Phosphorus 300 mg	

Choices/Exchanges: 1 1/2 Starch, 1 Nonstarchy Vegetable, 3 Lean Protein

GRILLED VEGGIE KEBABS

⏱ 45 minutes
🍲 10 minutes
△ 8 servings
▷ 1 skewer

THESE VEGGIE KEBABS MAKE A GREAT SIDE DISH WITH ANY SUMMER GRILLED MEAT RECIPE, INCLUDING THE CHIMICHURRI CHICKEN KEBABS ON PAGE 234. FEEL FREE TO EXPERIMENT WITH DIFFERENT VEGETABLES HERE, SUCH AS CHERRY TOMATOES, YELLOW SQUASH, OR GREEN AND ORANGE PEPPERS.

MARINADE

1/3	cup red wine vinegar
1/4	cup olive oil
2	teaspoons dried oregano
1/4	teaspoon ground black pepper

KEBABS

3	zucchini, sliced into rounds
1	red pepper, cut into 1-inch chunks
1	pound mushrooms, cut in half
1	medium red onion, cut into 1-inch chunks
8	metal skewers

1. In a medium bowl, whisk together marinade ingredients.
2. Place vegetables in bowl with marinade and toss to coat. Marinate 30 minutes.
3. Prepare indoor or outdoor grill. Skewer vegetables evenly on 8 skewers, alternating zucchini, pepper, mushrooms, and onion. Reserve leftover marinade.
4. Grill vegetables over medium heat 10–12 minutes, basting with reserved marinade and turning occasionally.

Nutrition Facts

Serves: 8
Serving Size: 1 skewer

Amount per serving
Calories — **100**

Calories from fat 60

Total fat 7.0 g

   Saturated fat 1.0 g

   Trans fat 0.0 g

Cholesterol 0 mg

Sodium 10 mg

Potassium 440 mg

Total carbohydrate 7 g

   Dietary fiber 2 g

   Sugars 5 g

Protein 3 g

Phosphorus 85 mg

Choices/Exchanges: 1 Nonstarchy Vegetable, 1 1/2 Fat

GREEK MEATBALLS

- ⏱ 10 minutes
- 🍚 23 minutes
- 🍽 5 servings
- 🍵 3 meatballs

LC

MEATBALLS ARE A QUICK AND EASY FOOD THAT IS FUN FOR ALL AGES. SERVE THESE MEATBALLS WITH A LARGE SALAD AND A WHOLE-WHEAT PITA FOR A COMPLETE MEAL.

1	pound 90% lean ground beef
3	green onions, sliced
1/4	cup finely chopped kalamata olives
1	tablespoon olive juice
2	tablespoons oats
1/2	teaspoon garlic powder
1/4	teaspoon dried oregano
3	tablespoons crumbled reduced-fat feta cheese
1/4	teaspoon ground black pepper
8	tablespoons prepared hummus

1. Preheat oven to 375°F.
2. In a medium bowl, mix together all ingredients except hummus. Shape into 15 balls (about 1 inch each).
3. Place meatballs on a baking sheet and bake 20 minutes. Turn oven to broil and broil 2–3 minutes to make crisp.
4. Place hummus in a small bowl. Dip meatballs in hummus.

MAKE IT GLUTEN-FREE: *Use certified gluten-free oats and confirm all other ingredients are gluten-free.*

Nutrition Facts

Serves: 5
Serving Size: 3 meatballs

Amount per serving
Calories **240**

Calories from fat 130	
Total fat 14.0 g	
Saturated fat 4.6 g	
Trans fat 0.6 g	
Cholesterol 60 mg	
Sodium 280 mg	
Potassium 390 mg	
Total carbohydrate 6 g	
Dietary fiber 2 g	
Sugars 2 g	
Protein 21 g	
Phosphorus 235 mg	

Choices/Exchanges: 1/2 Starch, 3 Lean Protein, 1 1/2 Fat

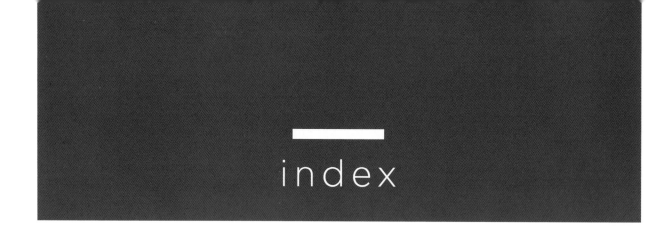

index

Note: Page numbers in **bold** refer to photographs.